RESEARCH AND PERSPECTIVES IN ENDOCRINE INTERACTIONS

Fondation Ipsen

D. Pfaff   C. Kordon
P. Chanson   Y. Christen   (Eds.)

Hormones
and Social Behavior

With 27 Figures, 13 in Color

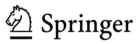 Springer

Donald W. Pfaff, Ph.D
Rockefeller University
Lab. Neurobiology & Behavior
1230 York Ave
New York, NY 10021
USA
e-mail: pfaff@rockefeller.edu

Claude Kordon, Ph.D
Institut Necker
156, rue de Vaugirard
75015 Paris
France
e-mail: kordon@necker.fr

Philippe Chanson, M.D.
Endocrinology
and Reproductive Diseases
University Hospital Bicêtre
78, rue du Général Leclerc
94275 Le Kremlin-Bicêtre
France
e-mail: philippe.chanson@
        bct.ap-hop-paris.fr

Yves Christen, Ph.D.
Fondation IPSEN
Pour la Recherche Thérapeutique
24, rue Erlanger
75781 Paris Cedex 16
France
e-mail: yves.christen@ipsen.com

ISBN 978-3-540-79286-4   e-ISBN 978-3-540-79288-8

DOI 10.1007/978-3-540-79288-8

Research and Perspectives in Endocrine Interactions ISSN 1861-2253

Library of Congress Control Number: 2008925348

© 2008 Springer-Verlag Berlin Heidelberg

Cataloging-in-Publication Data applied for Bibliographic information published by Die Deutsche Bibliothek
Die Deutsche Bibliothek lists this publication in the Deutsche Nationalbibliografie; detailed bibliographic data is available in the Internet at <http://dnb.ddb.de>.

Cover design: WMXDesign GmbH, Heidelberg, Germany
Typesetting and production: le-tex publishing services oHG, Leipzig, Germany

Printed on acid-free paper

9 8 7 6 5 4 3 2 1

springer.com

Preface

Social Bonding, a Product of Evolution: an Introduction to the Volume

Mechanisms underlying reproductive and maternal functions or coping represent the initial structuring force behind many social behaviors. They are accompanied by selective hormonal environments aimed at facilitating or stabilizing them. Sex and adrenal steroids are major players in the regulation of reproductive functions and coping challenges, but other hormones also participate in a variety of social behaviors (in particular, oxytocin and vasopressin, two phylogenetically very old moieties originally associated with maternal care and water balance) and are receiving increasing attention. Their role is highlighted in the present volume, which gathers contributions to the *Colloque Médicine et Recherche* "Hormones and Social Behavior" organized by the Fondation IPSEN in December 2007.

What is the key to understanding the rationale of hormonal substrates of behavior? Evolution, of course. Higher manifestations of social behavior have evolved from reproductive behavior, characterized by Ernst Mayr as "the leading edge of evolutionary change." As formulated by one contributor to this volume, however, "the evolutionary increase in neocortex seen in primates has induced a significant emancipation of behavior from hormonal determinants, and in parallel, an increasing role for intelligent social strategies" (Keverne 2008).

In so-called "lower" mammalian animals, many social behaviors are closely dependent upon the olfactory system, a component of autonomous regulation of such importance that it expresses a large proportion of all receptor genes present in the brain. When one looks at "higher" mammals such as primates, olfactory control becomes less stringent. Olfactory structures exhibit the same number of receptor genes, but a large number are transformed into non-coding "pseudogenes." In parallel, hormones initially targeted on physiological functions become increasingly associated with more diversified cognitive functions.

Consider oxytocin, one of two nonapeptides (along with vasopressin) concerned with fluid balance in the face of physiological challenges. Regarding social behaviors, oxytocin has evolved from an almost exclusive association with maternal care towards a role in the transmission of a "cultural" experience to offspring. Interestingly, this shift is facilitated by the capacity of oxytocin itself to induce glial plasticity around the very neurons that produce it, thus building temporary neuroanatomical barriers (Theodosis 2008) isolating its purely physiological actions from more behavioral ones.

Hormonal modulation is also an important determinant of anxiety, as shown for instance in a mice strain selected for a higher tendency to exhibit aggressive behavior and to overexpress vasopressin. During lactation, aggressiveness tends to become overprotective to the pups; it can be counteracted by administration of oxytocin. More generally, aggressiveness can be modulated in a gender-specific manner by androgens and estrogens (Neumann 2008). As far as anxiety is concerned, attempting to cope with its causes involves a two-step process that involves a balance between different hormones: exploration of coping behavior from a repertoire of available responses is facilitated by mineralocorticoids and oxytocin, whereas elimination of inappropriate responses depends more upon glucocorticoids and vasopressin (de Kloet et al. 2008).

The behavioral relevance of oxytocin has progressively extended to complex behaviors. The hormone is involved in the formation of discrete interpersonal bonds, as illustrated in the reproductive sphere by its capacity to stabilize lasting bonds in monogamous species (Olivier et al. 2008). On the other hand, sex hormones have a permissive role towards maternal mishandling in macaques, a relatively rare behavior in mammals. Mishandling also seems more likely to occur in animals presenting a greater polymorphism in the serotonin transporter gene. Epigenetic factors also facilitate this behavior, since, as also observed in humans, mishandled macaque infants develop a higher risk of becoming mishandlers themselves (Maestripieri 2008).

To what extent can one extrapolate these hormonal prerequisites to the brains and behaviors of humans? When investigating the management of trust and distrust in games designed to test a subjects reactions towards a stranger, the ability to trust was found to correlate with the activity of oxytocin (and vasopressin) neurons. The hormones have also been implicated in decision making relying on "altruistic" choices, i.e., responses in which subjects are challenged to sacrifice some of their own interests (Fehr 2008).

Neurohormone modulation of anxiety and social behavior involves recruitment of "arousal" capacities in the brain. Arousal triggers greater awareness towards anxiety, mostly by affecting three major parameters underlying social bonds: activity, sensitivity, and emotions. Interestingly, those parameters are precisely those that appear altered in autistic disorders (Choléris et al. 2008). In parallel, recent studies suggest that oxytocin neurons may be less active in autistic disorders (Neumann 2008, Maestripieri 2008, Olivier et al. 2008) and consequently less likely to compensate for decreased activity of "mirror neurons," whose decreased activity also been implicated in autism (Cattaneo et al. 2007).

The symposium also addressed sex-related behavioral disorders. A number of testable psychological symptoms are predictive of compulsive pedophilic behavior. Inhbition of testosterone secretion is usually quite effective in refraining manifestations of this disorder (Schober 2008). Based on brain imaging techniques, pedophilic trends can also be traced to a selective activation pattern of discrete brain structures (Stoléru 2008). On the other hand, sex hormones can act as aggravating or, in certain cases, protective factors towards behavioral consequences of alcohol ingestion (Eriksson 2008).

The evolutionary approach presented in this book provides clues to the relevance of social interactions as part of the natural selection process, for the survival of species, including ours. Proceeding further, as science often does, from the simple to the complex, and taking advantage of the wide pluridisciplinary range of the participants – coming from fields as diverse as molecular neuroscience, anthropology and psychology – a final question was raised as to whether biological substrates of complex social behaviors may also be relevant to moral issues characteristic of humans beings (Hauser and Young 2008): for instance, information aiming at decision making is not processed by the brain in the same way, whether or not a given situation is perceived as involving moral dilemmas. In fact, it could be argued (Pfaff and Adolphs 2008) that human social behavior mechanisms do not constitute a simple extension of other central nervous system regulatory functions but instead represent and require a different level of analysis. Understanding how social patterns are controlled by the brain may yield new insights into the nature of consciousness: human conscious experience depends upon a person being embedded in a complex social environment. According to this view, rational, moral behavior is a natural product of the human mind operating in social contexts and having been selected for during the process of human evolution.

Claude Kordon
Donald Pfaff
Philippe Chanson
Yves Christen

References

Cattaneo L, Fabbri-Destro M, Boria S, Pieraccini C, Monti A, Cossu G, Rizzolatti G (2007) Impairment of action chains in autism and its possible role in intention understanding. Proc Natl Acad Sci USA 104:17825–17830

Choleris E, Kavaliers M, Pfaff D (2008) Brain mechanisms theoretically underlying extremes of social behaviors: the best and the worst. In: Pfaff D, Kordon C, Chanson P, Christen Y (eds) Hormones and Social behaviour. Springer Verlag, Heidelberg, pp 13–25

de Kloet ER, Datson NA, Revsin Y, Champagne D, Oitzl MS (2008) Brain corticosteroid receptor function in response to psychosocial stressors. In: Pfaff D, Kordon C, Chanson P, Christen Y (eds) Hormones and Social behaviour. Springer Verlag, Heidelberg, pp 131–150

Eriksson CJP (2008) Role of alcohol and sex hormones on human aggressive behavior. In: Pfaff D, Kordon C, Chanson P, Christen Y (eds) Hormones and Social behaviour. Springer Verlag, Heidelberg, pp 177–185

Fehr E (2008) The Effect of Neuropeptides on Human Trust and Altruism: A Neuroeconomic Perspective. In: Pfaff D, Kordon C, Chanson P, Christen Y (eds) Hormones and Social behaviour. Springer Verlag, Heidelberg, pp 47–56

Hauser MD, Young L (2008) Modules, Minds and Morality. In: Pfaff D, Kordon C, Chanson P, Christen Y (eds) Hormones and Social behaviour. Springer Verlag, Heidelberg, pp 1–11

Keverne EB (2008) Impact of brain evolution on hormones and social behaviour. In: Pfaff D, Kordon C, Chanson P, Christen Y (eds) Hormones and Social behaviour. Springer Verlag, Heidelberg, pp 65–79

Maestripieri D (2008) Neuroendocrine mechanisms underlying the intergenerational transmission of maternal behavior and infant abuse in rhesus macaques. In: Pfaff D, Kordon C, Chanson P, Christen Y (eds) Hormones and Social behaviour. Springer Verlag, Heidelberg, pp 121–130

Neumann ID (2008) Brain oxytocin mediates beneficial consequences of close social interactions: from maternal love and sex. In: Pfaff D, Kordon C, Chanson P, Christen Y (eds) Hormones and Social behaviour. Springer Verlag, Heidelberg, pp 81–101

Olivier B, Chan JSW, Waldinger MD (2008) Serotonergic modulation of sex and aggression. In: Pfaff D, Kordon C, Chanson P, Christen Y (eds) Hormones and Social behaviour. Springer Verlag, Heidelberg, pp 27–45

Pfaff D, Adolfs R (2008) Social neuroscience: complexities to be unravelled. In: Pfaff D, Kordon C, Chanson P, Christen Y (eds) Hormones and Social behaviour. Springer Verlag, Heidelberg, pp 187–196

Schober J (2008) Aspects of Behavior in Pedophillic Sex Offenders Treated with Leuprolide Acetate. In: Pfaff D, Kordon C, Chanson P, Christen Y (eds) Hormones and Social behaviour. Springer Verlag, Heidelberg, pp 151–162

Stoléru S (2008) The brain, androgens, and pedophilia. In: Pfaff D, Kordon C, Chanson P, Christen Y (eds) Hormones and Social behaviour. Springer Verlag, Heidelberg, pp 163–175

Theodosis DT (2008) Hormones, brain plasticity and reproductive functions. In: Pfaff D, Kordon C, Chanson P, Christen Y (eds) Hormones and Social behaviour. Springer Verlag, Heidelberg, pp 103–120

Young LJ (2008) Molecular Neurobiology of the Social Brain. In: Pfaff D, Kordon C, Chanson P, Christen Y (eds) Hormones and Social behaviour. Springer Verlag, Heidelberg, pp 57–64

Table of Contents

List of Contributors

Adolphs, Ralph
California Institute of Technology, 331B Baxter Hall, CA 91125 Pasadena, USA

Champagne, D.
Division of Medical Pharmacology, Leiden/Amsterdam Center for Drug Research, LUMC, Gorlaeus Laboratory, Leiden University, PO Box 9502, 2300 RA Leiden, The Netherlands

Chan, Johnny S.W.
Department of Psychopharmacology, Utrecht Institute for Pharmaceutical Sciences and Rudolf Magnus Institute of Neuroscience, Utrecht University, Sorbonnelaan 36, 3584CA Utrecht, The Netherlands

Choleris, Elena
The Rockefeller University, New York, USA

Datson, N.A.
Division of Medical Pharmacology, Leiden/Amsterdam Center for Drug Research, LUMC, Gorlaeus Laboratory, Leiden University, PO Box 9502, 2300 RA Leiden, The Netherlands

de Kloet, E.R
Division of Medical Pharmacology, Leiden/Amsterdam Center for Drug Research, LUMC, Gorlaeus Laboratory, Leiden University, PO Box 9502, 2300 RA Leiden, The Netherlands

Eriksson, C.J. Peter
Department of Mental Health and Alcohol Research, National Public Health Institute, POB 33, 00251 Helsinki, Finland

Fehr, Ernst
University of Zurich, Institute for Empirical Research in Economics, Switzerland

Hauser, M.D.
Departments of Psychology, Human and Evolutionary Biology, Organismic & Evolutionary Biology, Harvard University, Cambridge, MA, 02138, USA

Kavaliers, Martin
The Rockefeller University, New York, USA

Keverne, E.B.
Sub-Department of Animal Behaviour, University of Cambridge, Madingley, Cambridge, CB23 8AA, UK

Maestripieri, Dario
Department of Comparative Human Development, The University of Chicago, Chicago, IL 60637, USA

Neumann, Inga D.
Department of Behavioural and Molecular Neuroendocrinology, University of Regensburg, Germany

Olivier, Berend
Department of Psychopharmacology, Utrecht Institute for Pharmaceutical Sciences and Rudolf Magnus Institute of Neuroscience, Utrecht University, Sorbonnelaan 36, 3584CA Utrecht, The Netherlands, and Yale University School of Medicine, Department of Psychiatry, New Haven, USA

Oitzl, M.S.
Division of Medical Pharmacology, Leiden/Amsterdam Center for Drug Research, LUMC, Gorlaeus Laboratory, Leiden University, PO Box 9502, 2300 RA Leiden, The Netherlands

Pfaff, Donald
The Rockefeller University Box 275, Department of Neurobiology and Behavior 1230 York Avenue, NY 10021-6399 New York, USA

Revsin, Y.
Division of Medical Pharmacology, Leiden/Amsterdam Center for Drug Research, LUMC, Gorlaeus Laboratory, Leiden University, PO Box 9502, 2300 RA Leiden, The Netherlands

Schober, Justine
Hamot Medical Center, Erie, PA, Department of Neurobiology and Behavior, The Rockefeller University, New York, NY, USA

Waldinger, Marcel D.
Department of Psychopharmacology, Utrecht Institute for Pharmaceutical Sciences and Rudolf Magnus Institute of Neuroscience, Utrecht University, Sorbonnelaan 36, 3584CA Utrecht, The Netherlands, and Haga-Hospital Leyenburg, Den Haag, The Netherlands

Stoléru, Serge
Inserm U742, 9 quai Saint-Bernard, 75005 Paris, France

Theodosis, Dionysia T.
INSERM U 862, Institut François Magendie, 146 Rue Léo Saignat, 33077 Bordeaux Cedex, France

Young, Larry J.
Center for Behavioral Neuroscience, Department of Psychiatry and Behavioral Sciences, and Yerkes National Primate Research Center, 954 Gatewood Road, Yerkes Primate Center, Emory University, Atlanta GA 30329, USA

Young, L.
Departments of Psychology, Harvard University, Cambridge, MA, 02138, USA

Modules, Minds and Morality

M.D. Hauser[1,2,3] and *L. Young*[1]

Summary

We here engage with a long-lasting debate in the cognitive sciences concerning domain-specific mechanisms for acquiring and processing different systems of knowledge, focusing on the problem of morality. We ask whether there are mechanisms that uniquely evolved in humans, and uniquely for the domain of morality. We discuss behavioral and neurophysiological evidence that bears on the role of emotions and mental state reasoning in moral cognition. Based on this evidence, we make a tentative, yet provocative, suggestion: what is unique to the moral domain is unlikely to be the mechanisms that underlie our emotional processing or folk psychology, but rather the ways in which these systems interface to create outputs that are distinctively moral.

We begin this essay talking about testes. We realize that this is an uncommon introduction, but we think that studies of testes provide an entry into a central question about the mind and thus the general focus of this essay: what evidence do we have for neuroanatomical specializations for distinct domains of knowledge? The study of testes reveals how you can get anatomical specialization based on particular social and ecological conditions.

In the early 1980s, Harcourt and colleagues (1981) made an extremely important discovery. If you plot testes size against the mating systems of monkeys and apes, you see a fascinating relationship: species with intense mating competition have larger testes than species with less intense mating competition. Thus, the polygynous chimpanzees have extremely large testes, whereas the monogamous gibbons have extremely small testes. In case you are curious, the size of human testes is closer to chimpanzees than gibbons, revealing what anthropologists have documented over the years: past and current human cultures are mostly polygynous, with monogamy largely a myth or recent cultural invention. The relationship between mating system and testes size is so tight that if you were walking in the woods and found a pair of detached testicles, you would be able to generate a confident prediction about this animal's mating system. The reason for this relationship falls out of standard Darwinian sexual selection: larger

---

[1] Department of Psychology
[2] Department of Human and Evolutionary Biology
[3] Department of Organismic & Evolutionary Biology, Harvard University, Cambridge, MA, 02138, USA, e-mail: mdh@wjh.harvard.edu

Pfaff et al.
Hormones and Social Behavior
© Springer-Verlag Berlin Heidelberg 2008

testes allow for greater sperm volume, which is critical in species where there is intense mating competition. Intense mating competition arises when there are few sexually receptive females and many sexually interested males.

Here we turn to the general problem of modularity and ask about the nature of domain-specific processing systems (Cosmides and Tooby 1994; Fodor 1983; Gallistel 1999; Sperber 1994) and, especially, the kind of neurophysiological evidence that bears on this problem. Specifically, we explore the moral domain and ask whether this system of knowledge is mediated by a specialized faculty or instead consists of a cluster of either domain-general or domain-specific, but non-moral, mechanisms for acquiring and acting upon moral knowledge (Hauser 2006; Stich 2006). Our road map is as follows. We begin with a brief discussion of face processing, as it provides perhaps one of the strongest cases to date of domain specificity. Though heated discussion continues over the strength of this claim, it is a useful example for our purposes as it clearly lays out the kinds of questions and evidence that must be addressed in making an argument for domain specificity. Second, we provide a framework for thinking about the moral domain that appeals to recent discussion of a different domain: language. In particular, we begin by discussing how theoretical and empirical work on language generates a set of fundamental questions that should be addressed by scholars focusing on any domain of knowledge, including morality. Third, we review recent research that highlights how neuroscientific findings contribute to our understanding of not only those processes that are critically involved in generating moral judgments but also the relative timing of such processes. Thus, we explore both the relative contribution of mental state reasoning and emotion and the timing of these processes relative to the delivery of a moral judgment. Many in-depth reviews have recently been written about some of these topics (Casebeer 2003; Greene and Haidt 2002; Haidt 2001, 2007; Hauser 2006; Moll et al. 2007), but here we attempt to put them together in a slightly different light.

Human Faces: An Illustrative Example of Domain Specificity

Studies of primate physiology, human infant development, adult psychophysics, neuroimaging and neuropsychology suggest that the primate brain has evolved a neural specialization for face processing (McKone et al. 2007). The idea here is that face processing, unlike other categorical distinctions, relies on within-category differences. That is, once the object is recognized as a face a process that appears to be domain specific in terms of the representations it handles, some other circuitry in the brain must assess whether it is male or female, same race or different race, and, if male and Caucasian, whether it is Fred, Mike, or Jim. To carry out this computation, the brain must assess subtle featural differences such as the distance between the eyes as well as their shape, the distance between the eyes and nose, the configuration of the nose and mouth, and so on. Evidence in favor of face specialization comes from studies showing, for example, selective breakdown in face recognition but not other objects (i.e., prosopagnosics), distinctive inversion effects in processing for faces as opposed to non-faces, and in fMRI studies, stronger activation for faces over non-faces in a particular cortical area (i.e., the fusiform face area; FFA). All of these data point to both sensory selectivity and domain specificity.

Though we align ourselves with those who argue in favor of the domain specificity of face processing, largely because of our reading of the comparative evidence reviewed by McKone and colleagues (2007), we raise here a recent debate because it sets up the way in which we want to think about morality, the target topic of this essay. In particular, Gauthier and Tarr (1997; Palmeri et al. 2004), among others, have responded to the claims about a domain-specific face area by suggesting that the circuitry, and its accompanying mechanisms, is instead dedicated to any within-category discrimination task that requires expertise. Thus, because we are face experts, this circuitry is engaged by faces. But it is also engaged when other categories involving expertise are perceived, including cars for automobile experts, birds for ornithologists, and even artificially constructed characters called "greebles" for greeble experts. This challenge raises two separate issues. First, as with any neural mechanism, we must separate questions of origins from questions of current function. Thus, it might be the case that the FFA evolved for face processing, because this was the only within-category discrimination task confronting nonhuman primates. Once humans evolved, other within-category distinctions emerged, creating a pressure for discrimination. Rather than building another circuit, our brains co-opted the FFA for novel problems of categorization involving expertise. If this is the right story, then we can still conclude that the FFA evolved for face processing but is presently used for both face processing and other tasks involving within-category discrimination.

The second issue is whether, both neurobiologically and psychologically, face processing shows different signatures from processing other objects. For example, in the literature reviewed by McKone et al. (2007), results suggest that the patterns uncovered for tests of holistic processing as well as the inversion effect are distinctively different for faces and other objects. More precisely, there is no holistic processing for objects of expertise (e.g., dogs), as well as weak to negligible inversion effects.

In summary, though the debate between domain specificity and expertise continues with respect to face processing, what we think is important about this debate is that it sets up testable hypotheses about how to explore the problem. In particular, it has generated a wealth of data from different populations (animals, human infants and adults), using different methods (single unit physiology, brain imaging, patient-based neuropsychology) to examine whether a given domain of knowledge is mediated by domain-specific or general mechanisms. We follow this lead in our approach to moral psychology.

The Ingredients of a Language Faculty

We begin by building on a distinction that has been made in discussions of language that in part parallels the issues raised in the previous section on faces and that we find useful as a heuristic into research on moral psychology (Hauser 2006; Mikhail 2000, 2007). In particular, in discussions of language, it is necessary to ask about those mechanisms that are involved in processing language but are not specific to language, as opposed to those mechanisms that are both involved in language and specific to it (Hauser et al. 2002). This distinction has been referred to as the faculty of language broad (FLB) as opposed to narrow (FLN). Thus, for example, when processing spoken language, our auditory system is involved, as are our systems of attention and memory.

But none of these systems is specific to language and thus count as a constituent of FLB. It is worth noting that, simply because a process is part of FLB, it does not mean it is peripheral or a merely minor contributor to the domain. Thus, if an individual incurs damage to circuitry involved in working memory, there will be difficulties in both language production and perception, due in part to the necessity of accessing working memory for embedding phrases and running the recursive operations that provide language's limitless expression. It is, of course, also the case that our memory systems constrain this recursive mechanism; that is, a recursive operation that iteratively embeds one phrase inside of another is not limited, but our capacity to understand and produce embedded phrases is limited to about three to four within a given sentence.

Concerning FLN, we are after mechanisms that are both uniquely human and unique to language. This definition sets up an empirical search that is comparative in terms of both phylogeny and domains of knowledge. Thus, finding a trait that is critical to language processing and unique to humans is only one part of the analysis. We must then move on to an examination of whether this trait is uniquely involved in language or deployed in other domains as well. Take, for example, the capacity for combinatorial operations over discrete entities. This is a capacity that is neither uniquely human nor unique to language. Many songbirds and whales have the capacity for rich combinatorics, repeating, and rearranging notes and motifs within their species-specific songs. This fact alone knocks out combinatorial operations from FLN and moves them into FLB. But, even if no other organism had this capacity, we can readily see the combinatoric mind in operation in many domains of human knowledge, including music, mathematics, the construction of artifacts, and so forth. At present, there is considerable controversy concerning what is "in" FLN. Hauser et al. (2002) put forward the hypothesis that FLN constitutes the mechanisms underlying narrow syntax as they interface with semantics and phonology. There are, of course, other options, including the possibility that FLN is restricted to the output representations of more domain-general mechanisms; for example, it is conceivable that neither the computations underlying syntax nor the conceptual representations subserving semantics are unique to language, but when these two systems interact, they generate language-specific representations. What we wish to emphasize here is that to understand any domain of knowledge we should engage in these questions and attempt to assess the relative modularity of the system, while keeping open the possibility that the domain in play lacks unique computational mechanisms, representing instead the synthetic integration of multiple mind-internal systems that output domain-specific material.

To give a sense of how such interface conditions might operate, consider a recent linguistic example and, specifically, the morpho-syntax of the singular-plural distinction. It is clear that no other system except language marks a distinction between singular and plural. Yet, it is possible that this distinction comes from an object-centered and non-linguistic conceptual distinction between one vs. many along with the phonological marking that this distinction mandates, as well as a structural rule from syntax that dictates where the morphology changes. Some empirical support for this idea comes from the observation that nonhuman primates have a set-based quantificational system that distinguishes one from many, but not many from many (Barner et al., in press). However, the singular-plural distinction in language appears to take this basic form and makes a seemingly odd change, at least from the perspective of objects. If you take the object "apple." you certainly have "1 apple" as opposed to "2, 10, 1,000,000 appleS." But you also have "0, 0.5, −1, and 1.0 appleS." Thus, the output of the interface between these systems generates representations that are unique to language and, thus, part of FLN. This is, at least, one interpretation, and it is possible that the same kind of interpretation can be applied to other domains, such as music (e.g., time and frequency discrimination interfacing with emotion) and morality (e.g., theory of mind, action perception, and emotion interfaces). At this stage, these issues are poorly understood, especially in terms of the specific mechanism that handles the interface and how systems with different representational formats combine to create new representations.

The Ingredients of a Moral Faculty

The distinction between FLB and FLN can readily be translated into the moral domain by asking which, if any, mechanisms are unique to humans and unique to morality? That is, which mechanisms fall under the classification of faculty of morality broad (FMB) and which under the classification of faculty of morality narrow (FMN)? As in the case of language, it is clear that several mechanisms involved in, for example, moral judgments are also involved in many other kinds of judgment, including attention, visual and auditory perception, and memory. We focus the remaining discussion on the role of two such mechanisms in moral judgment: mental state representation and emotional processes.

Folk Mental States

Recent conceptual and empirical studies of moral judgment (Borg et al. 2006; Cushman et al. 2006, submitted for publication; Dwyer 1999; Greene et al. 2001, 2004; Hauser et al. 2007; Knobe 2003a, b; Mikhail, in press) have targeted our folk psychological representations and, in particular, the mental states that comprise our theory of mind (e.g., beliefs, desires, intentions, goals). In particular, as behavioral and functional neuroimaging research suggests, moral situations trigger, at some level, an appraisal of mental states (Cushman et al. submitted for publication; Young et al. 2007): did the agent intend to harm the victim or was it accidental? What did the agent believe about his intended goal of helping another? Indeed, we judge intentional harms to be worse than the same harms brought about accidentally. Furthermore, brain regions previously associated with theory of mind in non-moral contexts (e.g., right temporo-parietal junction; rTPJ; Fletcher et al. 1995; Gallagher et al. 2000; Saxe and Kanwisher 2003) are recruited robustly during moral judgment (Young et al. 2007). Stating that moral scenarios trigger mental state attribution should not be misinterpreted as a claim that moral judgments always require an appeal to mental states. Consequentialism, to take one philosophical perspective, mandates that we restrict our moral considerations to outcomes as opposed to means. Our point here is that, when our intuitive moral judgments emerge, they will often derive from an inference about others' mental states.

In recent work attempting to understand the kinds of mental states that enter into our moral judgments and, in particular, whether there are specific principles that mediate our judgments, researchers have pointed to two specific distinctions that commonly emerge in philosophical and legal discussions (Borg et al. 2006; Cushman et al. 2006, submitted for publication; Hauser et al. 2007; Mikhail 2000, in press): 1) harm caused as a means to the greater good is worse than harm caused as a side-effect (doctrine of double effect; DDE) and 2) harm caused by action is worse than harm caused by omission) doctrine of doing and allowing; DDA]. This kind of evidence is not, however, sufficient to argue that these distinctions are exclusive moral principles, or part of FMN. It is possible, for example, that both distinctions are mediated by non-moral psychological processes (and thus, part of FMB), such as the relative transparency of the agent's intentions and causal responsibility for the outcomes that ensue. Follow-up work (Cushman et al., submitted for publication) using non-moral scenarios supports this more domain-general interpretation. In particular, differences between doing and allowing (DDA) are largely driven by differences in causal responsibility, whereas differences between means and side effects (DDE) are largely driven by the ascription of intentionality. These results suggest that at least some moral dilemmas are judged by recruiting non-moral, but folk, psychological representations.

Bringing the behavioral and physiological studies together, recent work using neuroimaging (Young et al. 2007) and repetitive transcranial magnetic stimulation (rTMS; Young et al., in preparation), suggests that the rTPJ is critically involved. For example, when people deliver judgments about the permissibility of an action, they take into account the protagonist's beliefs as well as the nature of the outcome. In these situations, fMRI results similarly reveal that belief attribution as subserved by rTPJ is critical for moral judgment. In cases of accidental harm, where beliefs and outcomes are mismatched, Young et al. also observed the most significant activation of the rTPJ, suggesting modulation of beliefs by the outcome. Further, there was significant activation in the anterior cingulate and precuneus, areas implicated in conflict resolution. Unclear at this stage is why the parallel case of belief-outcome mismatch - that is, attempted harm - failed to show a parallel pattern of activation in rTPJ and the conflict regions. Finally, when subjects undergo rTMS to the rTPJ, they were more likely to focus on the outcomes because, in these conditions, the suppression of rTPJ activation functionally resulted in a disruption of belief inference. A critical next step is to assess whether the interface between belief-based systems and outcome-based systems has a unique moral signature or whether its operation is similar in other, non-moral domains.

Emotional Processing

It is clear that emotions play a rather promiscuous role in a wide range of human mental life that is non-moral, such as the feeling of elation following a major scientific discovery, contentment following the consumption of an exceptional meal, anger in response to accidentally stubbing a toe, and fear in response to a snake. A number of arguments and empirical studies (Blair 1995, 1997; Blair et al. 1995; Damasio 1994, 2003; Haidt 2001, 2003, 2007; Hume 1739/1978; Moll et al. 2001, 2002, 2007; Nichols 2002, 2004; Prinz 2004) have recently championed the position that a subset of emotions, especially the highly social and self-other referencing emotions such as guilt, shame, loyalty, and empathy, are causally necessary for morality.

Here, we focus on two questions that have recently been illuminated by neurophys-iological studies. First, to what extent are emotional processes causally necessary for moral judgments? Though there has been considerable work on the role of emotion in moral judgment and behavior, our question is actually two separate ones: 1) when, in the course of detecting an event and making a decision about its moral content, do emotions play a role? and 2) given the temporal and causal role of emotion, are they equally important in all moral contexts and if not, which moral problems most critically recruit the emotions and their underlying neural circuitry?

Behavioral studies using emotional priming and hypnosis (Valdesolo and DeSteno 2006; Wheatley and Haidt 2006), together with imaging experiments with normals and neuropsychological studies with patient populations (e.g., psychopathy, individuals with damage to frontal regions), reveal deficits in moral judgments and behavior when the emotions are either heightened or flattened (Anderson et al. 1999; Blair 1995, 1997; Blair et al. 1995; Ciaramelli et al. 2007; Greene et al. 2001, 2004; Koenigs et al. 2007; Mendez et al. 2005; Moll et al. 2002, 2005, 2007). Our question concerns the diversity of moral situations in which emotions may or may not play a role. To explore this question, we carried out a study of individuals with adult-onset focal lesions to bilateral ventromedial prefrontal cortex (VMPC). These patients had been tested on an earlier battery of tasks tapping emotional experience and recognition, as well as social decision making. Overall, subjects showed a severe deficit with respect to the social emotions (guilt, embarrassment, empathy), flattened skin conductance in response to stimuli that normally evoke responses in non-patient populations, and poor decision making in socially relevant contexts. Based on these findings, and building off the perspective that emotions are the primary sources of our intuitive moral judgments, one would predict abnormal performance in generating permissibility of judgments.

To test this hypothesis, patients evaluated a series of moral scenarios, some of which featured relatively low-intensity emotions associated with "impersonal" harms (e.g., lying on a resume to improve career prospects), whereas others featured high-intensity, emotionally aversive "personal" harms (e.g., smothering a crying baby to escape detection and execution by enemy soldiers). As in previous fMRI studies (Greene et al. 2001, 2004), in a subset of the personal scenarios, an emotionally aversive harm was pitted against the "greater good." VMPC patients responded normally to the impersonal moral scenarios but, for the personal scenarios, the VMPC patients were significantly more likely to endorse committing an emotionally aversive harm if and only if a greater number of people would benefit – the utilitarian response. Importantly, in personal cases where the harm produced only self-benefit, VMPC patients were not more likely to endorse the harm, emphasizing the selectivity of the deficit and the need to carve the moral domain into multiple dimensions. A second lesion study, as well as studies of patients with blunted affect due to fronto-temporal dementia, confirmed this basic finding (Ciaramelli et al. 2007; Mendez et al. 2005). Together, these studies suggest that social emotions mediated by VMPC are indeed necessary for certain kinds of moral judgments, but by no means all.

Moral Specificity

Our goal in this essay has been to lay out a theoretical framework for thinking about the sources of our moral judgments, building on both an analogy to language (Dwyer 1999, 2004; Hauser 2006; Mikhail 2000, in press) and, more generally, current work in the cognitive sciences that aims to clarify the core architecture of particular domains of knowledge (Hirschfeld and Gelman 1994). We think it is important to distinguish between capacities that play a critical role in a particular domain but are not specific to it, as opposed to processes that are unique to a particular domain. This kind of distinction has played a central role in the core knowledge thesis that has been developed by Spelke (2000) and other developmental psychologists, targeting folk physics, mathematics, and psychology. It has played a more minor role in empirical studies of moral psychology.

At present, it is too early to decide any of these issues, but much of the published empirical work leads to the following tentative hypothesis: what is unique to the moral domain is not its individual components or processes but the ways in which these processes interface to both discriminate moral from non-moral social situations and to guide judgment and behavior. Take, for example, the distinction between intentional and accidental action. This is a folk psychological problem that is critical to the moral domain but clearly not specific to it. Moreover, it is a distinction that is shared with other nonhuman primates (Call et al. 2004; Lyons and Santos, in press; Wood et al. 2007) and appears to play some role in socially relevant contexts. For example, in a series of experiments on cotton-top tamarin monkeys, Hauser and colleagues (2003) have shown that individuals are more likely to reciprocate with individuals who intentionally give food to another than with individuals who selfishly obtain food but, as a byproduct, deliver food to another.

A similar account could be given for many of our emotions, including some highly suggestive and provocative studies of empathy-like behavior in primates and mice (de Waal 1996; Langford et al. 2006; Preston and de Waal 2002). As Trivers (1971) pointed out, selection for reciprocity would favor a cast of emotional responses that would support continued interactions with cooperators but lead to aggressive actions toward cheaters. Consequently, moral outrage and moralistic aggression emerge as the outcomes of an interface between the calculus of fairness and the emotions that both support and reinforce it. Thus, although an emotionally flattened human might be able to detect virtuous cooperators and sinful cheaters, she wouldn't be motivated to continue her relationship with the former or ostracize and punish the latter. Similarly, an emotionally motivated human who lacked the ability to detect intentions, beliefs and goals would find good and bad consequences differentially motivating but would find the accidents no different than the volitionally desired goals. In human evolution, perhaps uniquely, we acquired a capacity to connect our folk mental states up with our emotions, creating a distinctive moral domain.

References

Anderson SW, Bechara A, Damasio H, Tranel D, Damasio AR (1999) Impairment of social and moral behavior related to early damage in human prefrontal cortex. Nature Neurosci 2:1032–1037

Barner D, Wood J, Hauser MD, Carey S (2008) Evidence for a non-linguistic distinction between singular and plural sets in rhesus monkeys. Cognition, 107:603–622

Blair RJR (1995) A cognitive developmental approach to morality: investigating the psychopath. Cognition 57:1–29

Blair RJR (1997) Moral reasoning and the child with psychopathic tendencies. Personality Individual Differences 22:731–739

Blair RJR, Sellars C, Strickland I, Clark F, Williams AO, Smith M and L. Jones (1995) Emotion attributions in the psychopath. Personality Individual Differences 19:431–437

Borg JS, Hynes C, Van Horn J, Grafto, S, Sinnott-Armstrong W (2006) Consequences, action, and intention as factors in moral judgments: an fMRI investigation. J Cogn Neurosci 18:803–817

Call J, Hare B, Carpenter M, Tomasello M (2004) 'Unwilling' versus 'unable': chimpanzees' understanding of human intentional action. Devel Sci 7:488–498

Casebeer WD (2003) Moral cognition and its neural constituents. Nature Rev Neurosci 4:841–846

Ciaramelli E, Miccioli M, Ladavas E, di Pellegrino G (2007) Selective deficit in personal moral judgment following damage to ventromedial prefrontal cortext. Social Cogn Affect Neurosci 2:84–92

Cosmides L, Tooby J (1994) Origins of domain specificity: the evolution of functional organization. In: Hirschfeld LA, Gelman SA (eds) Mapping the mind: domain specificity in cognition and culture. Cambridge University Press, Cambridge, pp 85–116

Cushman F, Young L, Hauser MD (2006) The role of conscious reasoning and intuition in moral judgments: testing three principles of harm. Psychol Sci 17:1082–1089

Damasio A (1994) Descartes' error. Boston, MA, Norton

Damasio A (2003) Looking for Spinoza. New York, Harcourt Brace

de Waal FBM (1996) Good natured. Cambridge MA, Harvard University Press

Dwyer S (1999) Moral competence. In: Murasugi K, Stainton R (eds) Philosophy and linguistics. Westview Press, Boulder CO, pp 169–190

Dwyer S (2004) How good is the linguistic analogy. Retrieved February 25, 2004, from www.umbc.edu/philosophy/dwyer

Fletcher CD, Happe F, Frith U, Baker SC, Dolan RJ, Frith CD (1995) Other minds in the brain: a functional imaging study of "theory of mind" in story comprehension. Cognition 58:109–128

Fodor JA. (1983) The modularity of mind. Cambridge, MA, MIT Press

Gallagher HL, Happe F, Brunswick N, Fletcher PC, Frith U, Frith CD (2000) Reading the mind in cartoons and stories: an fMRI study of "theory of mind" in verbal and nonverbal tasks. Neuropsychologia 38:11–21

Gallistel CR (1999) The replacement of general purpose learning models with adaptively specialized learning modules. In: Gazzaniga MS (ed) The cognitive neurosciences 2nd Ed. Cambridge, MA, MIT Press, pp 1179–1191

Gauthier I, Tarr M (1997) Becoming a 'greeble' expert: exploring mechanisms for face recognition. Visual Res 37:1673–1682

Greene JD, Haidt J (2002) How (and where) does moral judgment work? Trends Cogn Sci 6:517–523

Greene JD, Sommerville RB, Nystrom LE, Darley JM, Cohen JD (2001) An fMRI investigation of emotional engagement in moral judgment. Science 293:2105–2108

Greene JD, Nystrom LE, Engell AD, Darley JM, Cohen JD (2004) The neural bases of cognitive conflict and control in moral judgment. Neuron 44:389–400

Haidt J (2001) The emotional dog and its rational tail: A social intuitionist approach to moral judgment. Psychol Rev 108:814–834

Haidt J (2003) The moral emotions. In: Davidson RJ, Scherer KR, Goldsmith HH (eds) Handbook of affective sciences. Oxford University Press, Oxford, pp 852–870

Haidt J (2007) The new synthesis in moral psychology. Science 316:998–1002

Harcourt AH, Harvey PH, Larson SG, Short RV (1981) Testes weight and breeding system in primates. Nature 293:55–57

Hauser MD (2006) Moral minds: how nature designed our sense of right and wrong. New York, Ecco/Harper Collins

Hauser MD, Chomsky N, Fitch WT (2002) The faculty of language: What is it, who has it, and how did it evolve? Science 298:1554–1555

Hauser MD, Chen MK, Chen F, Chuang E (2003) Give unto others: genetically unrelated cotton-top tamarins preferentially give food to those who altruistically give food back. Proc Royal Soc London, B 270:2363–2370

Hauser MD, Cushman F, Young L, Jin RK-X, Mikhail J (2007) A dissociation between moral judgments and justifications. Mind Lang 22:1–21

Hirschfeld LA, Gelman SA (eds) (1994) Mapping the mind: domain-specificity in cognition and culture. Cambridge, Cambridge University Press.

Hume D (1739/1978) A treatise of human nature. Oxford, Oxford University Press

Knobe J (2003a) Intentional action and side effects in ordinary language. Analysis 63:190–193

Knobe J (2003b) Intentional action in folk psychology: an experimental investigation. Phil Psychol 16:309–324

Koenigs M, Young L, Adolphs R, Tranel D, Hauser MD, Cushman F and Damasio A (2007) Damage to the prefrontal cortex increases utilitarian moral judgments. Nature 446:908–911

Langford DJ, Crager SE, Shehzad Z, Smith SB, Sotocinal SG, Levenstadt JS, Chanda ML, Levitin DJ, Mogil JS (2006) Social modulation of pain as evidence for empathy in mice. Science 312:1967–1970

Lyons D, Santos LR (2008) Intentional vs accidental actions in capuchins Developmental Science In press

McKone E, Kanwisher N, Duchaine BC (2007) Can generic expertise explain special processing for faces? Trends Cogn Sci 11:8–15

Mendez M, Anderson E, Shapira JS (2005) An investigation of moral judgment in frontotemporal dementia. Cogn Behav Neurol 18:193–197

Mikhail J (2007) Universal moral grammar: theory, evidence, and the future. Trends Cogn Sci 11:143–152

Mikhail JM (2000) Rawls' linguistic analogy: A study of the 'generative grammar' model of moral theory described by John Rawls in 'A theory of justice'. Unpublished PhD, Cornell University, Ithaca

Mikhail JM (2008) Rawls' linguistic analogy. New York, Cambridge University Press, in press

Moll J, Eslinger PJ, Oliviera-Souza R (2001) Frontopolar and anterior temporal cortex activation in a moral judgment task: preliminary functional MRI results in normal subjects. Arch Neuropsychiat 59:657–664

Moll J, Oliveira-Souza R, Eslinger PJ (2002) The neural correlates of moral sensitivity: a functional MRI investigation of basic and moral emotions. J Neurosci 27:2730–2736

Moll J, Oliveira-Souza R, Moll FT, Ignacio IE, Caparelli-Daquer EM, Eslinger PJ (2005) The moral affiliations of disgust. Cogn Behav Neurol. 18:68–78

Moll J, Zahn R, Oliveira-Souza RD, Krueger F, Grafman J (2007) The neural basis of human moral cognition. Nature Rev Neurosci 6:799–809

Nichols S (2002) Norms with feeling: toward a psychological account of moral judgment. Cognition 84:221–236

Nichols S (2004) Sentimental rules. New York, Oxford University Press

Palmeri TJ, Wong AC-N, Gauthier I (2004) Computational approaches to the development of perceptual expertise. Trends Cogn Sci 8:378–386

Preston S, de Waal FBM (2002) Empathy: its ultimate and proximate bases. Behav Brain Sci 25:1–72

Prinz JJ (2004) Gut reactions. New York, Oxford University Press

Saxe R, Kanwisher N (2003) People thinking about thinking people: the role of the temporo-parietal junction in "theory of mind". NeuroImage 19:1835–1842

Spelke ES (2000) Core knowledge. Am Psychologist 55:1233–1243

Sperber D (1994) The modularity of thought and the epidemiology of representations. In: Hirschfeld LA, Gelman SA (eds) Mapping the mind. Cambridge University Press, New York, pp 112–134

Stich S (2006) Is morality an elegant machine or a kludge? J Cognition Culture 6:181–189

Trivers RL (1971) The evolution of reciprocal altruism. Quart Revf Biol 46:35–57

Valdesolo P, DeSteno D. (2006) Manipulations of emotional context shape moral judgment. Psychol Sci 17:476–477

Wheatley T, Haidt J (2006) Hypnotically induced disgust makes moral judgments more severe. Psychol Sci 16:780–784

Wood J, Glynn DD, Phillips BC, Hauser MD (2007) The perception of rational, goal-directed action in nonhuman primates. Science 317:1402–1405

Young L, Cushman F, Hauser MD, Saxe R (2007) The neural basis of the interaction between theory of mind and moral judgment. Proc Natl Acad Sci 104:8235–8240

Brain Mechanisms Theoretically Underlying Extremes of Social Behaviors: The Best and the Worst

Elena Choleris[1], *Martin Kavaliers*[1], and *Donald Pfaff*[1]

Summary

The best, most pleasant forms of social behaviors amongst humans are characterized by a degree of altruism, sometimes reciprocal altruism, that has been encouraged universally by institutions that promote civil behavior. Here we review a surprisingly parsimonious neuroscientific theory of how humans manage to behave according to the "golden rule." This theory, while allowing the understanding of pro-social behavior, also leads to a consideration of the neural mechanisms underlying aggression and abnormal social behavior, such as autistic behavior. Here we theorize that damagingly high levels of inputs from ascending CNS arousal systems to the amygdala heighten social anxiety in a manner that increases the chance of autistic behavior.

Introduction

Among scientific theories, the most elegant are those that make very few initial assumptions and do not plead special conditions or abilities. To quote Albert Einstein: "A theory should be as simple as possible but not simpler." Below we propose a means of understanding how people behave in a reciprocally altruistic fashion (when they do). The theory is not predicated on special abilities of the human forebrain; rather, it depends on a *loss* of information, the easiest kind of neural and behavioral transformation to achieve.

Equally important, especially from the points of view of behavioral medicine and public health, are the disorders of social behavior. Knowing that the amygdala is involved in the generation of fear, and observing the behavior of autistic children, we believe that social anxiety may be involved in autism. High levels of arousal-related transmitters being released in the amygdala could account for an avoidance of normal social contact.

Implications of Loss of Social Information in Cortical Circuits

Evolutionary biologists have long considered the origins of reciprocal altruism, where an altruistic act is defined as one that benefits the recipient while having negative

---

[1] The Rockefeller University, New York, USA, e-mail: pfaff@rockefeller.edu

Pfaff et al.
Hormones and Social Behavior
© Springer-Verlag Berlin Heidelberg 2008

consequences on the fitness of the performer (reviewed in Lehmann and Keller 2006). Among humans, it appears that shibboleths associated with every religious system we have read (examples in Pfaff 2007) include a norm frequently referred to as the "golden rule" – I should behave toward you as I would have you behave toward me – and one of its consequences could be manifest as reciprocal altruism. The broad appearance of this ethical dictum among human societies encourages a search for its neurobiological underpinnings. Further, a mechanistic analysis is encouraged by the success of Axelrod and Hamilton (1981) in programming computers to display mutual cooperation. In their computer games, mutual cooperation got started spontaneously, thrived and resisted opposition. Axelrod's and Hamilton's success, taken together with the ubiquity of reciprocally altruistic behaviors amongst non-human primates, led us to theorize about mechanisms that could produce such behaviors.

A Theory in Four Steps

First, consider one person's, M's, action toward another, N. Before this act occurs, it is represented in M's brain, as every act must be. Motor acts being represented in one's own brain, so-called "corollary discharges," were conceived first in "reafferenz theory" (a neurophysiological theory that shows how the stability of the visual world is maintained during eye movements) and supported by a large body of experimental data (Held and Freedman 1963). Action representation to one's own brain remains of current interest in neuroscience (Cullen 2004; Sylvestre and Cullen 2006; Quiroga et al. 2006) and biophysics (Poulet and Hedwig 2006; McKinstry et al. 2006).

Second, this act will have consequences for N that M can predict and envision. Then comes the crucial step.

Third, to achieve a feeling consistent with Golden Rule behavior, then M blurs the difference between the other individual and himself to an abstract intermediate image. For example, in terms of face recognition, neurons (Gross et al. 1972) and inferotemporal cortical regions (Kanwisher et al. 1997) specialized for that function are well documented. Mechanisms for blurring, besides simply reducing cortical neuron reliability, include adding noise to the mechanism or altering temporal phases of inputs (Kanwisher N., personal communication). For example, simply reducing the efficiency of GABA-ergic inhibitory neurotransmission or increasing the efficiency of gap junction transmission would raise the overall level of cortical excitability to the point where noise could obscure the signals comprising facial or other images. As a result, instead of seeing the consequences of his act solely for the other individual, M sees them for himself. As an example posed for absolute clarity, if M had been planning on knifing N in the stomach, he loses the difference between N's body and his own. This loss of information is easy to posit because any one of the many steps required for the neurobiology of fear would provide the loss of information this theory supposes. As a result, the knifing is less likely to occur because he shares the other person's fear.

Additionally, the mirror neuron system (Rizzolatti and Craighero 2004) in the cerebral cortex may provide still another mechanism that permits a blurring of the difference between the person beginning an act and the target of that act.

Fourth, if the consequences of M's intended act are good for N, he does it; if the consequences for N are bad, then M does not do it. This decision rests not only upon fear mechanisms, as mentioned above, but also on positive, affiliative motivations, the bauplan of which is sex behavior, whose mechanisms are relatively well understood (chapters in Pfaff et al. 2002).

This explanation of an ethical decision by the would-be knifer has an attractive feature. Usually we have to recognize and remember differences between ourselves and others. However, the explanation of an ethical decision given here involves only the loss of information, not its acquisition or storage. The learning of complex information and its storage in memory are very hard to understand. However, the loss of information is easy to understand, because it only requires the breakdown of any single part of the complex memory-storage processes, whether it be an intricate biochemical adaptation, subtle synaptic modification or precise temporal pattern of electrical activity. Thus, dampening any one of the many mechanisms involved in memory can explain the blurring of identity required by this explanation of Golden Rule-related behavior. Leaving out any one of the mechanisms involved in social recognition or memory allows us to identify with the person toward whom we are about to act. Moreover, among the theoretical mechanisms described above, the individual mechanism left out could differ from species to species and from person to person and from occasion to occasion. In mechanistic terms, therefore, it is incredibly easy to achieve a sense of shared fate with another.

By extension, this parsimonious theory of how people can behave toward others as they would like themselves to be treated also predicts that, when the "blurring" does not occur, anti-social behaviors would be expressed. This theory thus leads to a consideration of the neurobiological bases of violence in the world, as well as a variety of CNS disorders that lead to pathologies of social behavior. Regarding aggression, comprehensive reviews have covered what we know about the neural, hormonal, genetic and environmental influence on agonistic behaviors in animals and people (Nelson 2006). Among the abnormalities of social behavior, we will treat CNS influences on the development of autism in the next section.

CNS Arousal Mechanisms Leading to Social Anxiety Leading to Autism

In humans, the proper processing and recognition of facial cues is crucial to the expression of normal social behavior. One of the hallmarks of autism and related disorders is an impairment of processing and recognition of facial expressions. Patients with Asperger's disorder and socio-emotional disorder are at increased risk of prosopagnosia, that is, the failure to recognize familiar faces (Barton et al. 2004). Furthermore, when faced with a face recognition task, adults with autism spectrum disorder utilize different face-scanning strategies (i.e., they look at the eyes and other inner features of faces less often than normal individuals) and fail to show proper activation of the fusiform face area and regions of the social brain, including the mirror neuron system and the amygdala. The degree of hypoactivation of these areas correlates with social symptoms of autism (Hadjikhani et al. 2007). When they do look at the eyes during facial discrimination tasks, autistic individuals show greater activation of the amygdala, suggesting increased emotional responses associated with gaze fixation (Dalton et al. 2005). Furthermore, when asked to identify the expression of feelings in photos of eyes, autistic patients' lower performance was associated with lower or no activation of the superior temporal gyrus and the amygdala (Davidson and Slagter 2000). It seems, thus, that autistic individuals' impaired social recognition is associated with impaired proper processing of social emotions by the amygdala. Also autistics appear not to obtain any rewarding or pleasurable responses from these human contacts.

Consistent with the non-human animal literature (Choleris et al. 2006), it appears that social recognition in humans is under the control of estrogens and their cognate receptors, estrogen receptors (ERs) alpha and beta. In this regard, there is a female advantage in facial processing and the recognition of emotional expressions (Hampson et al. 2006; Montagne et al. 2005) that is modulated by testosterone (van Honk and Schutter 2007). Augmented testosterone (and possibly reduced estradiol) reduces facial recognition and processing. This sex difference in facial recognition and processing has interesting parallels and implications for ERs and sex differences in autism.

A neuropeptide that has been involved in all of the estrogen-dependent social behaviors described above is the nonapeptide, oxytocin (OT). OT is produced in the hypothalamus and released in various areas of the brain as well as in the blood stream, thus exerting its effects both in the CNS and in the periphery (Gimpl and Fahrenholz 2001). Its release from dendrites as well as axons has been studied in some detail (reviewed in Landgraf and Neumann 2004). In particular OT is known to foster pro-social behaviors. including social recognition (Choleris et al. 2003, 2006, 2007; Fergusson et al. 2000, 2001), social learning (Popik and van Ree 1993), maternal (Pedersen et al. 1994; Young et al. 1997; Cho et al. 1999; Insel and Hulihan 1995; Razzoli et al. 2003) and sexual behaviors (Bancroft 2005; Carter 1992). OT is involved in social bonds – romantic and maternal love – even in humans (Bartel and Zeki 2004). Aggression, in contrast, is inhibited by OT administration (McCarthy 1990; Ferris 2005) and increased by blocking OT action (Lubin et al. 2003; Giovenardi et al. 1998). Mice whose gene for oxytocin has been rendered non-functional [oxytocin "knockout" (OTKO) mice] are more aggressive in both home cage (Winslow et al. 2000) and semi-natural environment testing conditions (Ragnauth et al. 2005).

OT and estrogens act in a linked manner, with OT activity being regulated by estrogens at two levels. First, production of OT is under the control of estrogens, as indicated by several pieces of evidence. Plasma OT levels and OT receptor (OTR) mRNA fluctuate with the estrous cycle in a manner consistent with fluctuations in circulating levels of estrogens (Bale et al. 1995; Sarkar et al. 1992; Ho and Lee 1992). More direct evidence shows that estrogen administration heightens the electrical excitability of OT-producing neurons in the paraventricular nucleus (PVN) of the hypothalamus. Second, the transcription of the gene for OTR is under estrogen control, with estrogen administration increasing the rate of transcription from the OTR gene (Quinones-Jenab et al. 1997). This effect is pronounced in the amygdala, which is relevant for the focus of this review, as highlighted below.

A Functional Genomic Network Supporting Social Recognition

The evidence that the risk of developing an autism spectrum disorder carries important genetic influences is overwhelming (Freitag 2007; Losh and Piven 2007; Hoekstra et al. 2007; Szatmari et al. 2007). Our concern is to use our and others' functional genomic evidence to look into the identification of specific genes contributing to autism's component functions: social recognition and the related function, social anxiety.

In this story, OT and OTR will play major parts, while vasopressin (VP) and its receptors will also provide interesting points. The release of oxytocin in the CNS – not only from synaptic endings but also from dendrites – in the hypothalamus and in the amygdala is thought to be of major importance for a variety of biologically adaptive social behaviors (Landgraf and Neumann 2004).

OT produced within neurons of PVN can be transported along axons into the amygdala, where significant levels of OTR are to be found (Elands et al. 1988; Yoshimura et al. 1993). There, both OT and VP affect neuronal excitability, with the two neuropeptides acting on distinct populations of cells (Huber et al. 2005; Terenzi and Ingram 2005). We have integrated OT actions in the amygdala with estrogenic effects there and its known neuroanatomy to formulate a 4-gene micronet theory that explains certain changes in social recognition in mice.

The involvement of OT in social recognition was initially demonstrated through pharmacological manipulations showing that administration of low levels of OT facilitates social recognition, whereas OT antagonists block it (Popik and Vetulani 1991; Popik et al. 1992, 1996). Later, studies with genetically modified mice showed that both male (Ferguson 2000) and female (Choleris et al. 2003) OTKO mice have a complete deficit in social recognition, even when tested with the more sensitive choice test paradigm (Choleris et al. 2006). OTRKO mice, too, are impaired in social recognition, further confirming the critical involvement of this system (Takayanagi et al. 2005). Further studies then pointed at the medial amygdala as the site of action of OT and OTR in the regulation of social recognition. The deficit of the OTKO male mice can be rescued by infusion of OT in the medial amygdala, whereas infusion of an OT antagonist inhibits social recognition in wild-type males (Ferguson 2001). Similarly, wild-type females that receive an antisense oligonucleotide targeting the mRNA of the OTR gene in the medial amygdala become completely impaired in social recognition (Choleris et al. 2007). The link with estrogens became apparent when it turned out that both ERα and ERβ knockout (α-ERKO and β-ERKO) mice were also impaired in social recognition (Choleris et al. 2003). When assessed with a more sensitive social discrimination test, this impairment was complete in the α-ERKO and only partial in the β-ERKO mice (Choleris et al. 2006). As in the α-ERKO and β-ERKO mice, OTKO mice showed impaired social recognition, as reflected in impaired ability to recognize and avoid parasitized conspecifics. The OTKO mice are also impaired in utilizing other mice as a source of information in mate choices and parasite avoidance.

OT involvement in social disorders has been demonstrated. Low OT plasma levels are observed in autistic patient populations (Modhal et al. 1998; Green et al. 2001), where altered oxytocin production from its prohormone precursor is shown (Green et al. 2001). Furthermore, in initial clinical trials, intravenous infusion of oxytocin ameliorated behavioral symptoms of autism in adult patients (Hollander et al. 2003). Alterations in the OT system are observed also in individuals affected with schizophrenia (Bernstein et al. 1998; Feifel and Reza 1999; Mai et al. 1993) and depression (Bernstein et al. 1998; Uvnäs-Moberg et al. 1999).

The specific impairment in social recognition of the α-ERKO, β-ERKO and OTKO mice prompted the proposal of a 4-gene micronet model to explain the action of estrogens on the oxytocinergic system in the regulation of this behavior. In this model,

ERβ regulates the production of OT in the PVN, whereas ERα controls the transcription of the gene for OTR in the medial amygdala which, in turn, receives and processes olfactory input of social relevance from the main and accessory olfactory systems (Dulac and Torello 2003; Johnston 2003). This model is supported by molecular biology studies and fully explains the behavior of the KO mice. First, ER-β is highly expressed in the mouse PVN, where ER-α is almost absent (Mitra et al. 2003), and directly regulates the production of OT (Patisaul et al. 2003). Accordingly, estrogen regulation of OT is inhibited in β-ERKO mice (Nomura et al. 2002b). Second, ERα is highly expressed in the amygdala (Mitra et al. 2003), where it is necessary for the induction of OTR (Young et al. 1998).

This model explains the behavioral results of the α-ERKO and β-ERKO mice in the more sensitive choice test paradigm (Choleris et al. 2006). The essentiality of ERα for OTR production in the amygdala (Young et al. 1998) explains the complete impairment of the α-ERKO mice, whereas the partial impairment of the β-ERKO mice (Choleris et al. 2006) can be explained by an ERβ-mediated upregulation of existing baseline production of OT in the PVN (Mitra et al. 2003). Accordingly, baseline OT levels and mRNA of the OT gene in the PVN of β-ERKO mice are normal, but they fail to respond to stimulation by estrogens (Nomura et al. 2002b). The baseline levels of OT likely allow for a certain degree of social discrimination in β-ERKO mice, which in normal mice can be enhanced following estrogens/ER-β mediated increase in OT production.

McCarthy and her colleagues (1996) have reported that oxytocin has anxiolytic properties if and only if estrogens are circulating in an adequately high concentration. This requirement for estrogens presumably is due to the strong influence of estrogens on oxytocin receptor gene transcription (Young et al. 1998). In fact, in females, blocking OT receptor activity in the brain increases anxiety-like behaviors in a manner that depends on the hormonal state of the female (Neumann et al. 2000a, 2000b). In the male, testosterone-dependent sexual activity can be followed by the reduction of anxiety due, at least in part, to the release of OT within the brain (Waldherr and Neumann, 2007).

Generalized CNS Arousal Mechanisms Related to Fear

It has been hypothesized that large numbers of ascending and descending neuronal systems involving the expression of more than 120 genes are involved in the adaptive regulation of CNS arousal (Pfaff 2006). Some of the initial need states leading to arousal, such as hunger, are quite specific. However, based on results of a meta-analysis using the mathematical statistical technique of principal components analysis, we have argued that there is a generalized arousal component, an "urarousal," that can account for as much as one-third of arousal-related behaviors (Garey et al. 2003). Of special interest for the present discussion are the effects of generalized arousal neurotransmitters in the amygdala.

Inputs to the amygdala from ascending systems that drive generalized arousal might be important for social anxiety, related to the recognition mechanisms just reviewed above, because this same brain region implicated in social recognition, the amygdala, is crucial for producing the emotion of fear. If signals from conditioned stimuli for fear do not reach the amygdala, then conditioned fearful responses do not occur (reviewed in LeDoux 2000; Rodrigues et al. 2004; Schafe et al. 2005). Likewise, if outputs from the amygdala are suppressed, for example under the influence of the prefrontal cortex), then fear is reduced. In fact, neuropharmacological approaches to the suppression of amygdaloid facilitation of fear are important not only for syndromes such as post-traumatic stress disorder but also, according to our theorizing below, to reduce the social anxiety of autism (Davis 2005; Ressler et al. 2004). The importance of the amygdala for fear, established in laboratory rodents, holds true for higher primates, including humans (Paton et al. 2006; Kalin et al. 2004; Phelps and LeDoux 2005). What are the relationships of these mechanisms to generalized arousal?

Frightening emotions and emotional memories will not operate correctly to raise fear in a biologically adaptive fashion if the entire CNS has not been aroused. James McGaugh and his colleagues have reported (Roozendaal et al. 2004; McIntyre and McGaugh 2005) that the proper operation of amygdaloid mechanisms related to fear depends on synaptic inputs releasing the arousal-related transmitters, norepinephrine and dopamine. For example, the laboratory of James McGaugh, at University of California at Irvine, reported that they trained rats in a task in which the animals had to avoid returning to a place where their feet had been shocked. Infusing a dopamine receptor antagonist into the lateral amygdala prevented peak performance of fear learning. Conversely, infusing dopamine itself or, for that matter, norepinephrine, into the amygdala enhanced retention of the learned fear response. Even additional shocks between training and testing – which would arouse the animal – increased subsequent fear responses. Thus, animals with low levels of generalized arousal are less likely to show high levels of learned fear responses.

Another arousal-supporting neurotransmitter, serotonin, is involved in the production of anxiety and fear. Serotonin-containing fibers reach the amygdala through long axonal projections from the median and dorsal raphe nuclei of the midbrain. Some of the most exciting work on genetic contributions to fear and anxiety has dealt with the serotonin transporter (5-HTT), the molecule responsible for the reuptake of serotonin from its synaptic cleft. It is now widely recognized that the gene encoding 5-HTT contains a 44 base-pair sequence that in some individuals is inserted, producing a long allele that has high transcriptional activity, whereas in other individuals it is deleted, producing a short allele that has less transcriptional activity. In cell cultures, this translates into a twofold greater rate of reuptake when the long allele is present. What does this mean for anxiety and fear and the amygdala. Three lines of evidence gathered so far show its importance. First, human subjects with one or two copies of the short allele exhibit greater amygdala neuronal activity, as assessed by functional magnetic resonance imaging (fMRI) responses to pictures of frightened or angry faces (Hariri et al. 2002). Second, subjects with a short allele show stronger coupling between amygdala and prefrontal cortex fMRI responses to aversive pictures (Heinz et al. 2005). Since this part of the cortex can act to suppress amygdaloid output, their increased correlation is of undoubted significance and the mechanism remains to be discovered. Third, as expected, patients with one or two copies of the short allele actually showed increased levels of anxiety-related traits, state anxiety and enhanced activation in the right amygdala to anxiety provocation (Furmark et al. 2004).

Hyperarousal Fostering Social Anxiety

There is little doubt that prolonged high levels of arousal are aversive. The Yerkes-Dodson law, supported by a century of research, states that task performance will consequently be reduced. This would be expected to include "social tasks" in which appropriate behavior with another individual is required.

There are at least three levels of mechanisms to discuss in dealing with the connection between hyperarousal and social anxiety. First, it is easy to think of long-lasting high levels of activity in the ascending arousal systems, including those mentioned above, as causing a socially anxious state. Second and more complex are the possible roles of the neuropeptides oxytocin and vasopressin themselves. They both affect the autonomic nervous systems, are both connected with the regulation of fluid balance in the body and are both involved in the regulation of smooth muscle contraction. The simplest formulation is to state that OT is more concerned with autonomic responses associated with reproduction in safe situations (lactation, delivery of babies), whereas VP is more important with emergency responses to threatening situations (dehydration, hemorrhage). Both of these physiological levels of hypothesis will benefit from comparisons among high-anxiety and low-anxiety lines of rats (Landgraf and Wigger 2002, 2003). Third is the most psychological level of exploration. It considers a "mismatch hypothesis" that social anxiety results in part from a feeling of lack of preparation for the social encounter. If we feel adequately prepared and if OT and VP levels are optimal, then we feel supported and social anxiety does not occur. If instead we are not adequately prepared and/or if OT and VP levels are not optimal, then we certainly will be hyperaroused and the anticipation of the social event, whatever it may be, will be anxiogenic.

Social Anxiety Fostering Autism

We theorize that imbalances among the levels of expression of certain genes in neurons within the amygdala or among expression of genes in CNS arousal pathways lead to the appearance of autism spectrum disorders. Already, the notion of strong amygdaloid involvement receives strong support from the literature. Ralph Adolphs and his colleagues (Spezio et al. 2007) have found that substantial damage to the amygdala reduces eye contact during conversations, following up earlier work (Adolphs et al. 2005) during which destruction of the amygdala in a human was found to have damaged the ability to respond to fearful expressions of others in a normal way. Conversely, scientists working with Andreas Meyer-Lindenberg (Kirsch et al. 2005) reported that human amygdaloid function is modulated by oxytocin, in that fear-inducing visual stimuli did not activate the amygdala in human subjects given intranasal applications of oxytocin. Thus we hypothesize that, in the amygdala, oxytocin action will reduce the potential for autism, whereas excess stimulation from ascending arousal pathways – typical perhaps with Asperberger's patients – will increase the likelihood of autism. Consistently, autistic children have enlarged amygdalar volumes (Schumann et al. 2004).

The possible role of ascending arousal systems, such as dopamine, norepinephrine and serotonin, in influencing the amygdala in such a manner as to increase social anxiety has received some support. All three of these neurotransmitters are imbalanced in autism (Penn et al. 2006). Likewise, there are a few studies showing opioid dysfunction in autistics, also summarized by Penn et al. (2006).

Outlook

In summary, we have presented parsimonious theories of brain mechanisms underlying some of the best forms of social behaviors and some of the worst: altruism and autism. Research to test the "image blurring" component of the hypothesis for reciprocal altruism could involve, for example, purposefully adding noise to the relevant sensory systems by blocking GABA inhibitory transmission. Experiments to test the arousal component leading to social anxiety might well include pharmacologic manipulation of the amygdala with respect to its noradrenergic, dopaminergic and serotonergic inputs. In both cases, laboratory neuroscience is speaking to matters of great public concern.

References

Adolphs R, Gosselin F, Buchanan TW, Tranel D, Schyns P, Damasio AR (2005) A mechanism for impaired fear recognition after amygdala damage. Nature 433:68–72

Axelrod R, Hamilton WD (1981) The evolution of cooperation. Science 211:1390–1396

Bale TL, Dorsa DM, Johnston CA (1995) Oxytocin receptor mRNA expression in the ventromedial hypothalamus during the estrous cycle. J Neurosci 15:5058–5064

Bancroft J (2005) The endocrinology of sexual arousal. J Endocrinol 186:411–427

Bartel A, Zeki S (2004) The neural correlates of maternal and Romantic love. Neuroimage 21:1155–1166

Barton JJS, Cherkasova M, Hefter R, Coz TA, O'Connor M, Manoach DS (2004) Are patients with social developmental disorders prosopagnostic? Perceptual heterogeneity in the Asperger and soci-emotional processing disorders. Brain 127:1706–1716

Bernstein HG, Stanarius A, Baumann B, Henning H, Krell D, Danos P, Falkai P, Bogerts B (1998) Nitric oxide synthase-containing neurons in the human hypothalamus: reduced number of immunoreactive cells in the paraventricular nucleus of depressive patients and schizophrenics. Neuroscience 83:867–875

Carter CS (1992) Oxytocin and sexual behavior. Neurosci Biobehav Rev 16:131–144

Cho MM, DeVries AC, Williams JR, Carter CS (1999) The effects of oxytocin and vasopressin on partner preferences in male and female prairie voles (Microtus ochrogaster). Behav Neurosci 113:1071–1079

Choleris E, Gustafsson JÅ, Korach KS, Muglia, LJ, Pfaff DW, Ogawa S (2003) An estrogen dependent micronet mediating social recognition: a study with oxytocin- and estrogen receptor α- and β-knockout mice. Proc Natl Acad Sci USA 100:6192–6197

Choleris E, Ogawa S, Kavaliers M, Gustafsson J-Å, Korach KS, Muglia LJ, Pfaff DW (2006) Involvement of estrogen receptor α, β and oxytocin in social discrimination: a detailed behavioral analysis with knockout female mice. Genes Brain Behav 5:528–539

Choleris E, Little SR, Mong JA, Puram SV, Langer R, Pfaff DW (2007). Microparticle based delivery of oxytocin receptor antisense DNA in the medial amygdala blocks social recognition in female mice. Proc Natl Acad Sci USA 104:4670–4675

Cullen K (2004) Sensory signals during active versus passive movement. Current Opin Neurobiol 14:698–670

Dalton KM, Nacewicz BM, Johnstone T, Schafer HS, Gernsbacher MA, Goldsmith HH, Alexander AL, Davidson RJ (2005) Gaze fixation and the neural circuitry of face processing in autism. Nature Neurosci 8:519–526

Davidson RJ, Slagter HA (2000) Probing emotion in the developing brain: functional neuroimaging in the assessment of the neural substrates of emotion in normal and disordered children and adolescents. Ment Retard Dev Disabil Res Rev 6:166–170

Davis M (2005) Searching for a drug to extinguish fear. Cerebrum 7:47–58

Dulac C, Torello, T. (2003) Molecular detection of pheromone signals in mammals: from genes to behaviour. Nature Rev Neurosci 4:551–562

Elands J, Beetsma A, Barberis C, de Kloet ER (1988) Topography of the oxytocin receptor system in rat brain. J Chem Neuroanat 293–302

Feifel D, Reza T (1999) Oxytocin modulates psychomimetic-induced deficits in sensorimotor gating. Psychopharmacology 141:93–98

Ferguson JN, Young LJ, Hearn EF, Matzuk MM, Insel TR, Winslow JT (2000) Social amnesia in mice lacking the oxytocin gene. Nature Genet 25:284–288

Ferguson JN, Aldag JM, Insel, TR, Young LJ (2001) Oxytocin in the medial amygdala is essential for social recognition in the mouse. J Neurosci 21:8278–8285

Ferris CF (2005) Vasopressin/oxytocin and aggression. Novartis Found Symp 268:190–198

Fichna J, Janecka A, Costentin J, Do Rego J-C.(2007) The endomorphin system and its evolving neurophysiological role. Pharmacol Rev 59:88–123

Freitag M (2007) The genetics of autistic disorders. Mol Psychiat, 12:2–22

Furmark T, Tillfors M, Garpenstrand H, Marteinsdottir I, Langström B, Oreland L, Fredrikson M (2004) Serotonin transporter polymorphism related to amygdala excitability and symptom severity in patients with social phobia. Neurosci Lett 362:189–192

Garey J, Goodwillie A, Frohlich J, Morgan M, Gustafsson JA, Smithies O, Korach KS, Ogawa S, Pfaff DW (2003) Genetic contributions to generalized arousal of brain and behavior. Proc Natl Acad Sci USA 100:11019–11022

Gimpl G, Fahrenholz F (2001) The oxytocin receptor system: structure, function, and regulation. Physiol Rev 81:629–683

Giovenardi M, Padoin MJ, Cadore LP, Lucion AB (1998) Hypothalamic paraventricular nucleus modulates maternal aggression in rats: effects of ibotenic acid lesion and oxytocin antisense. Physiol Behav 63:351–359

Green LA, Fein D, Modhal C, Feinstein C, Waterhouse L, Morris M (2001) Oxytocin and autistic disorder: alteration in peptide forms. Biol Psychiatr 50:609–613

Gross CG, Rocha-Miranda CE, Bender DB (1972) Visual properties of neurons in inferotemporal cortex of the macaque. J Neurophysiol 35:96–111

Hadjikhani N, Joseph RM, Snyder J, Tager-Flusberg H (2007) Abnormal activation of the social brain during face perception in autism. Human Brain Mapp 28:441–449

Hampson E, van Anders SM, Mullin LI (2006) A female advantage in the recognition of emotional facial expressions: test of an evolutionary hypothesis. Evol Human Behav 27:401–416

Hariri A, Mattay V, Tessitore A, Kolachana B, Fera F, Goldman D, Egan MF, Weinberger DR (2002) Serotonin transporter genetic variation and the response of the human amygdala. Science 297:400–404

Heinz A, Braus D, Smolka M, Wrase J, Puls I, Hermann D, Klein S, Grüsser SM, Flor H, Schumann G, Mann K, Büchel C (2005) Amygdala-prefrontal coupling depends on a genetic variation of the serotonin transporter. Nature Neurosci 8:20–23

Held R, Freedman S (1963) Plasticity in human sensorimotor control. Science 142:455–462

Ho ML, Lee JN (1992) Ovarian and circulating levels of oxytocin and arginine vasopressin during the estrous cycle in the rat. Acta Endocrinol (Copenhagen). 126:530–534

Hoekstra R, Bartels M, Verweij C, Boomsa D (2007) Heritability of autistic traits in the general population. Arch Pediatric Adolesc Med 161:372–377

Hollander E, Novotny S, Hanratty M, Yaffe R, DeCaria CM, Aronwitz BR, Mosovich S (2003) Oxytocin infusion reduces repetitive behaviors in adults with autistic and Asperger's disorders. Neuropsychopharmacology, 28:191–198

Huber D, Veinante, Stoop R (2005) Vasopressin and oxytocin excite distince neuronal populations in the central amygdala. Science 308:245–249

Insel TR, Hulihan TJ (1995) A gender-specific mechanism for pair bonding: oxytocin and partner preference formation in monogamous voles. Behav Neurosci 109:782–789

Johnston RE (2003) Chemical communication in rodents: from pheromones to individual recognition. J Mammal 84:1141–1162

Kalin NH, Shelton SE, Davidson RJ (2004) The role of the central nucleus of the amygdala in mediating fear and anxiety in the primate. J Neurosci 24:5506–5515

Kanwisher N, McDermott J, Chun MM (1997). The fusiform face area: a module in human extrastriate cortex specialized for face perception. J Neurosci 17:4302–4311

Kirsch P, Esslinger C, Chen Q, Mier D, Lis S, Siddhanti S, Gruppe H, Mattay VS, Gallhofer B, meyer-Linderberg A. (2005) Oxytocin modulates neural circuitry for social cognition and fear in humans. J Neurosci 5:11489–11493

Landgraf R, Neumann I (2004) Vasopressin and oxytocin release within the brain: a dynamic concept of multiple and variable modes of neuropeptide communication. Front Neuroendocrinol 25:150–176

Landgraf R, Wigger A (2002) High vs low anxiety-related behavior rats: an animal model of extremes in trait anxiety. Behav Genet 32:301–314

Landgraf R, Wigger A (2003) Born to be anxious: neuroendocrine and genetic correlates of trait anxiety in HAB rats. Stress 6:111–119

LeDoux J (2000) Emotion circuits in the brain. Ann Rev Neurosci 23:155–184

Lehmann L, Keller L (2006) The evolution of cooperation and altruism – a general framework and a classification of models. J Evol Biol 6:1365–1376

Losh M, Piven J (2007) Social cognition and the broad autism phenotype. J Child Psychol Psychiat 48:105–112

Lubin DA, Elliott JC, Black MC, Johns JM (2003) An oxytocin antagonist infused into the central nucleus of the amygdala increases maternal aggressive behavior. Behav Neurosci 117:195–201

Mai JK, Berger K, Sofroniew MW (1993) Morphometric evaluation of neurophysin-immunoreactivity in the human brain: pronounced inter-individual variability and evidence for altered staining patterns in schizophrenia. J Hirnforsch 34:133–154

McCarthy MM (1990) Oxytocin inhibits infanticide in female house mice (Mus domesticus). Horm Behav 24:365–375

McCarthy MM, McDonald CH, Brooks PJ, Goldman D (1996) An anxiolytic action of oxytocin is enhanced by estrogen in the mouse. Physiol Behav 60:1209–1215

McIntyre C, McGaugh J (2005) Memory-influencing intra-basolateral amygdala drug infusions modulate expression of Arc protein in the hippocampus. Proc Natl Acad Sci USA 102:10718–10723

McKinstry JL, Edelman GM, Krichmar JL (2006) A cerebellar model for predictive motor control tested in a brain-based device. Proc Natl Acad Sci USA 103:3387–3392

Mitra SW, Hoskin E, Yudkovitz J, Pear L, Wilkinson HA. Hayashi S, Pfaff DW, Ogawa S, Rohrer SP, Schaeffer JM, McEwen BS, Alves SE (2003) Immunolocalization of estrogen receptor β in the mouse brain: comparison with estrogen receptor α. Endocrinology 144:2055–2067

Modhal CM, Green LA, Fein D, Morris M, Waterhouse L, Feinstein C, Levin H (1998) Plasma oxytocin levels in autistic children. Biol Psychiatr 43:270–277

Montagne B, Kessels RP, Figerio E, De Haan EH, Perret DI (2005) Sex differences in the perception of affective facial expressions: do men really lack emotional sensitivity? Cogn Processing 6:136–141

Nelson RJ (Ed) (2006). Biology of aggression. New York: Oxford University Press

Neumann ID, Torner L, Wigger A (2000a) Brain oxytocin: differential inhibition of neuroendocrine stress responses and anxiety-related behaviour in virgin, pregnant and lactating rats. Neuroscience 95:567–575

Neumann ID, Wigger A, Torner L, Holsboer F, Landgraf R (2000b) Brain oxytocin inhibits basal and stress-induced activity of the hypothalamo–pituitary–adrenal axis in male and female rats: partial action within the paraventricular nucleus. J Neuroendocrinol 12:235–243

Nomura M, McKenna E, Korach KS, Pfaff DW, Ogawa S (2002a) Estrogen receptor-beta regulates transcript levels for oxytocin and arginine vasopressin in the hypothalamic paraventricular nucleus of male mice. Mol Brain Res 109:84–94

Nomura M, Durback L, Chan J, Gustafsson J-A, Smithies O, Korach KS, Pfaff DW, Ogawa S (2002b) Genotype/age interactions on aggressive behavior in gonadally intact estrogen receptor β-knockout (βERKO) male mice. Horm Behav 41:288–296

Patisaul HB, Scordalakes EM, Young LJ, Rissman EF (2003) Oxytocin, but not oxytocin receptor, is regulated by oestrogen receptor beta in the female mouse hypothalamus. J Neuroendocrinol 15:787–793

Paton JJ, Belova MA, Morrison SE, Salzmann CD. (2006) The primate amygdala represents the positive and negative value of visual stimuli during learning. Nature 439:865–870

Pedersen CA, Caldwell JD, Walker C, Ayers G, Mason GA (1994) Oxytocin activates the postpartum onset of rat maternal behavior in the ventral tegmental and medial preoptic areas. Behav Neurosci 108:1163–1171

Penn HE (2006) Neurobiological correlates of autism: a review of recent research. Child Neuropsychol 12:57–79

Pfaff D (2006) Brain arousal and information theory. Cambridge: Harvard University Press

Pfaff D (2007) The neuroscience of fair play. Washington: Dana Press

Pfaff D, Arnold A, Etgen A, Fahrbach S, Rubin R (2002) Hormones, brain and behavior (5 volumes). San Diego: Academic Press/Elsevier

Phelps E, LeDoux J (2005) Contributions of the amygdala ato emotion processing: From animal models to human behavior. Neuron 48:175–187

Popik P, van Ree JM (1993) Social transmission of flavored tea preferences: facilitation by a vasopressin analog and oxytocin. Behav Neur Biol 59:63–68

Popik P, Vetulani J (1991) Opposite action of oxytocin and its peptide antagonists on social memory in rats. Neuropeptides 18:23–27

Popik P, Vetulani J, van Ree JM (1992) Low doses of oxytocin facilitate social recognition in rats. Psychopharmacology 106:71–74

Popik P, Vetulani J, van Ree JM (1996) Facilitation and attenuation of social recognition in rats by different oxytocin-related peptides. Eur J Pharmacol 308:113–116

Poulet J, Hedwig B (2006). The cellular basis of a corollary discharge. Science 311:518–522

Quiñones-Jenab V, Jenab S, Ogawa S, Adan RAM, Burbach PH, Pfaff DW (1997) Effects of estrogen on oxytocin receptor messenger ribonucleic acid expression in the uterus, pituitary and forebrain of the female rat. Neuroendocrinology 65:9–17

Quiroga RQ, Snyder LH, Batista AP, Cui H, Andersen RA (2006). Movement intention is better predicted than attention in the posterior parietal cortex. J Neurosci 26:3615–3620

Ragnauth AK, Devidze N, Moy V, Finley K, Goodwillie A, Kow L-M, Muglia LJ, Pfaff DW (2005) Female oxytocin gene-knockout mice, in a seminatural environment, display exaggerated aggressive behavior. Genes Brain Behav 4:229–239

Razzoli M, Cushing BS, Carter CS, Valsecchi P (2003) Hormonal regulation of agonistic and affiliative behavior in female Mongolian gerbils (Meriones unguiculatus). Horm Behav 43:549–553

Ressler KJ, Rothbaum BO, Tannenbaum L, Anderson P, Graap K, Zimand F, Hodges L, Davis M (2004) Cognitive enhances as adjuncts to psychotherapy: use of D-cycloserine in phobic individuals to facilitate extinction of fear. Arch Gen Psychiatr 61:1136–1144

Rizzolatti G, Craighero L (2004). The mirror-neuron system. Annu Rev Neurosci 27:169–192

Rodrigues SM, Schafe GE, LeDoux JE (2004) Molecular mechanisms underlying emotional learning and memory in the lateral amygdala. Neuron 44:75–91

Roozendaal B, Hahn EL, Nathan SV, deQuervain DJ, McGaugh JL (2004) Glucocorticoid effects on memory retrieval require concurrent noradrenergic activity in hippocampus and basolateral amygdala. J Neurosci 24:8161–8169

Sarkar DK, Frautschy SA, Mitsugi N (1992) Pituitary portal plasma levels of oxytocin during the estrous cycle, lactation, and hyperprolactinemia. Ann NY Acad Sci 652:397–410

Schafe GE, Doyère V, LeDoux JE (2005) Tracking the fear engram: the lateral amygdala is an essential locus of fear memory storage. J Neurosci 25:10010–10014

Schumann CM, Hamstra J, Goodlin-Jones BL, Lotspeich LJ, Kwon H, Buonocore MH, Lammers CR, Reiss AL, Amaral DG (2004) The amygdala is enlarged in children but not adolescents with autism; the hippocampus is enlarged at all ages. J Neurosci 24:6392–6401

Spezio M, Po S, Castelli F, Adolphs R (2007) Amygdala damage impairs eye contact during conversations with real people. J Neurosci 27:3994–3997

Sylvestre PCullen K (2006) Premotor correlates of integrated feedback control for eye-head gaze shifts. J Neurosci 26:4922–4929

Szatmari P, Paterson AD, Zwaigenbaum L, Roberts W, Brian J, Liu XQ, Vincent JB, Skaug JL, Thompson AP, Senman L, Feuk L, Qian C, Bryson SE, Jones MB, Marshall CR, Scherer SW, Vieland VJ, Bartlett C, Mangin LV, Goedken R, Segre A, Pericak-Vance MA, Cuccaro ML, Gilbert JR, Wright HH, Abramson RK, Betancur C, Bourgeron T, Gillberg C, Leboyer M, Buxbaum JD, Davis KL, Hollander E, Silverman JM, Hallmayer J, Lotspeich L, Sutcliffe JS, Haines JL, Folstein SE, Piven J, Wassink TH, Sheffield V, Geschwind DH, Bucan M, Brown WT, Cantor RM, Constantino JN, Gilliam TC, Herbert M, Lajonchere C, Ledbetter DH, Lese-Martin C, Miller J, Nelson S, Samango-Sprouse CA, Spence S, State M, Tanzi RE, Coon H, Dawson G, Devlin B, Estes A, Flodman P, Klei L, McMahon WM, Minshew N, Munson J, Korvatska E, Rodier PM, Schellenberg GD, Smith M, Spence MA, Stodgell C, Tepper PG, Wijsman EM, Yu CE, Rogé B, Mantoulan C, Wittemeyer K, Poustka A, Felder B, Klauck SM, Schuster C, Poustka F, Bölte S, Feineis-Matthews S, Herbrecht E, Schmötzer G, Tsiantis J, Papanikolaou K, Maestrini E, Bacchelli E, Blasi F, Carone S, Toma C, Van Engeland H, de Jonge M, Kemner C, Koop F, Langemeijer M, Hijmans C, Staal WG, Baird G, Bolton PF, Rutter ML, Weisblatt E, Green J, Aldred C, Wilkinson JA, Pickles A, Le Couteur A, Berney T, McConachie H, Bailey AJ, Francis K, Honeyman G, Hutchinson A, Parr JR, Wallace S, Monaco AP, Barnby G, Kobayashi K, Lamb JA, Sousa I, Sykes N, Cook EH, Guter SJ, Leventhal BL, Salt J, Lord C, Corsello C, Hus V, Weeks DE, Volkmar F, Tauber M, Fombonne E, Shih A (2007) Mapping autism risk loci using genetic loci using genetic linkage and chromosomal rearrangements. Nature Genet 39:319–328

Takayanagi Y, Yoshida M, Bielsky IF, Ross HE, Kawamata M, Onaka T, Yanagisawa T, Kimura T, Matzuk MM, Young LJ, Nishimori K (2005) Pervasive social deficits, but normal parturition, in oxytocin receptor-deficient mice. Proc Natl Acad Sci USA 102:16096–16101

Terenzi M, Ingram CD (2005) Oxytocin-induced excitation of neurons in the rat central and medial amygdaloid nuclei. Neuroscience 134:345–354

Uvnäs-Moberg K, Björkstrand E, Hillegaart V, Ahlenius S (1999) Oxytocin as a possible mediator of SSRI-induced antidepressant effects. Psychopharmacology 141:95–101

van Honk J, Schutter DJLG (2007) Testosterone reduces conscious detection of signals serving social correction. Psychol Sci 18:663–667

Waldherr M, Neumann ID (2007) Centrally released oxytocin mediates mating-induced anxiolysis in male rats. Proc Natl Acad Sci USA 104:169681–16684

Winslow JT, Hearn EF, Ferguson J, Young LJ, Matzuk MM, Insel TR (2000) Infant vocalization, adult aggression, and fear behavior of an oxytocin null mutant mouse. Horm Behav 37:145–155

Yoshimura R, Kyama H, Tohyama M (1993) Localization of oxytocin receptor messenger ribonucleic acid in the rat brain. Endocrinology 133:1239–1246

Young LJ, Winslow JT, Wang Z, Gingrich B, Guo Q, Matzuk MM, Insel TR (1997) Gene targeting approaches to neuroendocrinology: oxytocin, maternal behavior, and affiliation. Horm Behav 31:221–231

Young LJ, Wang Z, Donaldson R, Rissman EF (1998) Estrogen receptor α is essential for induction of oxytocin receptor by estrogen. Neuroreport 9:933–936

Serotonergic Modulation of Sex and Aggression

Berend Olivier[1,2], *Johnny S.W. Chan*[1], and *Marcel D. Waldinger*[1,3]

Summary

The serotonergic system in the central nervous system (CNS) has complex interactions with many, if not all other neurotransmitter systems in the brain. Its localization, distribution and amazing receptor diversity makes it an appealing system for modulatory aspects in many basic behaviors, including sexual and aggressive behaviors. Notwithstanding decades of research into the putative role of the serotonin (5-HT) system in aggression and sex, no clear picture has emerged. In aggression, depending on state or trait, 5-HT is involved in either the performance or its termination. Application of drugs, and particular selective ligands for certain receptors, suggests a specific role for the (postsynaptic) 5-HT_{1B} and to a lesser extent, the 5-HT_{1A} receptor in the modulation of (offensive) aggression. In sexual behavior, the role of 5-HT is less well studied. Here, 5-HT_{1A} receptor activation and blockade of 5-HT_{2C} receptors are prosexual, whereas 5-HT_{1B} receptor activation is inhibitory. Selective serotonergic uptake inhibitors have no acute effects on sexual behavior but are inhibitory after chronic administration. The role of serotonin in aggression and sexual behavior most likely involves different, partly overlapping, neurochemical systems, suggesting that independent networks in both behavioral systems are differentially influenced by serotonergic tone influencing various 5-HT receptors.

Introduction to the Serotonergic System and 5-HT Receptors

The serotonergic neurotransmitter system is equipped with one endogenous ligand, 5-hydroxytryptamine (5-HT, serotonin), and has at least 14 structurally, functionally and pharmacologically distinct 5-HT receptor subtypes. These receptor subtypes can be assigned to one of seven families, namely 5-HT_{1-7} (Hoyer et al. 1994), and each receptor subtype appears to have a distinct and limited distribution in the central nervous system (CNS). Nonetheless, whether all these different receptor families and/or subtypes have their own distinct functions is unclear, although very likely. Importantly, in addition to

[1] Department of Psychopharmacology, Utrecht Institute for Pharmaceutical Sciences and Rudolf Magnus Institute of Neuroscience, Utrecht University, Sorbonnelaan 36, 3584CA Utrecht, The Netherlands
[2] Yale University School of Medicine, Department of Psychiatry, New Haven, USA, e-mail: b.olivier@pharm.uu.nl
[3] Haga-Hospital Leyenburg, Den Haag, The Netherlands

Pfaff et al.
Hormones and Social Behavior
© Springer-Verlag Berlin Heidelberg 2008

their postsynaptic distribution throughout the CNS, 5-HT$_1$ receptors are also located presynaptically as autoreceptors, where they regulate the activity of 5-HT neurons in the dorsal raphé nucleus (Stamford et al. 2000; Pineȳro and Blier 1999). Moreover, serotonergic transporter molecules (5-HTT) are present on serotonergic neurons (both somatodendritically and presynaptically), where they facilitate the re-uptake of 5-HT after cell firing-induced 5-HT release. Selective serotonin reuptake inhibitors (SSRI) inhibit this transporter and cause enhanced 5-HT levels in the synaptic cleft, leading to enhanced serotonergic neurotransmission.

The putative role of 5-HT in aggression and sexual behavior will be discussed in the following paragraphs. Traditionally, serotonergic activity can be lowered by applying neurotoxins, e.g., pCPA or 5,7-DHT, but also by manipulating the levels of the essential amino acid, l-tryptophan. Moreover, comparison of the activity of the 5-HT system in aggressive versus non-aggressive individuals or during the performance of aggressive acts can be used to study the role of 5-HT. Pharmacological tools and genetic modifications (gene knock out, knock in, overexpression) can be used to selectively engineer specific 5-HT receptors, thereby deciphering the specific roles of the various subsystems of the 5-HT system in the CNS.

5-HT and Aggression: Is 5-HT Inhibitory in Aggression?

The dogma about the relationship between 5-HT and aggression is that 5-HT inhibits aggression; this assertion is mainly derived from studies in which 5-HT levels in the brain were decreased by neurotoxic agents like pCPA or 5,7-DHT, which deplete 5-HT from serotonergic cells. Such an inverse relationship between 5-HT and aggression has been found in animals and humans, although in the latter measurements of 5-HT activity were based on cerebral spinal fluid (CSF) levels of its main metabolite, 5-HIAA. Notwithstanding severe criticisms of this parameter, for many years it was the only measure in humans reflecting (indirectly) the functional status of the 5-HT system. In animals, 5-HT and 5-HIAA can be measured directly in the brain and it could be assumed that the inverse relationship between functional serotonergic activity and aggression should easily be established. However, several contradictory results have been found, and even reports of a positive relationship between 5-HT and aggression occur. In humans, aggression is associated with suicidal behavior and both seem to be associated with low serotonergic function, although it is possible that both phenomena are independently regulated (Mann 2003).

Measurement of contents of 5-HT and 5-HIAA in postmortem brain tissue and determining a turnover rate from these two parameters was originally described to be lower in aggressive vs. non-aggressive mice (Giacalone et al. 1968), but recent studies also found no differences in the prefrontal cortex (Caramaschi et al. 2007). Successive measurements of CSF samples in humans more or less found a serotonergic hypofunction (Brown et al. 1979; Linnoila et al. 1983; Kruesi et al. 1990), although this 5-HT hypofunction or deficiency trait has been associated with impulsivity and risk-taking behavior rather than aggression per se (Mann 2003). A causal relationship between 5-HT activity and aggression or impulsivity cannot be derived from static measurements of 5-HT or 5-HIAA measurements in brain tissue or CSF. A functional role of serotonergic neurons in the initiation, execution and stopping of aggression

(Coccaro 1989; Miczek et al. 2002) still has to be established, although some progress has been made using in vivo microdialysis techniques in freely moving (aggressive) animals. This technique, however, lacks sufficient resolution because sample time (minutes) is still of a different magnitude than the actual behavior (seconds). Van Erp and Miczek (2000) measured extracellular 5-HT (and dopamine) release in 10-min samples in the nucleus accumbens (Nac) and prefrontal cortex (PFC) in rats before, during and after 10-min aggressive interactions with a male conspecific. During the agonistic interaction, no detectable change in 5-HT release was found in the NAc, but 5-HT levels were already decreased during fighting in the PFC. After the confrontation, 5-HT levels in the PFC remained lowered (compared to pre-confrontation baseline) for at least one hour, whereas 5-HT in the NAc was not affected. Dopamine levels were enhanced in both brain areas after (but not during) the aggressive confrontation. However, 5-IIT levels were decreased in the NAc of rats that had been conditioned to fight at a specific time each day over a 10-day period (Ferrari et al. 2003). In the latter experiments, heart rate and dopamine release were concurrently measured and both were raised in anticipation of the fight. Apparently, the actual performance of aggression can be dissociated from the anticipation of a fight, where dopamine plays an important role in the physiological and behavioral sequels around the performance and anticipation of aggression and serotonin seems to be particularly related to termination of aggression.

Measuring electrophysiological events in the serotonergic neurons during the performance of aggression would be very helpful in unraveling the precise role of the 5-HT system but seems technically challenging. Moreover, the 5-HT system is not one homogeneous mass of cells but extremely differentiated; the dorsal and median raphé nuclei projecting to the different areas of the forebrain are the most prominent sources of 5-HT neurons innervating areas involved in the initiation, performance and termination of aggressive behavior. Interestingly, no systematic studies have been performed thus far trying to delineate the role of the different 5-HT cell groups in various aspects of aggression, although local lesions or local application of drugs in the dorsal or median raphé nuclei have been performed. It is highly unlikely that all 5-HT cell groups are involved, and selective blockade or activation of individual cell groups in determining the role of 5-HT in aggression would be very fruitful.

A recent approach to unraveling the role of the 5-HT system in aggression is studying the differences between highly aggressive and lowly aggressive individuals (de Boer et al. 2003). These authors argue, based on the assumption that the individual level of (offensive) aggression of a rat is part of an individual coping strategy and thus an important indicator of a trait-like behavioral and physiological response pattern (Koolhaas et al. 2007). In their extensive studies on endophenotypes of highly aggressive and non-aggressive rodents, no inverse relationship between 5-HT activity and aggression was found, but a positive correlation was found between the level of trait-like aggression (high or low) and basal CSF concentrations of 5-HT and 5-HIAA (Van der Vegt et al. 2003). Apparently, normal offensive aggression is positively related to serotonergic neuronal activity, whereas an inverse relationship probably exists between 5-HT activity and impulse-like violent aggression (Coccaro 1989).

Thus a general pattern emerges where trait and state aggression are probably differentially regulated by the 5-HT system, although much more research is needed to substantiate this hypothesis (for recent discussion, see Ferrari et al. 2005).

5-HT Receptors

The 14 different 5-HT receptors and the 5-HTT enable the unraveling of the function and contribution of the different receptors in various aspects of aggression. To date, ligands are available for most receptors, including (partial) agonists and antagonists, although for some receptors no adequate tools are available. Since 5-HT$_{1\text{ and }2}$ receptors have been studied since the 1980s, research on the role of these receptors in aggression is most abundant. Recent overviews of the involvement of 5-HT receptors in aggression can be found in Olivier (2004, 2005).

5-HT$_1$ Receptors

Clinically, only one partial 5-HT$_{1A}$ receptor agonist, buspirone, has been available; its effect on aggression in humans is not very well described (Ratey et al. 1991; Kavoussi et al. 1997) but does not appear very promising. Preclinically, an extensive range of 5-HT$_{1A}$ receptor ligands is available (Olivier et al. 1999), and prototypic agonists like 8-OH-DPAT, flesinoxan and buspirone or antagonists like WAY100,635 have been used in aggression studies in animals.

   Although practically all studies report anti-aggressive effects of 5-HT$_{1A}$ receptor agonists in various species, these effects are not specific in the sense that anti-aggressive effects occur at doses that also compromise non-aggressive elements of the behavioral repertoire (Olivier et al. 1995; Miczek et al. 1998a,b). 5-HT$_{1A}$ receptor antagonists have no intrinsic effects on aggression but are able to antagonize the anti-aggressive effects of 5-HT$_{1A}$ receptor agonists (Miczek et al. 1998b; Mendoza et al. 1999; de Boer et al. 2000; de Boer and Koolhaas 2005). There is conflicting evidence whether 5-HT$_{1A}$ receptor agonists exert their anti-aggressive effects via pre- or postsynaptically located 5-HT$_{1A}$ receptors. Lesions of the raphe nuclei, removing 5-HT$_{1A}$ somatodendritic autoreceptors, did not prevent the anti-aggressive effects of eltoprazine (Sijbesma et al. 1991) or 8-OH-DPAT (Nikulina and Miczek 1999). However, eltoprazine is a mixed 5-HT$_{1A,1B}$receptor agonist and its anti-aggressive effects in 5,7-dihydroxytryptophan-lesioned rats might be due to activation of postsynaptic 5-HT$_{1B}$ receptors. In the Nikulina and Miczek (1999) study, the remaining 5-HT$_{1A}$ autoreceptors (there was a limited depletion of 5-HT in this study, suggesting a considerable number of intact 5-HT neurons after the 5,7-DHT insult) may be responsible for this effect. Infusion of 8-OH-DPAT and eltoprazine into the dorsal raphe nucleus (Mos et al. 1993) reduced aggressive behavior in rats but concomitantly reduced social interest and increased inactivity, indicative of a non-selective reduction of aggression. TFMPP, a more selective 5-HT$_{1B}$ receptor agonist than eltoprazine, had no effect under these conditions, suggesting that the non-specific reduction of aggression after 8-OH-DPAT and eltoprazine was caused by activation of serotonergic autoreceptors in the dorsal raphe nucleus. When these drugs were infused into the lateral ventricle, 8-OH-DPAT had no anti-aggressive effects, whereas eltoprazine and TFMPP had a very selective anti-aggressive effect, indicating that postsynaptic 5-HT$_{1A}$ receptors are not involved in the aggression-modulating effects of 5-HT$_{1A}$ receptor agonists and that the specific reduction in aggression is induced by activation of postsynaptically located 5-HT$_{1B}$ receptors (Mos et al. 1992). A strong argument against a specific role for 5-HT$_{1A}$ receptors in specific modulation of (offensive) aggression derives from studies where aggression was evoked by electrical stimulation in the hypothalamus of rats (Kruk et al.

1979). This kind of violent aggressive behavior towards a male conspecific, was not at all sensitive to 5-HT$_{1A}$ receptor agonists like 8-OH-DPAT, buspirone and flesinoxan (Olivier et al. 1994), even at extremely high doses. Apparently, by directly stimulating the neural substrate activating aggressive behavior, the role of the 5-HT$_{1A}$ receptor is minimal or non-existent, whereas 5-HT$_{1B}$ receptor agonists (TFMPP and eltoprazine) dose-dependently and behavior-specifically reduced this kind of "violent" aggression.

On the other hand, certain 5-HT$_{1A}$ receptor agonists from the benzodioxopiper-azine class (Olivier et al. 1999) seem to exert anti-aggressive effects via presynaptic 5-HT$_{1A}$ autoreceptors (de Boer et al. 2000; Van der Vegt et al. 2001; de Boer and Koolhaas 2005). Activation of presynaptic 5-HT$_{1A}$ autoreceptors leads to decreased firing of the 5-HT neuron and decreased release of 5-HT at the synaptic level. It seems unlikely that such a general reduction in 5-HT turnover, which affects all (pre- and postsynaptic) 5-HT receptors, would lead to such a specific reduction in aggression. Moreover, chronic administration of 5-HT$_{1A}$ receptor agonists leads to downregula-tion of 5-HT$_{1A}$ autoreceptors and subsequent increased cell firing and enhanced 5-HT release. On a chronic basis, the acute anti-aggressive effects would subside and even enhanced aggression might develop after chronic treatment. No chronic studies with 5-HT$_{1A}$ receptor agonists have been reported, but they are clearly needed to answer the acute vs. chronic effects of 5-HT$_{1A}$ receptor agonists on aggression.

The 5-HT$_{1B}$ receptor has been the focus of interest in the development of clinically relevant anti-aggressive agents, the so-called serenics (Olivier et al. 1990). The 5-HT$_{1B}$ receptor terminology has been confusing. The 5-HT$_{1B}$ receptor in rodents and humans,

Table 1. Summary of effects of psychoactive agents with selectivity for subtypes of serotonin receptors

5-HT principle	Resident-intruder mouse	Resident-intruder rat	Maternal aggression rat	Brain-induced aggression rat	Muricide rat	Defensive behavior mouse/rat
1A agonist	0 ▼	▼	▼	0	0	0
1A antagonist	0	0	0	0	0	0
1B agonist	+	+	+	+	+	0
1B antagonist	0	0	0	0	0	0
2A agonist	▼	▼	▼	-	▼	-
2A antagonist	▼	▼	-	0	▼	-
2C agonist	▼	▼	▼	-	-	-
2C antagonist	▼	▼	▼	-	-	-
3-agonist	0	0	-	-	0	-
3-antagonist	0	0	0	-	0	-
4,5,6-agonist/ antagonist	-	-	-	-	-	-
7-agonist	-	-	-	-	-	-
7-antagonist	0	-	-	-	-	-
Reuptake blockade	▼	▼	▼	0	0	0

0 = no effect on aggression; ▼ =non-specific reduction in aggression; + = specific reduction in aggression (serenic effect); - = not-tested. Data are based on our published and unpublished work (summarized in Olivier et al. 1990, 1995, 1994) and published data.

although exerting a similar function, differs in an essential amino acid in the ligand binding domain of the receptor, which leads to a dramatic difference in its pharmacological sensitivity and specificity (Hartig et al. 1996). Agonists for the rodent ($r5-HT_{1B}$) $5-HT_{1B}$ receptor are anti-aggressive and exert a serenic profile (Olivier et al. 1990), defined as a dose-dependent decrease in offensive aggression, without concomitant sedation, motor or sensory impairment that could explain the anti-aggressive effect. The early serenics (e.g., fluprazine, DU28412, DU 27725, eltoprazine, batoprazine; Olivier et al. 1990) were mixed $5-HT_{1A/1B}$ receptor agonists, leaving the $5-HT_{1A}$ receptor as an option for mediating (part of) the anti-aggressive effect, but more recently synthesized $5-HT_{1B}$ receptor agonists, including, for example, anpirtoline, CP-94,253 and zolmitriptan, were far more selective for this receptor and showed a similar, highly specific anti-aggressive effect, both in aggressive residential mice and in mice made more aggressive via low doses of alcohol or social instigation (Fish et al. 1999; de Almeida et al. 2001; Miczek and de Almeida 2001).

$5-HT_{1B}$ receptor knockout (KO) mice (Saudou et al. 1994) showed enhanced aggressive behavior (Saudou et al. 1994; Ramboz et al. 1995; Brunner and Hen 1997; Bouwknecht et al. 2001), but due to the low baseline aggression level of the genetic background (129Sv) strain, the "enhanced" aggression in the KO mice was still low. More recent studies (Pattij et al. 2003, 2004; Bouwknecht et al .2001) have implicated the $5-HT_{1B}$ receptor in impulsivity regulation rather than offensive aggression per se (Lesch and Merschendorf 2000). Olivier and coworkers suggested that the specific anti-aggressive effects of $5-HT_{1B}$ receptor agonists are modulated via postsynaptic $5-HT_{1B}$ receptors (Olivier et al. 1995; Olivier and Van Oorschot 2005). Such postsynaptic $5-HT_{1B}$ receptors are located as heteroreceptors on non-serotonergic neurons (including dopaminergic, cholinergic, and $GABA_A$-ergic neurons). These heteroreceptors, when activated by 5-HT, inhibit ongoing behavior, including aggression. Thus, $5-HT_{1B}$ receptor agonists inhibit those "aggression or impulsivity" modulating neurons, and removing the postsynaptic $5-HT_{1B}$ receptor (via null mutation of the $5-HT_{1B}$ receptor gene) removes this "brake," thereby facilitating various behaviors related to impulsivity, hyperactivity and aggression (Olivier and Young 2002). Based on the "hyperaggressive" $5-HT_{1B}$ receptor KO mouse and the anti-aggressive effects of $5-HT_{1B}$ receptor agonists, one could suggest that administration of $5-HT_{1B}$ receptor antagonists might lead to facilitation of aggression. However, all such antagonists appear silent, comparable to $5-HT_{1A}$ receptor antagonists, probably indicating that under normal, physiological conditions the serotonergic tone at post-synaptic $5-HT_{1B}$ receptors is not that strong.

5-HT$_2$ Receptors

Although $5-HT_2$ ligands have been synthesized and tested in aggression, these compounds are extremely difficult to typify in their specificity in aggression (for a nice review, see Miczek et al. 2002). The available agents for $5-HT_{2A \ and \ 2B}$ receptors are not that specific and, when tested, show anti-aggressive effects at similar doses that exert sometimes severe (sedating) side effects (Olivier et al. 1995; Sanchez et al. 1993). There is some evidence that $5-HT_{2A}$ receptor antagonists (e.g., risperidone) inhibit aggressive behavior in patients with various diagnoses, including, e.g., depression and schizophrenia. However, no specific evidence thus far points to a selective contribution of any $5-HT_2$ subtype receptor to aggression.

5-HT Transporter

Since the 5-HTT is only located on the serotonergic neuron (both in the synaptic terminal and the somatodendritic areas), its function is directly related to the feedback mechanisms involved in 5-HT neuron firing and 5-HT release. Because SSRIs block the uptake of 5-HT, the net effect after acute SSRI administration is probably a mild increase in 5-HT release at the synaptic terminal. After chronic administration, leading to down regulation of somatodendritic 5-HT$_{1A}$ autoreceptors and hence lowered inhibition of cell-firing and thus enhanced terminal 5-HT release, 5-HT is probably far more strongly enhanced than after acute administration. Therefore, acute and certainly chronic administration of SSRIs should lead to inhibition of aggression, based on the hypothesis that activation of postsynaptic 5-HT$_{1B}$ receptors mediates anti-aggressive effects. Clinical data seem to support this hypothesis (Cherek et al. 2002; Hollander 1999; Coccaro and Kavoussi 1997). However, SSRIs are not known as a mainstream treatment for aggressive pathology in humans (Goedhard et al. 2007). Preclinically, acute administration of SSRIs has anti-aggressive effects, although not in a behaviorally specific way (Olivier et al. 1995), which is not too surprising because the enhanced 5-HT activates all 5-HT receptors, and thus a plethora of effects might be expected. Chronic administration of SSRIs leads to contrasting effects: reductions in mice (Delina-Stula and Vassoet 1981) but increases in rats (Mitchell and Redfern 1997). Mutant mice and rats lacking the 5-HTT are less aggressive than their wild types (Holmes et al. 2003; Homberg et al. 2007b), in line with the notion that chronically elevated 5-HT release (Homberg et al. 2007a) is inhibitory on aggression.

In humans, a variation in the length of a repeat in the transcriptional control region of the 5-HT transporter (5HTTLPR) regulates expression of the transporter molecule and 5-HT uptake, with short alleles (s) resulting in lower activity than long (l) alleles and consequently resulting in lower 5-HT uptake. This polymorphism has been associated with various psychiatric conditions and a recent study (Reif et al. 2007) showed an association between the short allele 5HTT genotype and violence, but only in those patients with an adverse childhood environment. Such complex interactions between genetic variation in the 5-HT circuitry and certain environmental factors point to the complex causation of aggressive and violent behaviors, which are definitively not only dependent on the functioning of the serotonergic system (Miczek et al. 2007).

Miscellaneous Serotonergic Receptors

Although infrequent reports emerge on the possible role of other (5-HT$_{3,4,6,7}$) serotonergic receptors, it is unclear what role they might play. Early studies on 5-HT$_3$ receptor antagonists indicated an absence of any effects (Olivier et al. 1994; White et al. 1991; Sanchez et al. 1993). Some papers find some involvement of the 5-HT$_3$ receptor in aggression, but mostly under pharmacologically induced conditions, e.g., after cocaine in hamsters (Ricci et al. 2004, 2005), apomorphine in mice (Rudissaar et al. 1999) or alcohol in mice (McKenzie-Quirk et al. 2005). These contradicting results indicate that 5-HT$_3$ receptors do not play a big role in the modulation of aggression.

No data are available on the effects of 5-HT$_{4, 5 \text{ and } 6}$ receptor ligands on aggression, and there is only one publication (Navarro et al. 2004) showing no effect of the 5-HT$_7$ receptor antagonist SB269979.

Conclusions Regarding 5-HT and Aggression

Research on the status of the 5-HT system before, during and after the execution of aggression is showing an important role for serotonergic activity, although its definite contributions are still unknown. The research has pinpointed 5-HT_{1B} and 5-HT_{1A} receptors as key players in the modulation of aggression, probably with differential contributions of their respective auto- and heteroreceptors. The only serotonergic therapeutics available (SSRIs) are not presenting as very effective anti-aggressive agents (serenics), and the animal predictions of effective anti-aggressives ($5\text{-HT}_{1B/1A}$ receptor agonists) should be translated into human testing to judge the translational value of preclinical research.

5-HT and Sexual Behavior

Over the last decades an extensive body of research has indicated that central neurotransmitters such as dopamine and 5-HT and their receptors play an important role in the regulation of sexual behavior. Because excellent reviews exist concerning the role of central dopamine and central 5-HT in sexual behavior (Waldinger and Olivier 1998b; Olivier et al. 1998; Bitran and Hull 1987; Melis and Argiolas 1995; Hull et al. 1999, 2004), here we only briefly review the most important findings with regard to the role of serotonin in the regulation of sexual behavior of male mammals, with focus on the male rat (for extensive reviews, see Waldinger et al. 1998; Olivier et al. 1998; De Jong et al. 2006).

Animal Sexual Behavior

Increasing understanding of the neurobiology of normal and "pathological" sexual functioning has been derived from animal studies in which specific brain areas have been manipulated or animals have been challenged pharmacologically (for reviews, see Larsson and Ahlenius 1999; Pfaus 1999). Most of the current theoretical models of animal sexual functioning – and its underlying neurobiology – have been based on sexual behavior of laboratory rats (Hull and Dominguez 2007). Typically, in these experiments male rats are exposed to a receptive female and allowed to copulate for a certain period of time, or until ejaculation has occurred. Male rat sexual behavior is characterized by a series of mounts, either with or without vaginal intromission, that eventually will lead to ejaculation after a number of intromissions and duration of 2–10 min. A distinction can be made between appetitive and consummatory aspects of copulatory behavior, where latency until the first mount putatively reflects some of the appetitive aspects and sexual motivation (Ågmo 1999). Consummatory aspects of sexual behavior include intromission latencies, ejaculation latencies, mount frequencies and intromission frequencies and may all affect ejaculatory behavior.

5-HT, Serotonergic Receptors and Sexual Behavior

The importance of 5-HT in sexual behavior has been demonstrated by numerous studies showing that, for instance, lesions of the brainstem raphé nuclei (Albinsson et al. 1996) and 5-HT depletion (Tagliamonte et al. 1969) facilitate sexual behavior. On the other hand, administration of 5-hydroxytryptophan, the direct precursor of 5-HT, 5-HT itself and 5-HT releasers, such as MDMA and fenfluramine, has been shown to inhibit sexual behavior (Ahlenius et al. 1980; Dornan et al. 1991; Foreman et al. 1992; Gonzales et al. 1982). Altogether these findings suggest that a decrease in 5-HT neurotransmission may be involved in facilitation, whereas an increase in 5-HT neurotransmission may result in inhibition of sexual behavior.

Selective Serotonin Reuptake Inhibitors (SSRIs) and Sexual Behavior

The frequently reported sexual effects of SSRIs in men suggest an important role of 5-HT in human ejaculatory behavior. As described previously, in several human studies, we and others have demonstrated that various SSRIs, including paroxetine, sertraline and fluoxetine, are able to delay ejaculation in premature ejaculation (for review, see Waldinger 2002). Moreover these studies show that SSRIs exert only a minimal ejaculation delay in the first week that is often not clinically relevant. A clinically relevant ejaculation delay occurs gradually after 2–3 weeks of daily treatment. Interestingly, despite the putative similar underlying mechanism of action of SSRIs – briefly, preventing the reuptake of 5-HT, thereby elevating 5-HT levels – not all SSRIs delay ejaculation to the same extent. In humans, clomipramine and paroxetine have stronger ejaculation-delaying effects after 4 to 6 weeks of daily treatment than other SSRIs (Waldinger et al. 1998, 2001).

Acute and Chronic SSRI Administration in Male Rats

Analogous to the human situation, a distinction can be made in male rats between the effects of acute and chronic SSRI administration on ejaculation. Acute administration of various SSRIs, such as citalopram, clomipramine, paroxetine, sertraline, fluoxetine and fluvoxamine, did not delay ejaculation (Mos et al. 1999; Ahlenius and Larsson 1999; Matuszcyk et al. 1998). On the other hand, chronic administration of fluoxetine (Matusczyk et al 1998; Cantor et al. 1999; Frank et al. 2000) and paroxetine (Waldinger et al. 2001a,b) delayed ejaculation in male rats. Nonetheless, as in humans, not all SSRIs potently delayed ejaculation after chronic administration in male rats: fluvoxamine slightly affected some aspects of copulatory behavior but did not affect ejaculation (Waldinger et al. 2001a,b). It is unclear why the various SSRIs differ in their ability to delay ejaculation after chronic administration. The delay in onset of the therapeutic effect of SSRIs in depression and anxiety disorders has been related to adaptive changes of serotonergic autoreceptors (Haddjeri et al. 1998; Le Poul et al. 2000), and it is conceivable that the ejaculation-delaying effects of various SSRIs are due to differential adaptive changes of 5-HT receptors.

Ahlenius and Larsson (1999) studied the mechanism of SSRI-induced delay of ejaculation in more detail and showed that acute treatment with citalopram did not affect ejaculatory behavior. Co-administration of the 5-HT$_{1A}$ receptor antagonist WAY-100635 with citalopram strongly delayed ejaculation latencies, suggesting 5-HT$_{1A}$ receptor involvement in the effect of citalopram on ejaculation. De Jong et al. (2005) also showed that citalopram, acutely or chronically, did not inhibit sexual behaviour by itself but when combined with a sexually inactive dose of WAY100,635 completely abolished sexual behavior. Subsequently, it was found that the ejaculation-delaying effects of the combination of citalopram and WAY-100635 could be fully blocked by a selective 5-HT$_{1B}$ receptor antagonist, suggesting a role for this receptor subtype in the delay of ejaculation (Hillegaart and Ahlenius 1998). Interestingly, a previous study from the same laboratory also suggested a role for the 5-HT$_{1B}$ receptor in the delay of ejaculation. In this study it was shown that the 5-HT$_{1B}$ receptor agonist anpirtoline dose-dependently delayed ejaculation in rats

To summarize, the sexual side effects of SSRIs are still not fully understood. Nevertheless, some recent findings suggest that adaptive changes in the 5-HT system and its interactions with neuroendocrine systems may be responsible for their sexual effects.

Serotonin Receptor Agonists and Antagonists and Ejaculation in Male Rats

As described above, activation of 5-HT$_{1B}$ receptors has been associated with delaying ejaculation in male rats. 5-HT$_2$ receptors are also implicated in modulation of sexual activity, e.g., as shown by the 5-HT$_{2A/2C}$ receptor agonist DOI-induced inhibition of sexual behavior (Klint and Larsson 1995). On the other hand, several other studies have shown that 5-HT$_{2A/2C}$ receptor agonists generally inhibit sexual behavior by decreasing the number of animals that initiate copulation but do not affect ejaculation latencies in animals that do initiate copulation (Ahlenius and Larsson 1998; Klint et al. 1992; Watson and Gorzalka 1991). Thus, it appears that 5-HT$_2$ receptors in general inhibit sexual behavior but their precise role in the regulation of ejaculation is not entirely clear.

A facilitatory role in ejaculation has been ascribed to activation of 5-HT$_{1A}$ receptors, and various selective agonists for this receptor, such as 8-OH-DPAT (Ahlenius and Larsson 1991), FG-5893 (Anderson and Larsson 1994) and flesinoxan (Haensel and Slob 1997; Mos et al. 1991), potently facilitate sexual behavior and decrease ejaculation latencies. Nevertheless, the underlying mechanisms of the facilitatory effects of 5-HT$_{1A}$ receptor agonists are still unclear. A possible mechanism of action is the activation of presynaptic 5-HT$_{1A}$ receptors, which will lead to an inhibition of 5-HT neuronal firing and consequently result in facilitation of sexual behavior as described above. Alternatively, activation of postsynaptic 5-HT$_{1A}$ receptors may result in facilitation of sexual behavior. Evidence for a postsynaptic mechanism of action is provided by studies demonstrating that injection of 8-OH-DPAT directly into the medial preoptic area potently facilitated sexual behavior and lowered ejaculatory threshold (Matusczewich et al. 1999).

Animal Models of Premature and Retarded Ejaculation

Most of our current understanding of the anatomy and neurobiology of sexual behavior is based on animal studies using rats that are sexually experienced and display normal sexual behavior. Interestingly, the comparable ejaculation-delaying effects of SSRIs in humans and rats suggest high translational validity with regard to the regulation of ejaculation. Nevertheless, face validity is low when one tries to extend results obtained in rats that display normal sexual behavior to dysfunctions such as premature and retarded or even (an)-ejaculation. Over the last decades, several groups have studied rats that display hyposexual behavior, which are referred to, by different investigators, as sexually inactive, sluggish, impotent or non-copulating rats. Recent findings suggest

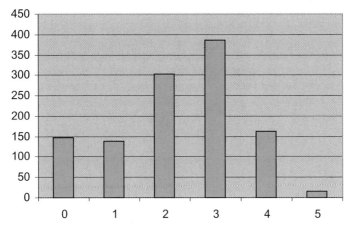

Fig. 1. Histogram displaying number of ejaculations during a 30-min mating test in a pooled population of male Wistar rats (total N > 1300), obtained from 15 subsequent experiments. The data were collected during the fourth mating test, representing stable sexual behavior. Male rats on either side of the Gaussian distribution were defined as "sluggish" (0–1 ejaculation), "normal" (2–3 ejaculations) and "rapid" ejaculators (4–5 ejaculations)

the presence of neurobiological differences associated with the hyposexual behavior that these rats display. On the other hand, hypersexual behavior can also be provoked pharmacologically. However, there are only a few studies of rats that are hypersexual by nature. Thus, investigating animals that do not display normal sexual behavior may help as understand the underlying neurobiological mechanisms and hopefully provide further insights into the etiology of ejaculatory dysfunctions.

In our laboratory we have found (Pattij et al. 2005; Olivier et al. 2006) that male outbred Wistar rats displayed sexual "endophenotypes." In subsequent cohorts of 100–120 male rats, we consistently found rats that displayed a very low (0–1), normal (2–3) or high (4–5) number of ejaculations in 30-min tests with a receptive female even after 4–8 training tests. The behaviour of these males seemed very stable, and we suggest the low-performing animals as putative models for delayed ejaculation in humans and the high-performing rats as models for premature ejaculation (Pattij et al. 2005; Olivier et al. 2006). Figure 1 shows the distribution of these endophenotypic sexual phenotypes in more than 1,300 male rats we have tested thus far.

These various endophenotypes are now the subject of pharmacological studies.

Studies with Rats Displaying Hyposexual Behavior

Early experiments in the 1940s demonstrated that rats reared in isolation were either not capable of achieving ejaculation or remained sexually inactive after repeated exposure to a receptive female (Beach 1942). In contrast, rats that were reared in groups with either same-sex or hetero-sex cage mates did not show these clear deficits in copulatory behavior. Importantly, in most but not all of the isolation-reared males, sexual performance gradually improved with experience. These early findings suggest that experience and learning play an important role in rat copulatory performance but apparently do not exclusively determine the ability to successfully copulate until

Table 2. Mean number of ejaculations, mounts and intromissions and ejaculation latency (in sec) for sexually naïve male rats during a 15-min test with a sexually active, estrus female

Drug (route)	Dose mg/kg	EF	MF	IF	EL (sec)
8-OH-DPAT (SC)	0	0.1	10.5	8.3	869
	0.1	1.5*	6.5*	7.6	351*
	0.2	1.9*	3.5*	5.1	187*
	0.4	1.7*	1.1*	1.1*	238*
Flesinoxan (IP)	0	0.3	13.9	12.2	854
	0.1	1.0*	7.9	13.4	636*
	0.3	1.3*	5.5*	9.8	459*
	1.0	1.8*	3.3*	8.2	281*
Buspirone (IP)	0	0.3	10.3	9.9	860
	3.0	1.2*	7.0	11.3	502*
	10.0	0.1	0.3*	1.8*	849
Ipsapirone (IP)	3.0	0.9(*)	7.9	11.3	502*
	10.0	1.5*	10.9	12.2	636*

All data are depicted as means. EF, ejaculation frequency; MF, mount frequency; IF, intromission frequency; EL, ejaculation latency. *significantly different ($P < 0.05$) from the corresponding vehicle (0 mg/kg) dose.

ejaculation. In early studies in our laboratory focussing on rats displaying different levels of sexual performance, we have tried to create hypo-sexual behavior in male rats by manipulating the level of sexual experience (Mos et al. 1990). To this end, we have studied the sexual behavior of 278 sexually naïve male Wistar rats in 15-min tests with an estrus female. Of those 278 males, 23 showed no sexual activity at all, i.e., no intromissions and at most one mount was scored during the test. Of the remaining 255 rats, 211 displayed sexual activity but failed to ejaculate during the test. The average ejaculation latency of the 44 ejaculating males was 620 ± 28 sec. If sexually naïve male rats were treated with 5-HT$_{1A}$ receptor agonists, they performed quite well (Table 2). In particular, the two full 5-HT$_{1A}$ receptor agonists, ($\pm$)-8-OH-DPAT and flesinoxan, enhanced sexual behavior to the level of sexually experienced male rats. The partial 5-HT$_{1A}$ receptor agonists, buspirone and ipsapirone, also facilitated sexual activity. These findings indicate that naïve male rats are able to perform sexual activities reminiscent of sexually experienced rats in a very short time interval. Apparently, sexually naïve rats may be influenced by certain factors that can be overcome by treatment with psychoactive drugs, at least 5-HT$_{1A}$ receptor agonists and (not shown here) α_2-adrenoceptor antagonists like yohimbine and idazoxan (Mos et al. 1990, 1991).

These pharmacological studies strongly suggest that neurobiological mechanisms underlie the differences observed in basal sexual behavior.

Studies with Rats Displaying Hypersexual Behavior

In contrast to studies focussing on rats that are hyposexual by nature, reports of rats that are hypersexual by nature are scarce. Nevertheless, numerous studies have indicated that a variety of selective pharmacological compounds, neurotransmitters and neuropeptides may facilitate sexual behavior (Bitran and Hull 1987; Argiolas 1999). Most interesting are those studies in which male rat sexual behavior is potently facilitated and in which the behavior shares some of the characteristics of human premature ejaculation. Indeed some of the clinical symptoms of premature ejaculation can be evoked pharmacologically in male rats. For instance, various selective $5\text{-}HT_{1A}$ receptor agonists have been shown to potently decrease ejaculation latencies and intromission and mount frequencies. Beside selective $5\text{-}HT_{1A}$ receptor agonists, a selective dopamine D_2 receptor agonist, SND-919 (Ferrari and Giuliani 1994), has also been shown to decrease ejaculation latencies in rats, although its effects were much less pronounced compared to the effects of $5\text{-}HT_{1A}$ receptor agonists.

In addition to pharmacological manipulations, tactile stimulation, such as shock and tail-pinching (Barfield and Sachs 1968; Wang and Hull 1980), facilitates ejaculatory behavior. Presumably these facilitatory effects are mediated by activation of the brain dopaminergic system (Leyton and Stewart 1996).

Conclusion Regarding 5-HT and Sexual Behavior

Research in humans and rats has indicated that modulating 5-HT levels in the CNS changes ejaculatory thresholds and associated sexual behavior. Activation of $5\text{-}HT_{1A}$ receptors and blockade of $5\text{-}HT_{2C}$ receptors facilitates sexual behavior, whereas activation of $5\text{-}HT_{1B}$ and $5\text{-}HT_2$ receptors inhibits it. SSRIs, that facilitate serotonin neurotransmission, inhibit sexual behavior but only after chronic administration. There is a paucity of data on the putative role of other 5-HT receptors in the modulation of sexual behavior.

Are the Serotonergic Systems Involved in Aggressive and Sexual Behavior (Dis)similar?

It is a widespread belief that aggressive and sexual behaviors share many underlying neurobiological, neurological, pharmacological and neuroendocrine mechanisms (Pedersen 2004). Newman (1999) suggested that the mechanisms underlying aggression are integrated in an extensive network involved in various forms of social interactions including sexual, aggressive and parental behaviors. The development of neurochemical systems within the CNS controlling these emotional bonds includes monoamines and several neuropeptides, systems typically involved in the regulation of aggressive and sexual behaviors. It is conceivable that such CNS systems are largely overlapping, including the 5-HT system. Considering the complex design of the 5-HT system in the CNS, with all its different 5-HT receptors at different locations and subserving different functions, it should not be surprising that they share some systems but might also differ in several aspects. The latter option seems to best fit observations of the role of the serotonergic system in aggressive and sexual behavior. Particularly, $5\text{-}HT_{1A}$ receptors seem to play a fundamentally opposite role in the modulation of sexual and aggressive behaviors, at least in rats. On the other hand, $5\text{-}HT_{1B}$ receptors seem to play a similar role in both systems. Comparable findings have been found using activation patterns in the brain after performance of sexual or aggressive behaviors (Veening et al. 2005). Moreover, there is support for anatomically segregated systems in the brain involved in various aspects of sexual/reproductive and defensive/offensive behaviors (Choi et al. 2005), pointing to the hard-wiring of such systems in the CNS. The question is whether the serotonergic system belongs to the hard-wired substrates underlying the often stereotyped and ritualistic behaviors in aggression and sex or if it belongs to putative modulatory systems that modulate ongoing behaviors and determine whether certain systems are on or off. Such "gate-control" mechanisms can be performed by the serotonergic system and, depending on the action performed, different parts of the serotonergic system might be involved. This highly speculative hypothesis might fit the tremendous amount of sometimes conflicting data about the role of the serotonergic system in aggression and sexual behavior.

References

Ahlenius S, Larsson K (1991) The effects of Benzodiazepines and 5-HT$_{1A}$ Agonists and Memory. In: Rodgers RJ, Cooper S (eds) 5-HT$_{1A}$ agonists, 5-HT$_3$ antagonists and benzodiazepines: their comparative behavioural pharmacology. J John Wiley and Sons, Chichester, pp 281–301

Ahlenius S, Larsson K (1998) Evidence for an involvement of 5-HT$_{1B}$ receptors in the inhibition of male rat ejaculatory behavior produced by 5-HTP. Psychopharmacology 137:374–382

Ahlenius S Larsson K (1999) Synergistic actions of the 5-HT$_{1A}$ antagonist WAY-100635 and citalopram on male rat ejaculatory behavior. Eur J Pharmacol 379:1–6

Ahlenius S Larsson K Svensson L (1980) Further evidence for an inhibitory role of central 5-HT in male rat sexual behavior. Psychopharmacology 68:217–220

Albinsson A, Andersson G, Andersson K, VegaMatuszczyk J, Larsson K (1996) The effects of lesions in the mesencephalic raphe systems on male rat sexual behavior and locomotor activity. Behav Brain Res 80:57–63

Andersson G, Larsson K (1994) Effects of FG-5893, a new compound with 5-HT$_{1A}$ receptor agonistic and 5-HT$_2$ antagonistic properties, on male-rat sexual-behavior. Eur J Pharmacol 255:131–137

Argiolas A (1999) Neuropeptides and sexual behaviour. Neurosci Biobehav Rev 23:1127–1142

Barfield RJ, Sachs BD (1968) Sexual behavior: stimulation by painful electrical shock to skin in male rats. Science 161:392–395

Beach FA (1942) Comparison of copulatory behavior of male rats raised in isolation, cohabitation, and segregation. J Genet Psychol 60:3–13

Bitran D, Hull EM (1987) Pharmacological analysis of male rat sexual behavior. Neurosci Biobehav Rev 11:365–389

Bouwknecht JA, Hijzen TH, Van der Gugten J, Maes RAA, Hen R, Olivier B (2001) Absence of 5-HT$_{1B}$ receptors is associated with impaired motor impulse control in male 5-HT$_{1B}$ knockout mice. Biol Psychiat 49:557–568

Brown GL, Goodwin FK, Ballenger JC, Goyer PF, Major LF (1979) Aggression in humans: correlates with cerebrospinal fluid amine metabolites. Psychiat Res 1:131–139

Brunner D, Hen R (1997) Insights into the neurology of impulsive behavior from serotonin receptor knockout mice. Ann. NY Acad Sci 836:81–105

Caramaschi D, De Boer SF, Koolhaas JM (2007) Differential role of the 5-HT$_{1A}$ receptor in aggressive and non-aggressive mice: an across-strain comparison. Physiol Behav 90:590–601

Cantor J, Binik I, Pfaus JG (1999) Chronic fluoxetine inhibits sexual behavior in the male rat: reversal with oxytocin. Psychopharmacology 144:355–362

Cherek DR, Lane SD, Pietras CJ, Steinberg JL (2002) Effects of chronic paroxetine administration on measures of aggressive and impulsive responses of adult males with a history of conduct disorder. Psychopharmacology 159:266–274

Choi GB, Dong HW, Murphy AJ, Valenzuela DM, Yancopoulos GD, Swanson LW, Anderson DJ (2005) Lhx6 delineates a pathway mediating innate reproductive behaviors from the amygdala to the hypothalamus. Neuron 46:647–660

Coccaro EF (1989) Central serotonin and impulsive aggression. Br J Psychiat 155:52–62

Coccaro EF, Kavoussi RJ (1997) Fluoxetine and impulsive aggressive behavior in personality-disordered subjects. Arch Gen Psychiat 54:1081–1088

De Almeida RMM, Nikulina E, Faccidomo S, Fish E, Miczek KA (2001) Zolmitriptan, a 5-HT$_{1B/1D}$ receptor agonist, alcohol, and aggression in male mice. Psychopharmacology 157:131–141

De Boer SF, Koolhaas JM (2005) 5-HT$_{1A}$ and 5-HT$_{1B}$ receptor agonists and aggression: A pharmacological challenge of the serotonin deficiency hypothesis. Eur J Pharmacol 526:125–139

De Boer SF, Lesourd M, Mocaer E, Koolhaas JM (2000) Somatodendritic 5-HT$_{1A}$ autoreceptors mediate the anti-aggressive actions of 5-HT(1A) receptor agonists in rats: an ethopharmacological study with S-15535, alnespirone, and WAY-100635. Neuropsychopharmacology 23:20–33

De Boer SF, Van der Vegt BJ, Koolhaas JM (2003) Individual variation in aggression of feral rodent strains: a standard for the genetics of aggression and violence. Behav Genet 33:485–501

Delina-Stula A, Vassout A (1978) The effects of antidepressants on aggressiveness induced by social deprivation in mice. Pharmacol Biochem Behav 14(Suppl 1):33–41

De Jong TR, Pattij T, Veening JG, Dederen PFJ, Waldinger MD, Cools AR, Olivier B (2005) Citalopram combined with WAY100635 inhibits ejaculation and ejaculation-related Fos immunoreactivity. Eur J Pharmacol 509:49–59

De Jong TR, Veening JG, Waldinger MD, Cools AR, Olivier B (2006) Serotonin and the neurobiology of the ejaculation threshold. Neurosci Biobehav Rev 30:893–907

Dornan WA, Katz JL, Ricaurte GA (1991) The effects of repeated administration of MDMA on the expression of sexual behavior in the male rat. Pharmacol Biochem Behav 39:813–816

Ferrari F, Giuliani D (1994) The selective D-2 dopamine-receptor antagonist eticlopride counteracts the ejaculatio-praecox induced by the selective D-2-dopamine agonist SND-919 in the rat. Life Sci 55:1155–1162

Ferrari PF, van Erp AMM, Tornatzky W, Miczek KA (2003) Accumbal dopamine and serotonin in anticipation of the next aggressive episode in rats. Eur J Neurosci 17:371–378

Ferrari PF, Palanza P, Parmigiani S, de Almeida RMM. Miczek KA (2005) Serotonin and aggressive behaviour in rodents and nonhuman primates: predispositions and plasticity. Eur J Pharmacol 526:259–273

Fish EW, Faccidomo S, Miczek KA (1999) Aggression heightened by alcohol or social instigation in mice: reduction by the 5-HT$_{1B}$ receptor agonist CP-94,253. Psychopharmacology 146:391–399

Foreman MM, Hall JL, Love RL (1992) Effects of fenfluramine and para-chloroamphetamine on sexual behavior of male rats. Psychopharmacology 107:327–330

Frank JL, Hendricks SE, Olson CH (2000) Multiple ejaculations and chronic fluoxetine: effects on male rat copulatory behavior. Pharmacol Biochem Behav 66:337–342

Giacalone E, Tansella M, Valzelli L, Garattini S (1968) Brain serotonin metabolism in isolated aggressive mice. Biochem Pharmacol 17:1315–1327

Goedhard LE, Stolker JJ, Heerdink ER, Nijman HL, Olivier B, Egberts TC (2006) Pharmacotherapy for the treatment of aggressive behavior in general adult psychiatry: A systematic review. J Clin Psychi 67:1013–24

Gonzales G, Mendoza L, Ruiz J, Torrejon J (1982) A demonstration that 5-hydroxytryptamine administered peripherally can affect sexual behavior in male rats. Life Sci 31:2775–2781

Haddjeri N, Blier P, De Montigny C (1998) Long-term antidepressant treatments result in a tonic activation of forebrain 5-HT$_{1A}$ receptors. J Neurosci 18:10150–10156

Haensel SM, Slob AK (1997) Flesinoxan: a prosexual drug for male rats. Eur J Pharmacol 330:1–9

Hartig PR, Hoyer D, Humphrey PP, Martin GR. (1996) Alignment of receptor nomenclature with the human genome: classification of 5-HT$_{1B}$ and 5-HT$_{1D}$ receptor subtypes. Tr Pharmacol Sci 17:103–105

Hillegaart V, Ahlenius S (1998) Facilitation and inhibition of male rat ejaculatory behaviour by the respective 5-HT$_{1A}$ and 5-HT$_{1B}$ receptor agonists 8-OH-DPAT and anpirtoline, as evidenced by use of the corresponding new and selective receptor antagonists NAD-299 and NAS-181. Br J Pharmacol 125:1733–1743

Hollander E (1999) Managing aggressive behavior in patients with obsessive-compulsive disorder and borderline personality disorder. J Clin Psychiat 60(S 15):38–44

Holmes A, Murphy DL, Crawley JN (2003) Abnormal behavioral phenotypes of serotonin transporter knockout mice: parallels with human anxiety and depression. Biol Psychiat 54:953–959

Homberg JR, Pattij T, Janssen MC, Ronken E, De Boer SF, Schoffelmeer AN, Cuppen E (2007a) Serotonin transporter deficiency in rats improves inhibitory control but not behavioural flexibility. Eur J Neurosci 26:2066–2073

Homberg JR, Olivier JD, Smits BM, Mul JD, Mudde J, Verheul M, Nieuwenhuizen OF, Cools AR, Ronken E, Cremers T, Schoffelmeer AN, Ellenbroek BA, Cuppen E (2007b) Characterization of the serotonin transporter knockout rat: a selective change in the functioning of the serotonergic system. Neuroscience 146:1662–76

Hoyer D, Clarke DE, Fozard JR, Hartig PR, Martin GR, Mylecharane EJ, Saxena PR, Humphrey PP (1994) International Union of Pharmacology classification of receptors for 5-hydroxytryptamine (Serotonin). Pharmacol Rev 46:157–203

Hull EM, Dominguez JM (2007) Sexual behavior in male rodents. Horm Behav 52:45–55

Hull EM, Lorrain DS, Du J, Matuszewich L, Lumley LA, Putnam SK, Moses J (1999) Hormone-neurotransmitter interactions in the control of sexual behavior. Behav Brain Res 105:105–116

Hull EM, Muschamp JW, Sata S (2004) Dopamine and serotonin: influences on male sexual behavior. Physiol Behav 83:291–307

Kavoussi R, Armstead P, Coccaro E (1997) The neurobiology of impulsive aggression. Psychiatry Clin North Am 20:395–403

Klint T, Larsson K (1995) Clozapine acts as a 5-HT$_2$ antagonist by attenuating DOI-induced inhibition of male rat sexual behaviour. Psychopharmacology 119:291–294

Klint T, Dahlgren IL, Larsson K (1992) The selective 5-HT$_2$ receptor antagonist amperozide attenuates 1-(2,5-dimethoxy-4-iodophenyl)-2-aminopropane-induced inhibition of male rat sexual behavior. Eur J Pharmacol 212:241–246

Koolhaas JM, De Boer SF, Buwalda B, van Rheenen K (2007) Individual variation in coping with stress: a multidimensional approach of ultimate and proximate mechanisms. Brain Behav Evol 70:218–226

Kruesi MJP, Rapoport JL, Hamburger S, Hibbs E, Potter WZ, Lenane M, Brown GR (1990) Cerebrospinal fluid monoamine metabolites, aggression, and impulsivity in disruptive behavior disorders of children and adolescents. Arch Gen Psychiat 47:419–426

Kruk MR, van der Poel AM, de Vos-Frerichs TP (1979) The induction of aggressive behaviour by electrical stimulation in the hypothalamus of male rats. Behaviour 70:292–322

Larsson K, Ahlenius S (1999) Brain and sexual behavior. Ann NY Acad Sci 877:292–308

Le Poul E, Boni C, Hanoun N, Laporte AM, Laaris N, Chauveau J, Hamon M, Lanfumey (2000) Differential adaptation of brain 5-HT$_{1A}$ and 5-HT$_{1B}$ receptors and 5-HT transporter in rats treated chronically with fluoxetine. Neuropharmacology 39:110–122

Lesch KP, Merschdorf U (2000) Impulsivity, aggression, and serotonin: a molecular psychobiological perspective. Behav Sci Law 18:581–604

Leyton M, Stewart J (1996) Acute and repeated activation of male sexual behavior by tail pinch: opioid and dopaminergic mechanisms. Physiol Behav 60:77–85

Linnoila M, Virkkunen M, Scheinin M, Nuutila A, Rimon R, Goodwin FK (1983) Low cerebrospinal fluid 5-hydroxyindole-acetic acid concentration differentiates impulsive from nonimpulsive violent behaviour. Life Sci 33:2609–2614

Mann JJ (2003) Neurobiology of suicidal behaviour. Nature Rev Neurosci 4:819–828

Matuszcyk JV, Larsson K, Eriksson E (1998) The selective serotonin reuptake inhibitor fluoxetine reduces sexual motivation in male rats. Pharmacol Biochem Behav 60:527–532

Matuszewich L, Lorrain DS, Trujillo R, Dominguez J, Putnam SK, Hull EM (1999) Partial antagonism of 8-OH-DPAT's effects on male rat sexual behavior with a D_2, but not a $5-HT_{1A}$, antagonist. Brain Res 820:55–62

McKenzie-Quirk SD, Girasa KA, Allan AM, Miczek KA (2005) $5-HT_3$ receptors, alcohol and aggressive behavior in mice. Behav Pharmacol 16:163–169

Melis MR, Argiolas A (1995) Dopamine and sexual behavior. Neurosci Biobehav Rev 19:19–38

Mendoza DL, Bravo HA, Swanson HH (1999) Antiaggressive and anxiolytic effects of gepirone in mice, and their attenuation by WAY-100,635. Pharmacol Biochem Behav 62:499–509

Miczek KA, Barros HM, Sakoda L, Weerts EM (1998a) Alcohol and heightened aggression in individual mice. Alcohol Clin Exp Res 22:1698–1705

Miczek KA, Hussain S, Faccidomo S (1998b) Alcohol-heightened aggression in mice: attenuation by $5-HT_{1A}$ receptor agonists. Psychopharmacology 139:160–168

Miczek KA, de Almeida RMMA (2001) Oral drug self-administration in the home cage of mice: alcohol-heightened aggression and inhibition by the $5-HT_{1B}$ agonist anpirtoline. Psychopharmacology 157:421–429

Miczek KA, Fish EW, de Bold JF, de Almeida RMM (2002) Social and neural determinants of aggressive behavior: pharmacotherapeutic targets at serotonin, dopamine and γ-aminobutyric acid systems. Psychopharmacology 163:434–458

Miczek KA, de Almeida RMM, Kravitz EA, Rissman EF, de Boer SF, Raine A (2007) Neurobiology of escalated aggression and violence. J Neurosci 27:11803–11806

Mitchell PJ, Redfern PH (1997) Potentiation of the time-dependent, antidepressant-induced changes in the agonistic behaviour of resident rats by the $5-HT_{1A}$ receptor antagonist, WAY-100635. Behav Pharmacol 8:585–606

Mos J, Olivier B, Bloetjes K, Poth M (1990) Drug-induced facilitation of sexual behaviour in the male rat: behavioural and pharmacological aspects. In: Slob AK, Baum MJ (eds) Psychoneuroendocrinology of growth and development. Rotterdam, Medicom Publishers, pp 221–232

Mos J, Van Logten J, Bloetjes K, Olivier B (1991) The effects of idazoxan and 8-OH-DPAT on sexual behaviour and associated ultrasonic vocalizations in the rat. Neurosci Biobehav Rev 15:505–515

Mos J, Olivier B, Poth M, van Aken H (1992) The effects of intraventricular administration of eltoprazine, 1-(3-trifluoromethylphenyl) piperazine hydrochloride and 8-hydroxy-2-(di-n-propylamino) tetralin on resident intruder aggression in the rat. Eur J Pharmacol 212:295–298

Mos J, Olivier B, Poth M, van Oorschot R, Van Aken H (1993) The effects of dorsal raphe administration of eltoprazine, TFMPP and 8-OH-DPAT on resident intruder aggression in the rat. Eur J Pharmacol 238:411–415

Mos J, Mollet I, Tolboom JTBM, Waldinger MD, Olivier B (1999) A comparison of the effects of different serotonin reuptake blockers on sexual behaviour of the male rat. Eur Neuropsychopharmacol 9:123–135

Navarro JF, Ibáñez M, Luna G (2004) Behavioral profile of SB 269970, a selective 5-HT (7) serotonin receptor antagonist, in social encounters between male mice. Methods Find Exp Clin Pharmacol 26:515–518

Newman SW (1999) The medial extended amygdala in male reproductive behaviour. A node in the mammalian social behaviour network. Ann NY Acad Sci 877:242–257

Nikulina EM, Miczek KA (1999) Post- vs. presynaptic sites of action of $5-HT_{1A}$ and $5-HT_{1B}$ receptor agonists in regulation of mouse aggressive behaviour. Behav Pharmacol 10:S67

Olivier B (2004) Serotonin and aggression. Ann NY Acad Sci 1036:382–92

Olivier B (2005) Serotonergic mechanisms in aggression. Novartis Found Symp 268:171–83

Olivier B, Young L (2002) Animal models of aggression. In: Davis KL, Charney D, Coyle JT, Nemeroff C (eds) Neuropsychopharmacology: the 5th generation of progress. Philadelphia, Lippincott, Williams & Wilkins, pp 1699–1708

Olivier B, van Oorschot R (2005) $5-HT_{1B}$ receptors and aggression: a review. Eur J Pharmacol 526:207–217

Olivier B, Mos J, Hartog J, Rasmussen DL (1990) Serenics: a new class of drugs for putative selective treatment of pathological destructive behaviour. Drug News Persp 3:261–271

Olivier B, Mos J, Raghoebar M, de Koning P, Mak M (1994) Serenics. Prog Drug Res 42:167–308

Olivier B, Mos J, van Oorschot R, Hen R (1995) Serotonin receptors and animal models of aggressive behaviour. Pharmacopsychiatry 28:80–90

Olivier B, van Oorschot R, Waldinger MD (1998) Serotonin, serotonergic receptors, selective serotonin reuptake inhibitors and sexual behaviour. Int Clin Psychopharmacol 13(suppl 6):S9–S14

Olivier B, Soudijn W, van Wijngaarden I (1999) The 5-HT$_{1A}$ receptor and its ligands: structure and function. Prog Drug Res 52:103–166

Olivier B, Chan JS, Pattij T, de Jong TR, Oosting RS, Veening JG, Waldinger MD (2005) Psychopharmacology of male rat sexual behavior: modeling human sexual dysfunctions? Int J Impot Res 18(Suppl 1):S14–S23

Pattij T, Van der Linde J, Groenink L, Broersen L, Van der Gugten J, Maes RAA, Olivier B (2003) Operant learning and differential-reinforcement-of-low-rate 36-sec responding in 5-HT$_{1A}$ and 5-HT$_{1B}$ receptor knockout mice. Behav Brain Res 141:137–145

Pattij T, Broersen L, Olivier B (2004) Impulsive-like responding in differential-reinforcement-of-low-rate 36-sec responding in mice depends on training history. Neurosci Lett 354:169–171

Pattij T, de Jong TR, Uitterdijk A, Waldinger MD, Veening JG, Cools AR, van der Graaf PH, Olivier B (2005) Individual differences in male rat ejaculatory behaviour: searching for models to study ejaculation disorders. Eur J Neurosci 22:724–734

Pedersen CA (2004) Biological aspects of social bonding and the roots of human violence. Ann NY Acad Sci 1036:106–127

Pfaus JG (1999) Neurobiology of sexual behavior. Curr Opin Neurobiol 9:751–758

Pineÿro G, Blier P (1999) Autoregulation of serotonin neurons: role in antidepressant drug action. Pharmacol Rev 51:533–591

Ramboz S, Saudou F, Amara DA, Belzung C, Segu L, Misslin R, Buhot MC, Hen R (1995) 5-HT$_{1B}$ receptor knock out-behavioral consequences. Behav Brain Res 73:305–312

Ratey J, Sovner R, Parks A, Rogentine K (1991) Buspirone treatment of aggression and anxiety in mentally retarded patients: a multiple-baseline, placebo lead-in study. J Clin Psychiat 52:159–162

Reif A, Rösler M, Freitag CM, Schneider M, Eujen A, Kissling C, Wenzler D, Jacob CP, Retz-Junginger P, Thome J, Lesch J-P, Retz W (2007) Nature and nurture predispose to violent behaviour: serotonergic genes and adverse childhood environment. Neuropsychopharmacology 32:2375–2383

Ricci LA, Grimes JM, Melloni Jr RH (2004) Serotonin Type 3 receptors modulate the aggression-stimulating effects of adolescent cocaine exposure in Syrian hamsters (Mesocricetus auratus). Behav Neurosci 118:1097–1110

Ricci LA, Knyshevski I, Melloni Jr RH (2005) Serotonin Type 3 receptors stimulate offensive aggression in Syrian hamsters. Behav Brain Res 156:19–29

Rudissaar R, Pruus K, Skrebuhhova T, Allikmets L, Matto V (1999) Modulatory role of 5-HT$_3$ receptors in mediation of apomorphine-induced aggressive behaviour in male rats. Behav Brain Res 106:91–96

Sanchez C, Arnt J, Hyttel J, Moltzen EK (1993) The role of serotonergic mechanisms in inhibition of isolation-induced aggression in male mice. Psychopharmacology 110:53–59

Saudou F, Amara DA, Dierich A, Lemeur M, Ramboz S, Segu L, Buhot MC, Hen R (1994) Enhanced aggressive behavior in mice lacking 5-HT$_{1B}$ receptor. Science 265:1875–1878

Sijbesma H, Schipper J, de Kloet ER, Mos J, van Aken H, Olivier B (1991) Postsynaptic 5-HT$_1$ receptors and offensive aggression in rats : a combined behavioural and autoradiographic study with eltoprazine. Pharmacol Biochem Behav 38:447–458

Stamford JA, Davidson C, McLaughlin DP, Hopwood SE (2000) Control of dorsal raphe 5-HT function by multiple 5-HT$_1$ autoreceptors: parallel purposes or pointless plurality? Tr Neurosci 23:459–465

Tagliamonte A, Tagliamonte P, Gessa GL, Brodie BB (1969) Compulsive sexual activity induced by p-chlorophenylalanine in normal and pinealectomized male rats. Science 166:1433–1435

Van der Vegt BJ, de Boer SF, Buwalda B, de Ruiter AJ, de Jong JG, Koolhaas JM (2001) Enhanced sensitivity of postsynaptic serotonin-1A receptors in rats and mice with high trait aggression. Physiol Behav 74:205–211

Van der Vegt BJ, Lieuwes N, Cremers TIFH, De Boer SF, Koolhaas JM (2003) Cerebrospinal fluid monoamine and metabolic concentrations and aggression in rats. Horm Behav 44:199–208

Van Erp MM, Miczek KA (2000) Aggressive behavior, increased accumbal dopamine and decreased cortical serotonin in rats. J Neurosci 15:9320–9325

Veening JG, Coolen LM, de Jong TR, Joosten HW, de Boer SF, Koolhaas JM, Olivier B (2005) Do similar neural systems subserve aggressive and sexual behaviour in male rats? Insights from c-Fos and pharmacological studies. Eur J Pharmacol 526:226–239

Waldinger MD (2002) The neurobiological approach to premature ejaculation (review article). J Urol 168:2359–2367

Waldinger MD, Olivier B (1998) Selective serotonin reuptake inhibitor-induced sexual dysfunction: clinical and research considerations. Int Clin Psychopharmacol 13(suppl 6):S27–S33

Waldinger MD, Hengeveld MW, Zwinderman AH, Olivier B (1998) Effect of SSRI antidepressants on ejaculation: a double-blind, randomized, placebo-controlled study with fluoxetine, fluvoxamine, paroxetine, and sertraline. J Clin Psychopharmacol 18:274–281

Waldinger MD, Plas A vd, Pattij T, Oorschot R v, Coolen LM, Veening JG, Olivier B (2001a) The SSRIs fluvoxamine and paroxetine differ in sexual inhibitory effects after chronic treatment. Psychopharmacology 160:283–289

Waldinger MD, Zwinderman AH, Olivier B (2001b) SSRIs and ejaculation: a double-blind, randomized, fixed-dose study with paroxetine and citalopram. J Clin Psychopharmacol 21:556–560

Wang L, Hull EM (1980) Tail pinch induces sexual behavior in olfactory bulbectomized male rats. Physiol Behav 24:211–215

Watson NV, Gorzalka BB (1991) DOI-induced inhibition of copulatory behavior in male rats: reversal by 5-HT$_2$ antagonists. Pharmacol Biochem Behav 39:605–621

White SM, Kucharik RF, Moyer JA (1991) effects of serotonergic agents on isolation-induced aggression. Pharmacol Biochem Behav 39:729–736

The Effect of Neuropeptides on Human Trust and Altruism: A Neuroeconomic Perspective

Ernst Fehr[1]

Summary

Neuroeconomics merges methods from neuroscience and economics to better understand how the human brain generates decisions in economic and social contexts. The emerging neuroeconomic approach (Camerer et al. 2005; Fehr et al. 2005; Glimcher and Rustichini 2004; Sanfey et al. 2006) seeks a microfoundation behind social and economic activity in neural circuitry, using functional magnetic resonance imaging (fMRI), transcranial magnetic stimulation (TMS), pharmacological interventions, and other techniques. Byproducts of such an ambitious program might include better understanding of individual pathologies in social behaviors, such as antisocial personality disorder or social phobia, and, more generally, poor individual decision-making abilities, including lacking the capacity to inhibit prepotent impulses. The approach may also provide insights into the effects of individual and social learning, empirical discipline of evolutionary modeling, and advice for how economic rules and institutions can be designed so that people react to rules in a socially efficient way.

Here we review the actual and predicted impact of neuropeptides such as oxytocin and vasopressin on human trust and altruism. Traditional economic analyses generally make the simplifying assumption that people are exclusively self-regarding; however, a large body of experimental evidence (Fehr and Fischbacher 2003) has been amassed indicating that many people exhibit social preferences, i.e., their preferred choices are based on a positive or negative concern for the welfare of others and on what other players believe about them. Social neuroeconomics (Fehr and Camerer 2007) tries to understand the brain processes that govern these regular deviations from purely self-interested behavior. Part of this endeavor concerns studying the impact of hormones on other-regarding behaviors and trust in other people's other-regarding behavior. Social neuroeconomics combines the tools of social

---

[1] University of Zurich, Institute for Empirical Research in Economics, e-mail: efehr@iew.uzh.ch

Pfaff et al.
Hormones and Social Behavior
© Springer-Verlag Berlin Heidelberg 2008

cognitive neuroscience (Adolphs 2003; Blakemore et al. 2004; Lieberman 2007) with well-structured tasks taken from economic theory. These tasks come equipped with benchmark theoretical predictions about rational play and the social efficiency of outcomes, which are useful for interpreting the results and cumulating regularity across studies.

Neuroeconomic Tools for Studying Social Preferences and Trust

The main tools for eliciting social preferences are simple one-shot games, such as the dictator game, the ultimatum game, or the third party punishment game (see below), that involve real monetary stakes and are played between anonymous interaction partners. In essence, an individual displays social preferences if he or she is willing to forgo his/her own material payoff for the sake of increasing or decreasing another individual's material payoff. For example, if an impartial observer (a "third party") in the third party punishment game is willing to punish a greedy dictator who gives nothing to the recipient (see below), and if the punishment is costly for the third party, his or her actions imply that he or she has a social preference.

Anonymity is important because it provides the conditions under which a baseline level of social preferences is observable. It is likely that face-to-face interactions change the strength and the pattern of social preferences, but this change can only be documented relative to the baseline. Moreover, a skeptic might argue that, because face-to-face interactions inevitably involve an individual's reputation, the observed behaviors represent a combination of social preferences and instrumental reputation seeking. The desire to acquire a reputation that is profitable in future interaction ("instrumental reputation seeking") is a purely self-regarding motive that has nothing to do with social preferences, i.e., it represents a confound. Therefore, the one-shot character and the anonymity in simple social preference experiments are crucial for the clean documentation of social preferences. Repeated interactions and a lack of anonymity are confounds that need to be eliminated if seeking a clean measure of social preferences.

In a "dictator" game (Kahneman et al. 1986; Mikula 1972), one player – the dictator – is given a sum of money that he can allocate between himself and another player, the recipient. The dictator game measures a positive concern for the recipient's material payoff that is independent of the recipient's behavior, because the recipient can take no actions. Empirically, dictator allocations are a mixture of 50% offers and 0% offers (i.e., the dictator keeps everything), and a few offers in between 50 and 0%, but the allocations are sensitive to details of how the game is described (Camerer 2003), the dictator's knowledge of who the recipient is (Eckel and Grossman 1996), and whether the recipient knows that he is part of a dictator game (Dana et al. 2006).

In an ultimatum game, the recipient can reject the proposed allocation (Güth et al. 1982). If she rejects it, both players receive nothing. Rejections are evidence of negative reciprocity (Rabin 1993), the motive to punish players who have treated you unfairly, or inequity aversion (Fehr and Schmidt 1999), which is a distaste for unfair outcomes. The amount a recipient loses by rejecting a proposed allocation serves as a measurement of the strength of these motives. Offers of less than 20% are rejected about half the time; proposers seem to anticipate these rejections and consequently offer on average approximately 40%. Cross-cultural studies, show that, across small-scale societies, ultimatum offers are more generous when cooperative activity and market trade are more common (Henrich et al. 2001).

In a third party punishment game, two players, the dictator A and the recipient B, participate in a dictator game (Fehr and Fischbacher 2004). A third player, the potential punisher C, observes how much A gives to B; C can then spend a proportion of his endowment on punishing A. This game measures to what extent "impartial" and "unaffected" third parties are willing to stick up for other players at their own expense, enforcing a sharing norm by punishing greedy dictators. Between 50 and 60% of the third parties punish selfish deviations from the equal split, suggesting that giving less than 50% in the dictator game violates a fairness norm. In principle, the third party punishment option can be used to measure economic willingness to punish violation of *any* social norm (e.g., a violation of etiquette, breaking a taboo, or making a linguistic slur). In Fehr and Fischbacher (2004), for example, the third party punishment game was used to document the existence of a "conditional cooperation" norm that prescribes cooperation conditional on others' cooperation.

In a trust or gift exchange game, two subjects, A and B, each have an initial endowment. A first decides whether to keep his endowment or to send it to B. Then B observes A's action and decides whether to keep the amount she received or send some of it back to A. In a trust game (Berg et al. 1995; Camerer and Weigelt 1988), the experimenter doubles or triples A's transfer, whereas the back transfer of player B is doubled or tripled in the gift exchange game (Fehr et al. 1993). Due to the multiplication of A's transfer or of B's back transfer, both players are better off collectively if A transfers money and B sends back a sufficient amount. This situation mimics a sequential economic exchange in the absence of contract enforcement institutions. B has a strong incentive to keep all the money and send none to A; if A anticipates this behavior, however, there is little reason to transfer, so a chance for mutual gain is lost. Empirically, As invest about half of their endowment in the trust game and Bs repay about as much as player A invested (Camerer 2003). Player As invest less than they do in risky choices with chance outcomes, however, indicating a pure aversion to social betrayal and inequality (Bohnet and Zeckhauser 2004).

In a public goods game (Ledyard 1995), players have a token endowment they can simultaneously invest in any proportion into a private project or a public project. Investment into the public project maximizes the aggregate earnings of the group, but each individual can gain more from investing into the private rather than the public project. Typically, players begin by investing half their tokens on average (many invest either all or none). When the game is repeated over time, with feedback at the end of each decision period, investments decline until only a small fraction (about 10%) of the players invest anything. The prisoners' dilemma (PD) game is a special case of a public goods game with two players and only two actions (cooperate or defect) for each player. When players are also allowed to punish other players at a cost to themselves, many players who invested punish the players who did not invest, which encouraged investment and led players close to the efficient solution in which everyone invested (Fehr and Gächter 2002).

The Impact of Oxytocin on Human Trust

The neuropeptide oxytocin (OT) plays a central role in non-human mammals in behavioral regulation in general and in positive social interactions in particular. Aside from its well-known physiological functions in milk letdown and during labor, OT receptors are distributed in various brain regions associated with behavior (Huber et al. 2005; Landgraf and Neumann 2004), including pair bonding, maternal care, sexual behavior and the ability to form normal social attachments (Carter 1998; Insel and Young 2001; Uvnas-Moberg 1998). Thus, OT seems to permit animals to overcome their natural avoidance of proximity and thereby facilitates approach behavior. Given the fact that OT appears to promote social attachment and affiliation in non-human mammals, Kosfeld et al. (2005) hypothesized that OT might also promote prosocial approach behavior – such as trust – in humans. Research has shown that neuropeptides cross the blood-brain barrier after intranasal administration (Born et al. 2002), providing a useful method for studying the central nervous effects of OT in humans (Heinrichs et al. 2004). Therefore, Kosfeld et al. (2005) used a double-blind study design to compare trusting behavior in a group of subjects who received a single dose of intranasal OT with that of subjects in a control group that received placebo.

They analyzed the impact of exogenously administered OT on individuals' decisions in a trust game with real monetary stakes (Berg et al. 1995; Bohnet and Zeckhauser 2004; Camerer and Weigelt 1988; Fehr et al. 1993) in which the investors could send 0, 4, 8 or 12 money units (MUs) to the trustee. Both the investor and the trustee had an endowment of 12 MUs. The experimenter tripled any amount sent by the investor, so that the trustee subsequently received three times the amount sent. Then, the trustee decided how much money to send back to the investor. The back transfer was on a 1:1 basis, i.e., it was not tripled. In this experiment, the investor's risk is due to the uncertainty of the trustee's behavior, i.e., a social interaction with a specific trustee constitutes the risk, which raises the question whether OT helps humans overcome a general aversion against risks or whether OT specifically affects trusting behavior in social interactions. To answer this question, Kosfeld et al. conducted a risk experiment in which the investor faced the same choices as in the trust game but where a random mechanism and not a trustee's decision determined the investor's risk. The random mechanism in the risk experiment replicated the trustees' decisions in the trust experiment. Therefore, the investors faced exactly the same risk as in the trust experiment; however, their transfer decisions were not embedded in a social interaction because there were no trustees in the risk experiment.

The investors' behavior in the risk experiment did not differ across the OT and placebo groups. There was also no significant difference in the comparison of the placebo group in the trust experiment with the OT and placebo groups in the risk experiment. However, the group of investors in the trust experiment who received OT exhibited significantly different transfer behavior relative to all other groups. Thus, OT increased the investors' transfer levels in the trust experiment but not in the risk experiment. In fact, only 10% of the subjects with OT chose the maximal transfer level in the risk experiment whereas 45% chose the maximal level in the trust experiment. Therefore, the differences between the OT group in the trust experiment and the OT group in the risk experiment were highly significant, suggesting that OT specifically affects trust in interpersonal interactions.

The Impact of OT on Generosity

Which mechanisms might be involved in the effect of OT on trusting behavior? One possibility is that OT causes a general increase in the investors' prosocial inclinations. which implies that it should not only affect the investors' prosocial behavior but also that of the trustees. If this conjecture were true, those trustees who were given OT should have made higher back transfers at a given transfer level than the trustees who received placebo. However, trustees given OT did not exhibit higher back transfers (see Fig. 1 below). Thus, OT did not increase the general inclination to behave prosocially. Rather, OT specifically affected investors' trusting behavior. One might hypothesize that the differing impact of OT on investors' and trustees' behavior is related to the fact that investors and trustees faced rather different situations. In particular, investors had to make the first step; they had to "approach" the trustee by transferring money. In contrast, the trustees could condition their behavior on the investors' actions. Thus, the psychology of trust is important for investors whereas the psychology of strong reciprocity (Gintis et al. 2003) or generosity is relevant for trustees.

A recent paper (Zak et al. 2007) confirmed that OT has no effect on generosity. The authors conducted a dictator game and administered OT intranasally to half of

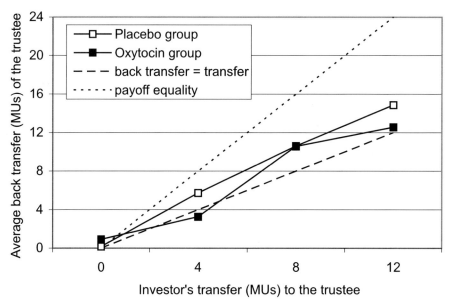

Fig. 1. Trustees' average back transfer for different levels of investors' transfers of money units (MUs) in the OT and placebo groups. The dotted line shows the level of the back transfer necessary to achieve payoff equality between the investor and the trustee. The broken line shows the level of the back transfer equal to the investor's transfer to the trustee. The trustees' back transfers were on average slightly higher than the amount sent by the investor. Trustees of both substance groups made higher back transfers for higher transfer levels of the investors. However, there is no statistically significant difference in back transfers between the OT and placebo groups

the subjects. In the dictator game, the dictator's transfer to the recipient measures unconditional generosity. OT did not affect the dictators' transfers to the recipients, thus indicating that unconditional generosity towards the recipients was unaffected. In addition, the authors conducted an ultimatum game and found that the OT subject in the role of a proposer made significantly higher offers to the responder. One possible interpretation of this result is that OT has an impact on the subject's ability to take the perspective of others. Alternatively, OT could make subjects more fearful of rejections in the ultimatum game because it causes a dislike of social conflict. It could also be the case that OT interacted with a special design feature in this study: the subjects in this study made decisions as a dictator in the dictator game, as a proposer in the ultimatum game and as a responder in the ultimatum game. Subjects made these decisions before they knew which role they ultimately would play. Perhaps, the OT effect on proposer behavior in the ultimatum game reflects an interaction between the imposed role reversal in the ultimatum game (which might enhance perspective taking) and the substance itself. The authors interpreted their finding in terms of an empathy-increasing effect of OT. Future research will have to show which of these interpretations, if any, is true.

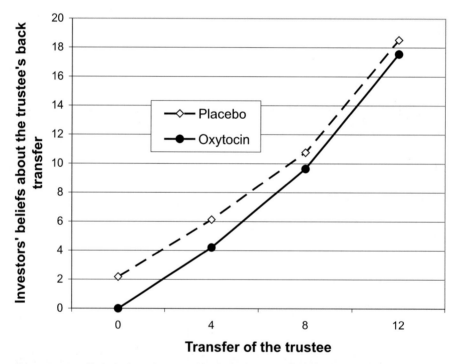

Fig. 2. Investors' beliefs about the average back transfer for different levels of investors' transfers in the OT and placebo groups. The broken line shows the belief in the placebo group. The thick line shows the belief in the OT group. However, there is no statistically significant difference in beliefs between the OT and placebo groups

The Impact of OT on Beliefs About the Trustees' Trustworthiness

Another mechanism behind OT's effect on trust could be based on subjects' beliefs. Perhaps OT rendered subjects more optimistic about the likelihood of a good outcome. To examine this question, Kosfeld et al. (2005) measured the investor's subjective expectation about the trustee's back transfer after every transfer decision. However, if anything, the placebo investors were more optimistic than were the OT investors, although these differences were small and statistically insignificant (see Fig. 2).

Does OT Reduce Betrayal Aversion?

Thus, OT does not affect risk-taking in non-social situations; neither does it affect the trustees' generosity nor make the investors more optimistic about the trustees' generosity. Based on these results, Kosfeld et al. (2005) hypothesized that OT helped subjects to overcome their betrayal aversion in social interactions. This explanation is consistent with the differing impact of OT across the trust and risk experiments and it is further

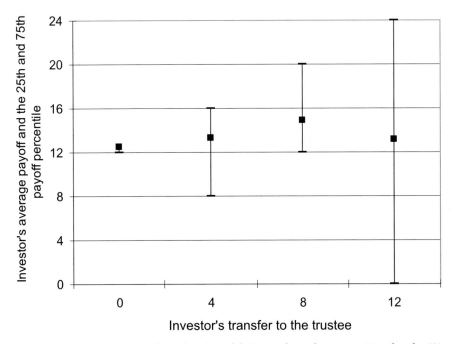

Fig. 3. Investors' average payoff as a function of their transfer to the trustee. Note that the OT and the placebo investors faced the same trustees. Thus they faced the same objective risk and they earned on average the same amount of money at any given transfer level. The figure shows that at a transfer level of 12, the investors earned less on average than if they had transferred only 4 or 8 MUs, but the risk of earning less than the endowment of 12 was much higher in case of a maximal transfer of 12

supported by the fact that investors faced a considerable betrayal risk: an increase in the transfer level from 4 or 8 MUs to 12 MUs decreased the investor's average payoff slightly, whereas it increased the objective risk of very low back transfers by the trustee.

Thus, OT may have an effect on trust because it reduces the subject's fear of being betrayed. This interpretation of OT's effect on trust in terms of betrayal aversion may be seen in the light of animal studies that indicate that an increased central nervous system availability of OT facilitates approach behavior by linking the overcoming of social avoidance with the activation of brain circuits implicated in reward (Insel and Shapiro 1992; Young et al. 2001).

Which Brain Circuitry Might Mediate OT's Effect on Trust?

Previous findings from neuroimaging and lesion studies suggest that subcortical brain structures, such as the amygdala and brainstem effector sites, which process fear, danger, and perhaps also risk of social betrayal, are involved in trusting behaviors. The amygdala has been shown to exhibit increased activation in social avoidance and phobia (Stein et al. 2002; Tillfors et al. 2001) and while viewing untrustworthy faces (Winston et al. 2002). Decreased amygdala activation has also been linked to genetic hypersociability (Meyer-Lindenberg et al. 2005), and lesion studies have indicated that patients with bilateral amygdala damage are impaired in judging the trustworthiness of other people's faces. These patients all judged other people to look more trustworthy and more approachable than did normal viewers (Adolphs et al. 1998). Finally, during the processing of fearful stimuli, subjects receiving OT have reduced amygdala activation and reduced connectivity of the amygdala with brainstem regions involved in automatic fear reactivity (Domes et al. 2007; Kirsch et al. 2005). This finding is in agreement with a recent animal study that demonstrates in vitro that OT acts on the central amygdala by inhibiting excitatory information from the amygdala to brainstem sites mediating the autonomic fear response (Huber et al. 2005b). Given that the amygdala is crucially involved in the processing of risks arising in social situations, one might hypothesize that OT affects the amygdala response to these social risks, thereby facilitating prosocial approach behavior – such as trust. A recent paper (Baumgartner et al. 2008) shows that this is indeed the case.

Concluding Remarks

Research on the impact of neuropeptides on important human social behaviors has just begun. The toolbox of methods available in experimental economics is indeed vast; a number of existing studies imply that neuropeptides and other hormones might play a key role in social behavior. For example, the animal literature on vasopressin suggests that it is important for altruistic punishment of third parties or for rejection behavior in the ultimatum game. Studying the impact of hormones in clean behavioral experimental paradigms is, of course, always only the first step towards a deeper understanding of the neurobiology of such behaviors. Combining behavioral hormone studies with fMRI to examine how the different hormones affect the neural network involved (such as in

Baumgartner et al. 2008) in these behaviors is also important. It may even be possible in some cases to affect this neural circuitry more directly with transcranial magnetic stimulation (Knoch et al. 2006). Thus, the opportunity for combining experimental techniques from economics and neuroscience offers exciting prospects.

References

Adolphs R (2003) Cognitive neuroscience of human social behaviour. Nature Rev Neuroscience 4:165–178

Adolphs R, Tranel D, Damasio AR (1998) The human amygdala in social judgment. Nature 393:470–474

Baumgartner T, Heinrichs M, vonLanthen A, Fischbacher U, Fehr E (2008) Oxytocin shapes the neural circuitry of trust and trust adaption. Neuron 58, May 2008

Berg J, Dickhaut J, McCabe K (1995) Trust, reciprocity and social history. Games and economic behavior 10:122–142

Blakemore SJ, Winston J, Frith U (2004) Social cognitive neuroscience: where are we heading? Trends Cogn Sci 8:216–222

Bohnet I, Zeckhauser R (2004) Trust, risk and betrayal. J Econ Behav Org 55:467–484

Born J, Lange T, Kern W, McGregor GP, Bickel U, Fehm HL (2002) Sniffing neuropeptides: a transnasal approach to the human brain. Nature Neurosci 5:514–516

Camerer CF (2003) Behavioral game theory – experiments in strategic interaction. Princeton University Press, Princeton

Camerer C, Weigelt K (1988) Experimental tests of a sequential equilibrium reputation model. Econometrica 56:1–36

Camerer C, Loewenstein G, Prelec D (2005) Neuroeconomics: how neuroscience can inform economics. J Econ Lit 43:9–64

Carter CS (1998) Neuroendocrine perspectives on social attachment and love. Psychoneuroendocrinology 23:779–818

Dana J, Cain DM, Dawes RM (2006) What you don't know won't hurt me: Costly (but quiet) exit in dictator games. Org Behav Human Decision Proc 100:193–201

Domes G, Heinrichs M, Glascher J, Buchel C, Braus DF, Herpertz SC (2007) Oxytocin attenuates amygdala responses to emotional faces regardless of valence. Biol Psychiat 62:1187–90

Eckel C, Grossman P (1996) Altruism in anonymous dictator games. Games Econ Behav 16:181–191

Fehr E, Camerer CF (2007) Social neuroeconomics: the neural circuitry of social preferences. Trends Cogn Sci 11:419–427

Fehr E, Fischbacher U (2003) The nature of human altruism. Nature 425:785–791

Fehr E, Fischbacher U (2004) Third-party punishment and social norms. Evol Human Behav 25:63–87

Fehr E, Gächter S (2002) Altruistic punishment in humans. Nature 415:137–140

Fehr E, Schmidt KM (1999) A theory of fairness, competition, and cooperation. Quart J Econ 114:817–868

Fehr E, Kirchsteiger G, Riedl A (1993) Does fairness prevent market clearing? An experimental investigation. Quart J Econ 108:437–459

Fehr E, Fischbacher U, Kosfeld M (2005) Neuroeconomic foundations of trust and social preferences: Initial evidence. Am Econ Rev 95:346–351

Gintis H, Bowles S, Boyd R, Fehr E (2003) Explaining altruistic behavior in humans. Evol Human Behav 24:153–172

Glimcher PW, Rustichini A (2004) Neuroeconomics: the consilience of brain and decision. Science 306:447–452

Güth W, Schmittberger R, Schwarze B (1982) An experimental analysis of ultimatum bargaining. J Econ Behav Org 3:367–388

Heinrichs M, Meinlschmidt G, Wippich W, Ehlert U, Hellhammer DH (2004) Selective amnesic effects of oxytocin on human memory. Physiol Behav 83:31–38

Henrich J, Boyd R, Bowles S, Camerer C, Fehr E, Gintis H, McElreath R (2001) In search of homo economicus: behavioral experiments in 15 small-scale societies. Am Econ Rev 91:73–78

Huber D, Veinante P, Stoop R (2005) Vasopressin and oxytocin excite distinct neuronal populations in the central amygdala. Science 308:245–248

Insel TR, Shapiro LE (1992) Oxytocin receptor distribution reflects social organization in monogamous and polygamous voles. Proc Natl Acad Sci USA 89:5981–5985

Insel TR, Young LJ (2001) The neurobiology of attachment. Nature Rev Neurosci 2:129–136

Kahneman D, Knetsch JL, Thaler R (1986) Fairness as a constraint on profit seeking: entitlements in the market. Am Econ Rev 76:728–741

Kirsch P, Esslinger C, Chen Q, Mier D, Lis S, Siddhanti S, Gruppe H, Mattay VS, Gallhofer B, Meyer-Lindenberg A (2005) Oxytocin modulates neural circuitry for social cognition and fear in humans. J Neurosci 25:11489–11493

Knoch D, Pascual-Leone A, Meyer K, Treyer V, Fehr E (2006) Diminishing reciprocal fairness by disrupting the right prefrontal cortex. Science 314:829–832

Kosfeld M, Heinrichs M, Zak P, Fischbacher U, Fehr E (2005) Oxytocin increases trust in humans. Nature 435:673–676

Landgraf R, Neumann ID (2004) Vasopressin and oxytocin release within the brain: a dynamic concept of multiple and variable modes of neuropeptide communication. Front Neuroendocrinol 25:150–176

Ledyard J (1995) Public Goods: A survey of experimental research. In: Kagel J, Roth AE (eds), Handbook of experimental economics. Princeton University Press, Princeton, pp 111–194

Lieberman MD (2007) Social cognitive neuroscience: a review of core processes. Annu Rev Psychol 58:259–289

Meyer-Lindenberg A, Hariri AR, Munoz KE, Mervis CB, Mattay VS, Morris CA, Berman KF (2005) Neural correlates of genetically abnormal social cognition in Williams syndrome. Nature Neurosci 8:991–993

Mikula G (1972) Reward allocation in dyads regarding varied performance ratio. Zeit Sozialpsychol 3:126–133

Rabin M (1993) Incorporating fairness into game theory and economics. Am Econ Rev 83:1281–1302

Sanfey AG, Loewenstein G, McClure SM, Cohen JD (2006) Neuroeconomics: cross-currents in research on decision-making. Trends Cogn Sci 10:108–116

Stein MB, Goldin PR, Sareen J, Zorrilla LT, Brown GG (2002) Increased amygdala activation to angry and contemptuous faces in generalized social phobia. Arch Gen Psychiat 59:1027–1034

Tillfors M, Furmark T, Marteinsdottir I, Fischer H, Pissiota A, Langstrom B, Fredrikson M (2001) Cerebral blood flow in subjects with social phobia during stressful speaking tasks: a PET study. Am J Psychiat 158:1220–1226

Uvnas-Moberg K (1998) Oxytocin may mediate the benefits of positive social interaction and emotions. Psychoneuroendocrinology 23:819–835

Winston JS, Strange BA, O'Doherty J, Dolan RJ (2002) Automatic and intentional brain responses during evaluation of trustworthiness of faces. Nature Neurosci 5:277–283

Young LJ, Lim MM, Gingrich B, Insel TR (2001) Cellular mechanisms of social attachment. Horm Behav 40:133–138

Zak PJ, Stanton AA, Ahmadi S (2007) Oxytocin increases generosity in humans. PLoS ONE 2, e1128

Molecular Neurobiology of the Social Brain

Larry J. Young[1]

Summary

There is growing evidence that social cognitive processes, such as the processing of social cues, social recognition, and social bonding, are regulated by distinct neural mechanisms in the brain. In particular, the neuropeptides oxytocin and vasopressin are emerging as key modulators of social cognition and behavior. This chapter focuses on comparative studies using monogamous and non-monogamous species of voles, as well as genetically engineered mice, that have contributed to our understanding of the roles of these peptides and the genes encoding their receptors in the regulation of social behavior. These studies suggest that variation in the regulation of neuropeptide receptor genes contributes to variation in social function and behavior, an observation that has implications for psychiatric disorders characterized by deficits in the social domain, including autism spectrum disorders (ASD) and schizophrenia.

Introduction

Animal models are critical for understanding the molecular, cellular and neurobiological mechanism underlying social behavior (Lim et al. 2005; Lim and Young 2006). For example, early studies in rats and sheep revealed a critical role for the neuropeptide oxytocin in the regulation of affiliative behavior, maternal motivation and mother-infant bonding (Pedersen and Prange 1979; Witt et al. 1992; Kendrick et al. 1997). More recently, Microtine rodents, or voles, have provided even more insights into the role of neuropeptides and other neurotransmitter systems in the regulation of complex social behaviors, such as social bonding and parental care (Young and Wang 2004). Prairie voles are highly social and socially monogamous, with mates forming enduring social attachments, or pair bonds (Getz and Carter 1996). In contrast, montane and meadow voles are relatively asocial and do not form any social attachments between mates (Jannett 1980). Behavioral pharmacological studies have revealed that oxytocin, and the related neuropeptide, arginine vasopressin, facilitate partner preference formation, the laboratory proxy for pair bond formation (Young and Wang 2004). The remainder of this chapter discusses in detail the studies examining the neural mechanisms by

---

[1] Center for Behavioral Neuroscience, Department of Psychiatry and Behavioral Sciences, and Yerkes National Primate Research Center, Emory University School of Medicine, Atlanta GA 30329, e-mail: lyoun03@emory.edu

Pfaff et al.
Hormones and Social Behavior
© Springer-Verlag Berlin Heidelberg 2008

which these neuropeptides facilitate social bond formation, explore the mechanisms underlying the species differences and individual variation in social behavior, and discuss the implications of these findings in relation to human social behavior and psychopathology.

Oxytocin and Vasopressin: Social Neuropeptides

Oxytocin and vasopressin (aka antidiuretic hormone) are nine-amino acid peptides produced in the hypothalamus and are best known for their peripheral functions regulating uterine contractions, lactation, and kidney function (Gainer and Wray 1994; Burbach et al. 2006). Peripheral oxytocin and vasopressin are secreted into the blood circulation from magnocellular hypothalamic neurons that project directly to the posterior pituitary. Peripherally released peptide hormones do not influence behavior, since they are excluded from the central nervous system by the blood-brain barrier. Oxytocin and vasopressin are also released within the brain, independent of peripheral release, where they activate their receptors located in specific brain nuclei (Ludwig and Leng 2006). It is these centrally released neuropeptides that modulate social behavior in animal models.

Neuropeptide Regulation of Social Bonding in Monogamous Rodents

As mentioned above, prairie voles are highly social and monogamous rodents that form life-long social attachments between mates, and they have become an important animal model for understanding the regulation of normal social function. In the laboratory, social bond formation is assessed using a "partner preference" test (Williams et al. 1994). The partner preference test is performed in a three-chambered arena in which the "partner" is loosely tethered in one chamber, a novel, or "stranger" individual with the same stimulus value as the partner is tethered in the opposite chamber, and the experimental animal is allowed to freely move through all three chambers, including a central, neutral chamber. During a three-hr test, both male and female prairie voles will spend significantly more time with the partner than the stranger following 24 hours of cohabitation with mating. In contrast, non-monogamous montane and meadow voles spend most of the time in the central, neutral chamber and do not differentiate between the partner and stranger. Pharmacological manipulations can be performed during the cohabitation period to elucidate the mechanisms underlying social bonding.

In female prairie voles, a central infusion of oxytocin facilitates partner preference formation after an abbreviated cohabitation period (Williams et al. 1994). Likewise, a selective oxytocin receptor antagonist prevents mating-induced partner preference formation (Insel and Hulihan 1995). In male prairie voles, vasopressin appears to play a more important role in social bond formation. Infusion of a vasopressin stimulates partner preference formation in the absence of mating, whereas a selective V1a vasopressin receptor antagonist prevents partner preference formation following mating (Winslow et al. 1993). In addition to stimulating social bonds between mates, oxytocin facilitates maternal care in female prairie voles and vasopressin stimulates paternal care in male prairie voles (Wang et al. 1994; Olazabal and Young 2006).

Species Differences in Neuropeptide Receptor Distribution and Social Behavior

Comparative neuroanatomical studies between the monogamous prairie voles and non-monogamous montane and meadow voles have revealed underlying species differences that likely account for the differences in social behavior. While the distribution of oxytocin and vasopressin peptides are similar across these species, there are marked species differences in the localization of the receptors for these peptides (Young and Wang 2004; Fig. 1). For example, prairie voles have high densities of oxytocin receptors in the nucleus acumbens (NAcc) whereas montane and meadow voles do not. Likewise, prairie voles have high densities of vasopressin receptors in the ventral pallidum, a major output nucleus of the NAcc; the non-monogamous species do not. The NAcc and ventral pallidum are major components of the dopamine mesolimbic reward pathway, which is also involved in the actions of drugs of abuse and addiction. To determine whether the receptors in these regions are involved in the regulation of social bond formation, site-specific infusions of neuropeptide antagonists were performed.

Infusion of a selective oxytocin receptor antagonist into the NAcc, but not into the adjacent caudate putamen, blocks partner preference formation in female prairie voles (Young et al. 2001; Fig. 1). Likewise, a selective V1a vasopressin receptor antagonist infused into the ventral pallidum, but not into the amygdala or thalamus, prevents mating-induced partner preference formation in male prairie voles (Lim and Young 2004). Other studies demonstrate that V1a receptors in the lateral septum are

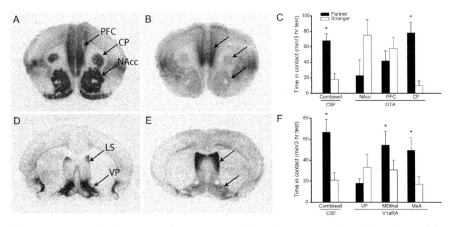

Fig. 1. Oxytocin and V1a vasopressin receptor regulation of pair bonding in prairie voles. Prairie voles (A) have high densities of oxytocin receptors (OTR) in the nucleus accumbens (NAcc) and caudate putamen (CP) compared to non-monogamous montane voles (B). Both species have OTR in the prefrontal cortex (PFC). (C) A selective OTR antagonist infused bilaterally into the NAcc or PFC, but not into the CP, blocks partner-preference formation in female prairie voles. Male prairie voles (D) have high densities of V1a vasopressin receptors (V1aR) in the ventral pallidum (VP) compared to montane voles (E). LS, lateral septum. (F) Infusion of a selective V1aR antagonist (V1aRA, 0.05 ng/side in 1 μl) into the VP, but not into the mediodorsal thalamus (MDthal) or medial amygdala (MeA), prevents mating-induced partner preference formation in male prairie voles. Scale bar = 1 mm. Reprinted from Young and Wang 2004

also critical for partner-preference formation in males (Liu et al. 2001). Furthermore, dopamine D2 receptors in the NAcc are also critical for partner-preference formation in both males and females (Aragona et al. 2003; Liu and Wang 2003). These studies demonstrate that the oxytocin and vasopressin receptor systems, through an interaction with the mesolimbic dopamine system, mediate social bond formation in prairie voles.

The comparative studies between monogamous and non-monogamous voles, along with the pharmacological studies mentioned above, suggest that species differences in the expression of oxytocin and vasopressin receptors in the reward pathway underlie the species differences in social bonding behavior. To test this hypothesis, viral vector experiments were performed to manipulate the expression of V1a receptors in male meadow voles, which do not form partner preferences (Lim et al. 2004). Briefly, an adeno-associated viral vector (AAV) containing the prairie vole vasopressin receptor under the control of a neuron-specific promoter was infused into the ventral pallidum of male meadow voles. This procedure resulted in an elevation of vasopressin receptor expression in the ventral pallidum only, to a level comparable to that of prairie voles. Remarkably, these genetically transformed meadow voles were capable of displaying partner preferences. This study demonstrates the principle that variation in neuropeptide receptor expression in the brain can produce variation in complex social behavior.

A Neural Model of Social Bonding

In rats and mice, oxytocin and vasopressin have been implicated in the facilitation of social recognition. Social recognition refers to the ability of an animal to recognize a familiar individual. Oxytocin knockout mice, which do not express any oxytocin, suffer from severe social amnesia and thus cannot recognize individuals that they have encountered previously (Ferguson et al. 2000). An infusion of oxytocin into the amygdala of these mutant mice prior to social exposure restores social recognition abilities (Ferguson et al. 2001). Likewise, V1a vasopressin knockout mice display social amnesia, which is rescued by re-expressing the receptor in the lateral septum using viral vector-mediated gene transfer (Bielsky et al. 2004, 2005). These studies suggest that oxytocin and vasopressin play a large role in the neural processing of social stimuli that is necessary for distinguishing individuals, a process that should be critical for social bond formation. These observations suggest a potential neural model to explain their role in social bonding. It has been suggested that social bonding results from the simultaneous activation of reward and reinforcement mechanisms, which involve dopamine, and the mechanisms underlying individual recognition through the processing of social cues, which involve oxytocin and vasopressin (Young and Wang 2004). If correct, the convergent activation of these brain mechanism results in a conditioned "partner" preference, in which the rewarding aspects of mating are associated with the social signature of the partner. The presence of the oxytocin and vasopressin receptors in the reinforcement centers of the brain promotes this association, whereas the absence of the receptors in non-monogamous species prevents this association.

Molecular Mechanisms Underlying Diversity in Social Behavior

Comparative genetic analyses have revealed potential genetic mechanisms that may underlie some aspects of natural variation in social behavior. A comparison of the genomic V1a vasopressin receptor gene (*avpr1a*) in the monogamous prairie and non-monogamous montane vole revealed that, while the coding regions of the genes were highly homologous, a highly repetitive element in the promoter of the gene differed significantly between the species (Young et al. 1999). Specifically, the prairie vole *avpr1a* promoter has a 430 bp microsatellite sequence located ~760 bp upstream of the transcription start site that is absent in the montane vole. Transcription assays in cell culture suggest that this variation in promoter sequence is sufficient to result in cell-type specific differences in gene expression, suggesting that it may be responsible for species differences in gene expression (Hammock and Young 2004). Further comparative studies in several other vole species suggest that the presence or absence of this element does not predict social organization in voles; nevertheless, more subtle variation in this microsatellite does appear to be associated with variation in vasopressin receptor expression in the brain (Fink et al. 2006; Young and Hammock 2007).

Microsatellite elements are composed of highly repetitive DNA sequences that are evolutionarily unstable (Kashi and King 2006). Instability in such elements has been implicated in diseases such as fragile X and Huntington's disease. Within prairie voles, individual variation in this element has been associated with individual variation in social behavior. In one study, breeding pairs of prairie voles were selected based on the length of the microsatellite in the *avpr1a* promoter. Breeding pairs that were homozygous for short or long versions of the microsatellite were created and the behavior of the parents and their offspring was analyzed. This study revealed that male prairie voles with relatively short microsatellites provided less extensive paternal care, were less interested in social stimuli, and were less likely to form social attachments than male prairie voles with longer microsatellites (Hammock and Young 2005). Furthermore, males with short or long microsatellite elements differed in the density of vasopressin receptor binding in specific brain regions. These studies reveal that polymorphisms in the vasopressin receptor gene promoter, *avpr1a*, are a potential source for variation in vasopressin receptor gene expression and social behavior.

Implications for Human Behavior

The human brain has oxytocin and vasopressin receptors, and the localization of these receptors in limbic brain regions suggests that they may be involved in regulating social behavior in humans (Loup et al. 1991). There are now several studies suggesting that these peptides may contribute to the regulation of social cognition in humans. For example, intranasal oxytocin infusions have been shown to enhance "trust" in economic-based games (Kosfeld et al. 2005). Furthermore, intranasal oxytocin enhances the ability to infer emotional states of others based on subtle facial expression (Domes et al. 2007). Brain imaging studies have revealed that oxytocin alters amygdala activity in response to socially relevant visual stimuli (Kirsch et al. 2005). There is also evidence that the oxytocin system may be involved in autism. For example, autistic individuals have been reported to have lower circulating plasma levels of oxytocin than healthy subjects (Modahl et al. 1998). Gene association studies have provided further evidence for a role, albeit modest, in the etiology of autism (Wu et al. 2005). Finally, intranasal oxytocin was recently reported to enhance some aspects of social cognition in autistic individuals (Hollander et al. 2007).

Genetic studies also suggest that variation in the human vasopressin receptor gene (AVPR1a) may also contribute to variation in human social cognition. The human AVPR1a contains three microsatellite elements, each of which is polymorphic. There have been three independent studies that reported modest associations between polymorphisms in the AVPR1a promoter and autism spectrum disorders, with one study specifically implicating this gene in the mediation of social skills (Kim et al. 2001; Wassink et al. 2004; Yirmiya et al. 2006). Other studies have suggested that variation in this gene contributes to variation in non-pathological social behavior (Kim et al. 2001; Wassink et al. 2004; Bachner-Melman et al. 2005a,b; Yirmiya et al. 2006).

Conclusion

The studies outlined here demonstrate the utility of using a comparative animal model approach to understand the neural mechanisms underlying complex social behavior. Studies in rats, sheep, mice and voles all suggest that oxytocin and vasopressin play important roles in regulating social cognition and behavior. The studies in voles provide insights into the neurobiological mechanism by which these peptides regulate social behaviors such as pair bonding and provide a mechanism underlying natural variation in behavior. Finally, there is some evidence that these findings in rodents can be translationally relevant to human cognition and behavior (Bartz and Hollander 2006; Lim and Young 2006). Future studies involving genetic analysis, pharmacological manipulations and brain imaging studies will further elucidate the role of these neuropeptides in regulating the human social brain.

References

Aragona BJ, Liu Y, Curtis TJ, Stephan FK, Wang ZX (2003) A critical role for nucleus accumbens dopamine in partner preference formation of male prairie voles. J Neurosci 23:3483–3490
Bachner-Melman R, Zohar AH, Bacon-Shnoor N, Elizur Y, Nemanov L, Gritsenko I, Ebstein RP (2005a) Link Between Vasopressin Receptor AVPR1A Promoter Region Microsatellites and Measures of Social Behavior in Humans. J Indiv Differ 26:2–10
Bachner-Melman R, Dina C, Zohar AH, Constantini N, Lerer E, Hoch S, Sella S, Nemanov L, Gritsenko I, Lichtenberg P, Granot R, Ebstein RP (2005b) AVPR1a and SLC6A4 gene polymorphisms are associated with creative dance performance. PLoS Genet 1:e42
Bartz J, Hollander E (2006) The neuroscience of affiliation: Forging links between basic and clinical research on neuropeptides and social behavior. Horm Behav 50:518–528
Bielsky IF, Hu S-B, Szegda KL, Westphal H, Young LJ (2004) Profound impairment in social recognition and reduction in anxiety in vasopressin V1a receptor knockout mice. Neuropsychopharmacology 29:483–493
Bielsky IF, Hu SB, Ren X, Terwilliger EF, L.J. Y (2005) The V1a vasopressin receptor is necessary and sufficient for normal social recognition: a gene replacement study. Neuron 47:503–513

Burbach P, Young LJ, Russell J (2006) Oxytocin: synthesis, secretion and reproductive functions. In: Neill JD (ed) Physiology of reproduction. Third Edition. Amsterdam: Elsevier pp 3055–3127

Domes G, Heinrichs M, Michel A, Berger C, Herpertz SC (2007) Oxytocin improves "mind-reading" in humans. Biol Psychiat 61:731–733

Ferguson JN, Young LJ, Hearn EF, Insel. TR, Winslow JT (2000) Social amnesia in mice lacking the oxytocin gene. Nature Genet 25:284–288

Ferguson JN, Aldag JM, Insel TR, Young LJ (2001) Oxytocin in the medial amygdala is essential for social recognition in the mouse. J Neurosci 21:8278–8285

Fink S, Excoffier L, Heckel G (2006) Mammalian monogamy is not controlled by a single gene. Proc Natl Acad Sci USA 103:10956–10960

Gainer H, Wray W (1994) Cellular and molecular biology of oxytocin and vasopressin. In: Knobil E, Neill JD (eds) The physiology of reproduction New York: Raven Press, pp 1099–1129

Getz LL, Carter CS (1996) Prairie-vole partnerships. Am Scient 84:56–62

Hammock EAD, Young LJ (2004) Functional microsatellite polymorphisms associated with divergent social structure in vole species. Mol Biol Evol 21:1057–1063

Hammock EAD, Young LJ (2005) Microsatellite instability generates diversity in brain and sociobehavioral traits. Science 308:1630–1634

Hollander E, Bartz J, Chaplin W, Phillips A, Sumner J, Soorya L, Anagnostou E, Wasserman S (2007) Oxytocin increases retention of social cognition in autism. Biol Psychiat 61:498–503

Insel TR, Hulihan T (1995) A gender-specific mechanism for pair bonding: oxytocin and partner preference formation in monogamous voles. Behav Neurosci 109:782–789

Jannett FJ (1980) Social dynamics of the montane vole *Microtus montanus*, as a paradigm. The Biologist 62:3–19

Kashi Y, King DG (2006) Simple sequence repeats as advantageous mutators in evolution. Trends Genet 22:253–259

Kendrick KM, Costa APCD, Broad KD, Ohkura S, Guevara R, Levy F, Keverne EB (1997) Neural control of maternal behavior and olfactory recognition of offspring. Brain Res Bull 44:383–395

Kim S, Young LJ, Gonen D, Veenstra-VanderWeele J, Courchesne R, Courchesne E, Lord C, Leventhal BL, Cook EH, Insel TR (2001) Transmission disequilibrium testing of arginine vasopressin receptor 1A (AVPR1A) polymorphisms in autism. Mol Psychiat 7:503–507

Kirsch P, Esslinger C, Chen Q, Mier D, Lis S, Siddhanti S, Gruppe H, Mattay VS, Gallhofer B, Meyer-Lindenberg A (2005) Oxytocin modulates neural circuitry for social cognition and fear in humans. J Neurosci 25:11489–11493

Kosfeld M, Heinrichs M, Zak PJ, Fischbacher U, Fehr E (2005) Oxytocin increases trust in humans. Nature 435:673–676

Lim MM, Young LJ (2004) Vasopressin-dependent neural circuits underlying pair bond formation in the monogamous prairie vole. Neurosci 125:35–45

Lim MM, Young LJ (2006) Neuropeptidergic regulation of affiliative behavior and social bonding in animals. Horm Behav 50:506–517

Lim MM, Wang Z, Olazábal DE, Ren X, Terwilliger EF, Young LJ (2004) Enhanced partner preference in promiscuous species by manipulating the expression of a single gene. Nature 429:754–757

Lim MM, Bielsky IF, Young LJ (2005) Neuropeptides and the social brain: Potential rodent models of autism. Int J Dev Neurosci 23:235–243

Liu Y, Wang ZX (2003) Nucleus accumbens dopamine and oxytocin interact to regulate pair bond formation in female prairie voles. Neuroscience 121:537–544

Liu Y, Curtis JT, Wang ZX (2001) Vasopressin in the lateral septum regulates pair bond formation in male prairie voles (*Microtus ochrogaster*). Behav Neurosci 115:910–919

Loup F, Tribollet E, Dubois-Dauphin M, Dreifuss JJ (1991) Localization of high-affinity binding sites for oxytocin and vasopressin in the human brain. An autoradiographic study. Brain Res 555:220–232

Ludwig M, Leng G (2006) Dendritic peptide release and peptide-dependent behaviours. Nature Rev Neurosci 7:126–136

Modahl C, Green LA, Fein D, Morris M, Waterhouse L, Feinstein C, Levin H (1998) Plasma oxytocin levels in autistic children. Biol Psychiat 43:270–277

Olazabal DE, Young LJ (2006) Oxytocin receptors in the nucleus accumbens facilitate "spontaneous" maternal behavior in adult female prairie voles. Neuroscience 141:559–568

Pedersen CA, Prange AJ, Jr. (1979) Induction of maternal behavior in virgin rats after intracerebroventricular administration of oxytocin. Proc Natl Acad Sci USA 76:6661–6665

Wang Z, Ferris CF, De Vries GJ (1994) Role of septal vasopressin innervation in paternal behavior in prairie voles (Microtus ochrogaster). Proc Natl Acad Sci USA 91:400–404

Wassink TH, Piven J, Vieland VJ, Pietila J, Goedken RJ, Folstein SE, Sheffield VC (2004) Examination of AVPR1a as an autism susceptibility gene. Mol Psychiat 9:968–972

Williams JR, Insel TR, Harbaugh CR, Carter CS (1994) Oxytocin administered centrally facilitates formation of a partner preference in prairie voles (*Microtus ochrogaster*). J Neuroendocrinol 6:247–250

Winslow J, Hastings N, Carter CS, Harbaugh C, Insel T (1993) A role for central vasopressin in pair bonding in monogamous prairie voles. Nature 365:545–548

Witt DM, Winslow JT, Insel TR (1992) Enhanced social interactions in rats following chronic, centrally infused oxytocin. Pharm Biochem Beh 43:855–861

Wu S, Jia M, Ruan Y, Liu J, Guo Y, Shuang M, Gong X, Zhang Y, Yang X, Zhang D (2005) Positive association of the oxytocin receptor gene (OXTR) with autism in the Chinese Han population. Biol Psychiat 58:74–77

Yirmiya N, Rosenberg C, Levi S, Salomon S, Shulman C, Nemanov L, Dina C, Ebstein RP (2006) Association between the arginine vasopressin 1a receptor (AVPR1a) gene and autism in a family-based study: mediation by socialization skills. Mol Psychiat 11:488–494

Young LJ, Wang Z (2004) The neurobiology of pair bonding. Nature Neurosci 7:1048–1054

Young LJ, Hammock EA (2007) On switches and knobs, microsatellites and monogamy. Trends Genet 23:209–212

Young LJ, Nilsen R, Waymire KG, MacGregor GR, Insel TR (1999) Increased affiliative response to vasopressin in mice expressing the vasopressin receptor from a monogamous vole. Nature 400:766–768

Young LJ, Lim M, B.Gingrich, Insel TR (2001) Cellular mechanisms of social attachment. Horm Behav 40:133–148

Impact of Brain Evolution on Hormones and Social Behaviour

E.B. Keverne[1]

Summary

In mammals, the social behaviour of males and females reflects their different lifetime reproductive strategies. Reproductive success in males is determined by the outcome of competition with other males, the dominant males mating with as many females as possible. Hence, males rarely form strong social relationships and male coalitions are typically hierarchical, with emphasis upon aggressive rather than affiliative behaviour. Females have a different strategy. They invest in the production of relatively few offspring, with reproductive success being determined by the quality of care and the ability to enable infant survival beyond the weaning age. Females, therefore, form strong social bonds with their infants and their female-female relationships are affiliative, especially among matrilineal kin who often assist with infant care. In a minority of mammalian populations (less than 5%), a promiscuous male strategy is not an option, owing to the low population density of females. In this situation, males and females form a partner preference (bond), defending their partners against intruders and both parents participating in infant care (Kleiman 1997). The questions addressed in this chapter concern the hormonal mechanisms that underpin these female-bonded social relationships and how the evolutionary development of the neocortex in large-brained primates has impacted on the role of "bonding" as being an integral adjunct of physiological homeostasis.

Introduction

The neural template for hormonal influences on social behaviour has been thoroughly investigated in small-brained mammals. Considerable attention has been given to the monogamous vole and the role of the neurohormones, oxytocin (OT) and vasopressin, in activating the reward mechanisms of the brain that are involved in establishing partner recognition and selective bonding. However, monogamy is relatively rare among mammals, and a more appropriate starting point for understanding social relationships at a mechanistic level is in the conserved mechanisms that underpin the reciprocal

---

[1] Sub-Department of Animal Behaviour, University of Cambridge, Madingley, Cambridge, CB23 8AA, UK, e-mail: ebk10@cam.ac.uk

Pfaff et al.
Hormones and Social Behavior
© Springer-Verlag Berlin Heidelberg 2008

bonding between mother and infant. Many mammalian adaptations have evolved, including placentation milk provisioning, homeothermy and intensive maternal care, to ensure the mother-infant bond has become a very significant biological relationship. The high levels of prenatal resource investment by female placental mammals and their unique ability to produce milk devolved the priority for parental care to the female. Infants were rendered special to females by the deployment of brain reward mechanisms that were linked to hormonal state and recognition systems, primarily olfactory, that ensured the successful nurturing of offspring.

The placenta has made a notable contribution to the way hormones shape the mother-infant relationship. The placenta is an endocrine organ in its own right, and through production and regulation of hormones by the placenta, the foetus determines its own destiny (Keverne 2006). Progesterone is the steroid hormone that dominates pregnancy and primes the female brain for promotion of maternal behaviour, increased maternal feeding and suppression of sexual behaviour (Fig. 1). Oestrogen levels, which increase towards the end of pregnancy, are also indirectly dependent on the placenta for conversion of progesterone to androgen, which then serves as the precursor for aromatisation to oestrogen. Progesterone and oestrogen are steroids that readily enter the blood-brain barrier and prime the brain's OT neurons and receptors. OT is produced by the hypothalamic parvocellular neurons that activate maternal behaviour, while the magnocellular neurons produce OT that is released from the posterior pituitary and is important for parturition and milk letdown. High levels of progesterone promote OT synthesis but inhibit neural firing and hence OT release (Keverne and Kendrick 1992). Around the time of parturition, the falling levels of progesterone and increasing levels of oestrogen promote synthesis of OT receptors in the brain (Broad et al. 1999). Having been synthesised in hypothalamic neurons, OT is released in the brain at parturition to facilitate olfactory recognition of offspring and thereby promote specific maternal bonding.

Although OT-based affiliative bonding is likely to have evolved in mammals to activate maternal care and reinforce the mother-infant bond, other female affiliative interactions in rodents are also regulated by OT. In the monogamous prairie vole,

Placental regulated steroids - effects on maternity

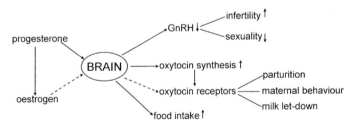

Fig. 1. Steroid hormones, notably progesterone and its aromatisation via androgen to oestrogen in the foetus, prime the brain for various components of maternalism and act directly to promote feeding and inhibit reproduction

Microtus ochrogaster, females form an enduring "pair bond" dependent on a specific olfactory partner preference induced by mating (Williams et al. 1992). A series of recent studies have demonstrated that the release of OT from the hypothalamus post-mating in prairie voles enables a female to form this exclusive olfactory partner preference (Williams et al. 1994; Lim et al. 2004b). Given that evolution is conservative, it is not surprising that many forms of social relationships have devolved from the mechanistic foundation that subserve mother-infant bonding. Indeed, there are many conserved similarities between mother-infant bonding and monogamy in prairie voles; both are triggered by an olfactory input (odour of infant or mate), both occur spontaneously after the release of OT, and both require vaginal-cervical stimulations (via parturition or mating) for this to be activated. Intriguingly, work with mice carrying mutations in the gene encoding OT confirm that this peptide hormone is crucial for social recognition, as these mutant mice are unable to form olfactory memories for conspecifics (Ferguson et al. 2000, 2001).

Olfaction and Social Reward

The brain's oxytocinergic system, together with olfactory recognition, underpins the formation of female social relationships, be they with mates, offspring or kin. The formation of these relationships requires familiarity, which for kin is brought about by prolonged contact and grooming. For completely novel stimuli, such as strange males or newly born offspring, overcoming neophobia is of some significance. It is, therefore, noteworthy that OT knockout mice that fail to form recognition memories also exhibit altered anxiety levels (Winslow et al. 2000; Amico et al. 2004). Hormones are also important in the context of mate recognition. The formation of familiar sexual relationships involves sexual activity, which can only occur when the female is in oestrus; offspring recognition requires parturition linked to the hormones of pregnancy. Both pregnancy and oestrus provide an endocrine context for the synthesis of OT and OT receptors. Oestrogen acts through the oestrogen receptors, ERα and ERβ; ERβ is expressed in the hypothalamic neurons that synthesize OT (Mitra et al. 2003), whereas ERα is required for the synthesis of OT receptors in the amygdala (Young et al. 1998). Interestingly, both ERα and the ERβ knockout mice are similarly impaired in social recognition tests, as observed in the OT knockout mice (Ferguson et al. 2001; Choleris et al. 2003). Hence, in the context of oestrus and parturition, the female's brain undergoes radical reorganisation with respect to the synthesis of OT and its receptor. The key areas of the brain associated with social recognition and preference are the olfactory bulb, the amygdala and the nucleus accumbens (Liu and Wang 2003).

Although the olfactory bulb has no oxytocinergic terminals, there is an abundance of OT receptors. This mismatch of terminals with receptors is functionally addressed by the neurohumoral release of OT into cerebrospinal fluid at parturition and mating. These significant biological events produce the changes in sensitivity, synaptic efficacy and neural firing in the olfactory bulb that are integral to the olfactory learning process for social familiarity (Keverne 1999; Brennan 2001). Hence, OT infusions into the cerebral ventricles enable social olfactory memory in rats (Dluzen et al. 2000), whereas OT infusions in the olfactory bulb reversibly influence both the frequency and the amplitude of excitatory postsynaptic currents at the reciprocal dendrodendritic synapses important for olfactory learning (Osaka et al. 2001). Moreover, OT infusions into the amygdala, a primary relay for olfactory processing, restore the ability to make social recognition in OT knockout mice (Ferguson et al. 2001). The amygdala has reciprocal connections with the NAcc, a structure that shows enhanced levels of Fos-IR and increased dopamine (DA) transmission in rats following exposure to biologically significant odours (Pfaus and Heeb 1997). OT receptors are particularly notable in both the shell and the core of the NAcc and have been implicated, together with DA release, in pair bond formation in the monogamous female vole (Liu and Wang 2003; Fig. 2). Moreover, if the socially relevant behaviour is experienced in the same context as neutral odours, and presumably other social sensory cues, a conditioned association of these second order cues as attractive with behaviourally rewarding properties will develop (Kippin et al. 2003). This association of odour cues with social reward is facilitated in the non-monogamous species by infusions of receptor agonists for the OT neuropeptide and also for the dopamine D2 receptor, whereas OT antagonists block odour-induced partner preferences in the monogamous species (Lim et al. 2004a). Mating at oestrus provides a means of imprinting olfactory recognition of conspecifics. These sensory cues acquire behaviourally rewarding properties

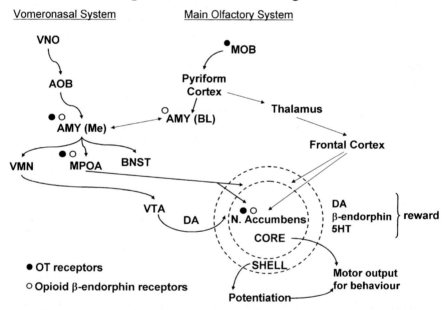

Fig. 2. The circuitry processing olfaction and pheromones is given special status by the neuropeptides regulating maternal behaviour and reward, with enhanced activity at a number of relays for this sensory input to the nucleus accumbens.
VMN – ventro-medial nucleus, MPOA – medial pre-optic area, VTA – ventral tegmental area, AMY – amygdala, **Me – Medial, (verify si bien transcript par Astrid)** BNST – bed nucleus of stria terminalis, VNO – vomeronasal organ, DA – dopamine, MOB – main olfactory bulb, AOB – accessory olfactory bulb

through connections with the NAcc, which further serves as a template for conditioning other secondary sensory cues. Hence, the expansion of features that become familiar and rewarding consolidates selective individual recognition for conspecifics with many common features and few differences. Thus a common biology linked to olfaction underpins many aspects of mammalian social behaviour in small-brained mammals.

The Role of Mammalian Olfactory Systems in Social Bonding

Olfaction is the primary sensory modality in small-brained mammals, coordinating and engaging their social behaviour. Thus, in the context of mother-infant bonding, the hormones of pregnancy induce the synthesis of oxytocin receptors in the olfactory and vomeronasal projection pathways (accessory and main olfactory bulbs, medial amygdala, and medial preoptic area; Fig. 2) as well as oxytocin and dopamine receptors in the nucleus accumbens, an area of the brain concerned with social and many other aspects of reward (Broad et al. 2006). Thus, if socially relevant behaviour occurs together with an individual's odour, a conditioned association can develop that enhances the attractiveness and memory of these familiar odours.

Small-brained mammalian rodents clearly have a well-developed sense of smell that is integral to determining sex differences in reproductive behavioural strategies (Keverne 2002). Indeed, the largest gene family in the mouse genome, >1000 out of 25,000 genes (Zhang and Firestein 2002), is given over to encoding receptors for olfactory molecules. In addition, some 300 genes code for vomeronasal receptors, which respond to non-volatile odours (pheromones), such as those odours found in urine and amniotic fluid that are key to sociobehaviour (Dulac and Axel 1995; Herrada and Dulac 1997). These receptors represent the first processing stage of the vomeronasal (or "accessory") olfactory system, which is the major pheromone chemosensory system in small-brained mammals (Brennan and Keverne 2004; Keverne 2002). This chemosensory system is distinct from the main olfactory system, which is present in all mammals and processes volatile airborne odours. However, it has been shown that a very small subset of these olfactory receptors do respond to peptide fractions (Liberles and Buck 2006), a property normally associated with vomeronasal organ (VNO) receptors. These peptides are probably binding proteins found in olfactory gland secretions and important for the transport of aquaphobic compounds through the watery mucous. The importance of the vomeronasal system for sociobehaviour in rodents, as reported earlier, has been illustrated in studies with mice carrying mutations in the vomeronasal genes coding for pheromone detection (V1r gene family; Del Punta et al. 2002) and receptor transduction (e.g., V2r gene family and V2r TRP2 ion channel; Stowers et al. 2002). Female mice lacking this VNO receptor ion channel fail to engage the behaviours that illustrate mother-infant bonding. They spend little time in the nest with their offspring and fail to protect them by aggressively excluding intruders from the nest area (Kimchi et al. 2007).

Although it appears from comparative genome studies that ancestral primates could process olfactory information via the vomeronasal system, this ability became vestigial 23 million years ago in the ancestry of modern-day New World and Old World primates and apes (Liman and Innan 2003; Zhang and Webb 2003). Further evidence for functional degeneracy comes from comparative phylogenetic analysis of the genes that encode olfactory receptors in marmoset monkeys (Whinnett and Mundy 2003). These studies have estimated from sequence disruptions that >30% of olfactory receptor genes are non-functional pseudogenes in non-human primates, rising to >60% in the human genome (Gilad et al. 2003, 2004). Coupled with these genetic changes, there has also been a dramatic reduction in the relative size of the olfactory cortex, from 65% of total cortex in insectivorous and rodent mammals to little more than 4% in Old World primates (Stephan et al. 1982).

The decline in olfactory processing has, in part, been driven by the need of large-brained Old World primates to gather their social and foraging information from visual cues as they evolved from nocturnal to diurnal lifestyles. Arguably, the most significant visual change in Old World primates was the evolution of trichromacy (Surridge and Mundy 2002; Surridge et al. 2003), which occurred at approximately the same time as the pseudogenization of the Old World primate vomeronasal genome (Webb et al. 2004). This change also coincided with the development of colourful sexual adornments that signal reproductive receptivity in females and dominance in males and a transition to vision as the dominant sensory system. Sexual behaviour was no longer restricted by oestrus and most sexual interactions became non-reproductive, but served for sexual bonding. Postpartum maternal care extended mother-infant bonding beyond the period of suckling when infant mobility required the complex visual recognition of faces at a distance. Indicative of this dramatic shift in the regulation of sociobehaviours from the reliance on olfactory information in small-brained rodents to visual information in Old World primates is the negative correlation found between the size of an area of the brain central to relaying visual information (the lateral geniculate nucleus) and that which relays chemosensory information (the olfactory bulb; Barton 1998).

These important anatomical changes in the evolutionary remodelling of the mammalian brain have been crucial to the reorganisation of reproductive strategies. In addition to the pseudogenization of vomeronasal and olfactory receptor genes, the downregulation of gonadal and placental hormones in determining sexual and maternal care has given way to an upregulation in social determinants of behaviour. Castrated male primates continue to show a sexual interest in females years after gonadectomy (Michael and Wilson 1973) but lose sexual interest within days of losing dominance and social status (Keverne 1992). Reproductive strategies are therefore very complex and embedded in social learning and the social structure of the group in which primates live. Moreover, delaying the onset of puberty and extending the period of postnatal care have enabled extensive growth and enlargement of the neocortex. In Old World female primates, unlike small-brained rodents, sexual behaviour is not restricted to a few hours determined by oestrus; neither do females require the hormones of pregnancy to become maternal. Hence, female sexual activity is not primarily reproductive since most occurs outside the fertile ovulatory period. Moreover, in the context of maternalism, non-pregnant females play an important role in infant care, which extends way beyond the infant's weaning period. Parenting and alloparenting are lifetime occupations for social living primates, an evolutionary development that has produced a profound impact on the brain.

Social Complexity, Neuropeptides and Brain Reward

Primates differ from other mammals in the complexity of their social interactions, and unlike other mammals, these interactions are not restricted to periods of prime biological significance, such as parturition and mating. Across primate taxa there are many different mating systems and affiliations, but it is the Old World monkey societies that are notably recognised for the complexity of their social organisation (Dunbar 1992). Throughout primate evolution there has been a general trend of increasing brain size relative to body size, driven largely by the requirement to process this increasingly complex social information (Dunbar 1998). For instance, baboons have both the largest relative neocortex size of any Old World primate species and the largest group size. This brain expansion has not been isometric but shows that different brain regions have evolved at different rates. In particular, the primate visual cortex has become especially enlarged, comprising up to 50% of total neocortex (Van Essen et al. 1992). It has also become increasingly complex, with several areas devoted to the differential processing of visual information such as facial expression (Perrett et al. 1992), including the evolution of some areas such as the middle temporal visual area that are non-homologous to cortical areas in other small-brained mammals (Ghazanfar and Santos 2004). The importance of vision in regulating primate social behaviour is evident from studies of feral primates, where the majority of primate social time is devoted simply to monitoring other individuals, whereas primate social group size correlates with increases in the number of neurons relaying visual information to the cortex (lateral geniculate nucleus; Barton 1998). Among the highly social Old World monkeys, it is females, rather than males, who form stable cohesive groups that are maintained over successive generations, with social rank of daughter, but not sons, being inherited from mothers (Wrangham 1980; Bergman et al. 2003). This finding is particularly well illustrated from extensive records of a 16-year study of baboons, where those females that are more social (those who are groomed more frequently by others) have higher infant survival and reproductive success (Silk et al. 2003). Such social behaviour is linked to the biology of reward, since grooming stimulates the release of beta-endorphins in the monkey brain. This peptide is released in small-brained mammals during sex and parturition acting as a rewarding enforcer of behaviour, but in primates, this peptide has acquired the distinctive function of rewarding social encounters, thereby forming the "social glue" of these complex societies (Keverne et al. 1989). Indeed, the number of grooming relationships is one of the most powerful predictors of neocortex size in primates (Kudo and Dunbar 2001). Social behaviour has thus had a powerful impact on the evolutionary expansion of those cortical areas of the brain concerned with decision taking and reward, which is not surprising since many of these decisions are related to social reward.

In order for social reward to have gained such power in cortical expansion, it has been necessary for maternal care in particular to become emancipated from hormonal determinants. Indeed, unlike small brain rodents, maternal behaviour in monkeys is no longer closely tied into physiological homeostasis and the strong dependence on hormones. Post-partum rodents return to oestrous within 72 hours after removing their pups whereas female baboons have been seen to continue carrying and grooming their dead offspring for months after death. Moreover, older sisters and maternal relatives participate in offspring care without having undertaken pregnancy and parturition. Mothers themselves are thus not required to delay their next pregnancy until their offspring are fully mature in brain development. Hence the advantage of the extended family network seen in Old World primates. Expansion of the neocortex releases maternal care from the restrictive confines of hormonal determinants, which benefits infant survival by further enabling non-parturient females to participate in offspring care and at the same time gain experience in mothering under the watchful eye of the matriarch.

Opioids and Primate Infant Attachment

The early development (first 10 weeks) of social behaviour in monkeys occurs primarily in the context of interactions with the mother. These early social interactions are almost totally under the mother's control, in terms of both the amount and kinds of interaction permitted with others in the group. By 40 weeks of age, infants are considerably more independent from their mother, and much of their behaviour is oriented towards peers. Nevertheless, mothers continue to monitor their infants and quickly intervene in response to risks arising during play (Simpson et al. 1989). The mother and her matriarch serve as a secure base from which the infant can obtain contact and grooming while developing and strengthening its social bonds with peers and other kin.

Administration of opioids has been shown to reduce the distress shown by infants of various species when separated from their mothers (Panksepp et al. 1997). For example, the opiate agonist morphine reduces distress vocalization rates in chicks, puppies, and rhesus monkeys. Processes involving opioid brain reward may therefore play a role in infant attachment, but to what extent is this the same mechanism that is deployed in development of social behaviour as well as in maternal bonding? This question has been investigated in a study of young rhesus monkeys given acute treatment with the opioid receptor blocker, naloxone, and observed in their natal group (Martel et al. 1995). Naloxone increases the duration of affiliative infant-mother contact and the amount of time the infants spend on the nipple. These effects occur even at one year of age, when the mothers are no longer lactating. Indeed, feeding is unaffected by naloxone treatment of infants, but play activity decreases and their distress vocalizations increase. Moreover, the opioid system in both infant and mother coordinates intimate contact during reunion (Kalin et al. 1995). These findings may be interpreted in terms of opiate receptor blockade reducing the "positive affect" that has accrued from the attachment relationship with mother and, as a result of which, the young infant returns to mother as the established secure base.

Opioids and Maternal Bonding

In addition to increasing OT synthesis in the brain, the hormones of pregnancy induce pro-opiomelanocortin synthesis, the precursor of the endogenous opioid, β-endorphin. It has been suggested that the activation of the endogenous opioid system at parturition and during suckling promotes the positive affect arising from maternal behaviour. In the early postpartum period, a mother's social interactions are almost exclusively with her infant, and opiate receptor blockade in the mother has marked effects on this relationship.

Studies on naloxone treatment of postpartum rhesus monkey mothers living in social groups have addressed the importance of opioids in maternal bonding. Naloxone treatment reduces the mothers' caregiving and protective behaviour shown towards their infants. In the first weeks of life, when infant retrieval is normally very high, naloxone-treated mothers neglect their infants and show little retrieval even when the infant moves a distance away. As the infants approach eight weeks of age, when a strong grooming relationship normally develops between mother and infant, mothers treated with naloxone fail to develop such a grooming relationship. Moreover, these mothers permit other females to groom their infants, whereas saline-treated controls are very possessive and protective of their infants (Martel et al. 1993).

The infant is not rejected from suckling, but the naloxone-treated mother's possessive preoccupation with the infant declines. She is not the normal attentive caregiver, and mother-infant interactions are invariably initiated by the infant. It is clear, therefore, that primates and other mammals have in common the involvement of endogenous opioids in maternal care, but the consequences of opioid blockade in small-brained mammals are much greater for the biological aspects of maternal behaviour. In rodents and sheep, interference with the endogenous opioid system severely impairs maternal behaviour, including suckling, whereas monkeys neglect their infant's social bonding but still permit suckling. These differences may reflect the degree of emancipation from endocrine determinants that maternal behaviour has undergone in Old World primates, and the importance of social reward activating the "bonding" mechanism.

Infant primates, both human and non-human, are highly susceptible to social perturbations in maternal care. The infant's developing brain requires social stimulation from a mother committed to providing the emotional rewards of suckling, huddling and grooming. It is clear that the process of infant socialization benefits from this close relationship and, because this occurs during early brain development, mother-infant separations are likely to have long-term consequences (Hinde et al. 1978). Indeed, in adults, extreme consequences for subsequent social relationships and maternal bonding occur if as infants they have been separated from their mothers and reared with peers (Suomi and Harlow 1975; Kraemer et al. 1991). Nursery-reared rhesus monkeys deprived of a maternal upbringing demonstrate reduced OT secretion and social behaviour but show increased aggressive and stereotypical behaviours. Increased stereotypical behaviours are often classically associated with the disruption of frontal cortical function and often result from an inability to suppress inappropriate behavioural responses (Winslow et al. 2003). Four years after experiencing separations from their mothers early during development, squirrel monkeys generate differences in emotional behaviour, stress physiology and development of the brain, notably in the medial prefrontal cortex (mPFC). Behavioural tests have subsequently shown these monkeys to be impaired in reward-related memory tasks (Lyons and Schatzberg 2003). Electrophysiological recordings from normal adult monkeys have shown the mPFC mediates the achievement of goals (Matsumoto and Tanaka 2004). The precise involvement of the prefrontal cortex in reward-related behaviour has also been examined in humans using imaging techniques (Fig. 3). Interestingly, the detection of unfavourable outcomes, response conflict and decision uncertainty elicit overlapping clusters of activation foci in the mPFC (Ridderinkhof et al. 2004). Choosing between actions associated with uncertain rewards and punishments in humans is mediated by neural circuitry involving frontal cortex, anterior cingulated and striatum (Rogers et al.

2004). Showing alternating videos of the own child versus that of a stranger to mothers provoked the greatest signal contrasts in the mPFC and orbito-frontal cortex. These distinctions required face recognition and emotional processing which correlated with activation in the visual cortex, temporal pole and amygdala (Ranote et al. 2004).

Discussion

The proximate determinants of mammalian social behaviour have their evolutionary origins in the mechanisms that subserve maternal care. Variations on this theme are exemplified across small-brained mammals, where the most important selective social bonds are seen between mother and offspring and between partners that mate. A great deal of attention has been given to "bonding" in the monogamous prairie vole, which has provided a tendency to focus on the peptides OT and vasopressin and the expression of their receptor genes as being evolutionarily conserved for "bonding." This mechanistic focus has been very important and influential but has not taken account of the broader aspects of biology that apply to small-brained mammals in general and parental care in particular. A comparison of mammalian maternal care and monogamous bonding reveals three common components of the biology that are

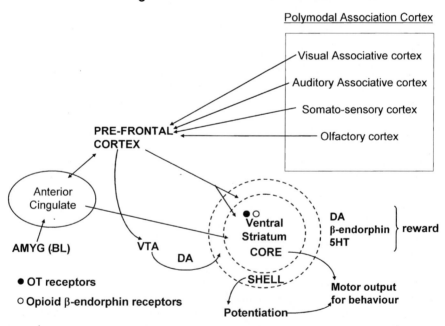

Fig. 3. The pre-frontal cortex dominates activation of the ventral striatum, processing a complexity of association cortical inputs in determining reward for motor output. Projections via the amygdala and anterior cingulate also provide pre-frontal cortex (medial pre-frontal) with emotional context

important: 1) hormonal priming by the foetal placenta for maternal care, cf. hormonal priming for oestrus by male pheromones in the vole; 2) vaginal-cervical stimulation at parturition, cf. vaginal-cervical stimulation at mating in the vole; and 3) olfactory recognition of offspring, cf. olfactory recognition of mating partner in the monogamous vole. Both maternal bonding and sexual bonding involve oxytocin in the female, a nine amino acid peptide that takes its evolutionary origins from vasotocin, which is also nine amino acids long. By the substitution of one amino acid, vasotocin has produced vasopressin, which in the male vole is required for "bonding," whereas the brain receptor distribution for both peptides has a focus on the nucleus accumbens and ventral pallidum. These neural structures form an integral part of the brain's social reward circuitry, which in small-brained mammals receives a primary input from olfactory circuitry.

Olfactory recognition is integral to sexual bonding in the monogamous prairie vole and integral to offspring recognition and maternal care in rodents as well as selective bonding in ungulates. Indeed, the selectivity of bonding through olfaction is extremely robust in ungulates, which forcibly reject all infants but their own with which they have bonded. The sexual bonding described for prairie voles is more akin to partner preference, since both males and females will and do mate with others given the opportunity. Monogamous pair bonding is also very rare among mammals (<5%), whereas maternal bonding applies to all mammals and, at a mechanistic level, probably formed the foundations from which all other social and bonded relationships, including monogamy, evolved.

Mammalian brain evolution recapitulated the reciprocal interplay between social bonding and maternal bonding. Evolutionary biologists hypothesise that increases in primate brain size have been driven by the selection pressures arising from living in social groups. Social living required an ability to predict how an individual's behaviour will impact differentially on other members of the group according to social status and how others, in turn, will react to this behaviour. However, since social cohesion and group continuity occurs through the matriline, field biologists often refer to the social group as being female bonded. To evolve brains as large as those seen in Old World primates and hominids, most of brain development has needed to be postponed to the post-natal period to facilitate the birth process. Such extensive periods of brain growth and maturation have required alloparental as well as maternal care, which has in turn required a degree of emancipation from the requirement for pregnancy hormones to determine maternal care. Maternal kin, including older sisters and aunts, can participate in offspring care and protection, thereby enhancing their own maternal skills, while the infant's brain is growing and maturing in a social environment, exposure to which will "imprint" important social skills. Equally important is provision of an attachment figure, primarily mother, which provides a secure base from which infants explore and develop other social relationships.

Understanding brain evolution is crucial to the realisation of what hormonal studies on small-brained mammals can and cannot inform us about primate, including hominid, brain and social behaviour. We already know from studies of animals with small brains that epigenetic processes are activated by the social environment. High levels of prosocial mothering (licking and grooming) produce offspring that also display the same prosocial behaviour, even if these offspring have been cross-fostered from a strain of mothers differing in a genetic background that produces low levels of these behaviours. Extending primate brain development and maturation into an equally extensive post-natal social environment has introduced an additional period for such epigenetic modifications in determining the social functioning of the adult brain. Those epigenetic mechanisms that are activated by hormones, as part of physiological homeostasis, and shape the in-utero and early post-natal development of the brain, are but a first stage that is important to all mammals. The second stage, namely extensive post-natal development, is especially important to large- brained mammals, ensuring that the brain is exposed to a social environment that equips it to function well during a lifetime of social interactions.

References

Amico J, Mantella R, Vollmer R, Li X (2004) Anxiety and stress responses in female oxytocin deficient mice. J Neuroendocrinol 16:319–324

Barton R (1998) Visual specialization and brain evolution in primates. Proc Biol Sci 265:1933–1937

Bergman T, Beehner J, Cheney D, Seyfarth R (2003) Hierarchical classification by rank and kinship in baboons. Science 302:1234–1236

Brennan P (2001) The vomeronasal system. Cell Mol Life Sci 58:546–555

Brennan P, Keverne EB (2004) Something in the air? New insights into mammalian pheromones. Curr Biol 14:R81–R89

Broad KD, Levy F, Evans F, Kimura T, Keverne EB, Kendrick KM (1999) Previous maternal experience potentiates the effects of parturition on oxytocin receptor mRNA expression in the paraventricular nucleus. Eur J Neurosci 11:3725–3737

Broad KD, Curley JP, Keverne EB (2006) Mother-infant bonding and the evolution of mammalian social relationships. Phil Trans Roy Soc B 361:2199–2214

Choleris E, Gustafsson J, Korach K, Muglia L, Pfaff D, Ogawa S (2003) An estrogen-dependent four-gene micronet regulating social recognition: a study with oxytocin and estrogen receptor-α and -β knockout mice. Proc Natl Acad Sci USA 100:6192–6197

Del Punta K, Leinders-Zufall T, Rodriquez I, Jukam D, Wysocki, CJ, Ogawa S, Zufall F, Mombaerts P (2002) Deficient pheromone responses in mice lacking a cluster of vomeronasal receptor genes. Nature 419:70–74

Dluzen D, Muraoka S, Engelmann N, Ebner K, Langraf R (2000) Oxytocin induces preservation of social recognition in male rats by activating α-adrenoceptors of the olfactory bulb. Eur J Neuroci 12:760–766

Dulac C, Axel R (1995) A novel family of genes encoding putative pheromone receptors in mammals. Cell 83:195–206

Dunbar RIM (1992) Neocortex size as a constraint on group six in primates. J Human Evol 20:469–493

Dunbar RIM (1998) Primate social systems. Chapman and Hall, London

Ferguson JN, Young, LJ, Hearn EF, Matzuk MM, Insel TR, Winslow JT (2000) Social amnesia in mice lacking the oxytocin gene. Nat Genet 25:284–288

Ferguson J, Aldag J, Insel T, Young L (2001) Oxytocin in the medial amygdala is essential for social recognition in the mouse. J Neuroci 21:8278–8285

Ghazanfar A, Santos L (2004) Primate brains in the wild: the sensory bases for social interactions. Nat Rev Neurosci 5:603–616

Gilad Y, Man P, Paabo S, Lancet D (2003) Human specific loss of olfactory receptor genes. Proc Natl Acad Sci USA 100:3324–3327

Gilad Y, Wiebe V, Przeworski M, Lancet D, Paabo S (2004) Loss of olfactory receptor genes coincides with the acquisition of full trichromaic vision in primates. PLoS Biol 2:E5

Herrada V, Dulac C (1997) A novel family of putative pheromone receptors in mammals with a topographically organized sexually dimorphic distribution. Cell 90:763–773

Hinde RA, Leighton-Shapiro ME, McGinnis L (1978) Effects of various types of separation experience on rhesus monkeys 5 months later. J Child Psychol Psychiat 19:199–211

Kalin NH, Sheldon SE, Lynn DE (1995) Opiate systems in mother and infant primates coordinate intimate contact during reunion. Psychoneuroendocrinology 7:735–742

Keverne EB (1992) Primate social relationships: Their determinants and consequences. In: Slater PJB, Rosenblatt JS, Beer C, Milinski M (eds) Advances in the study of behaviour. Academic Press, San Diego, pp 1–37

Keverne EB (1999) The vomeronasal organ. Science 286:716–720

Keverne EB (2002) Pheromones, vomeronasal function, and gender-specific behaviour. Cell 108:735–738

Keverne EB (2006) Trophoblast regulation of maternal endocrine function and behaviour. In: Moffett A, Loke C, McLaren A (eds) Biology and pathology of trophoblast. Cambridge University Press, Cambridge, pp 368–411

Keverne EB, Kendrick KM (1992) Oxytocin facilitation of maternal behavior. Ann NY Acad Sci 652:83–101

Keverne EB, Martenz ND, Tuite B (1989) β-endorphin levels in the cerebrospinal fluid of monkeys influenced by grooming relationships. Psychoneuroendocrinology 14:155–161

Kimchi T, Xu J, Dulac C (2007) A functional circuit underlying male sexual behaviour in the female mouse brain. Nature 448:1009–1014

Kippin T, Cain S, Pfaus J (2003) Estrous odors and sexually conditioned neutral odors activate separate neural pathways in the male rat. Neuroscience 117:971–979

Kleiman D (1977) Monogamy in mammals. Q Rev Biol 52:39–69

Kraemer GW, Ebert MH, Schmidt DE, McKinnery WT (1991) Strangers in a strange land: a psychobiological study of infant monkeys before and after separation from real or inanimater mothers. Child Dev 62:548–566

Kudo H, Dunbar R (2001) Neocortex size and social network size in primates. Anim Behav 62:711–722

Liberles SD, Buck LB (2006) A second class of chemosensory receptors in the olfactory epithelium. Nature 442:645–650

Lim MM, Young LJ (2004) Vasopressin-dependent neural circuits underlying pair bond formation in the monogamous prairie vole. Neuroscience 125:35–45

Lim M, Murphy A, Young L (2004a) Ventral striatopallidal oxytocin and vasopressin V1a receptors in the monogamous prairie vole (Microtus ochragaster). J Comp Neurol 468:555–570

Lim MM, Wang Z, Olazabal DE, Ren X, Terwilliger EF, Young LJ (2004b) Enhanced partner preference in a promiscuous species by manipulating the expression of a single gene. Nature 429:754–757

Liman ER, Innan H (2003) Relaxed selective pressure on an essential component of pheromone transduction in primate evolution. Proc Natl Acad Sci USA 100:3328–3332

Liu Y, Wang Z (2003) Nucleus accumbens oxytocin and dopamine interact to regulate pair bond formation in female prairie voles. Neuroscience 121:537–544

Lyons DM, Schatzberg AF (2003) Early maternal availability and prefrontal correlates of reward-related memory. Neurobiol Learn Mem 80:97–104

Martel FL, Nevison CM, Rayment FD, Simpson MJ, Keverne EB (1993) Opioid receptor blockade reduces maternal affect and social grooming in rhesus monkeys. Psychoneuroendocrinology 18:307–321

Martel FL, Nevison CM, Simpson MDA, Keverne EB (1995) Effects of opioid receptor blockade on the social behaviour of rhesus monkeys living in large family groups. Dev Psychobiol 28:71–84

Matsumoto K, Tanaka K (2004) The role of the medial prefrontal cortex in achieving goals. Curr Opin Neurobiol 14:178–185

Michael RP, Wilson MI (1973) Effects of castration and hormone replacement in fully adult male rhesus monkeys. Endocrinology (Baltimore) 95:150–159

Mitra S, Hoskin E, Yudkovitz J, Pear L, Wilkinson J, Hayuashi S, Pfaff D, Ogawa S, Rohrer S, Schaeffer J et al. (2003) Immunolocalization of estrogen receptor β in the mouse brain: comparison with estrogen receptor. Endocrinology 144:2055–2067

Osaka Y, Otrsuka T, Taniguchi M, Oka T, Kaba H (2001) Oxytocin enhances presynaptic and post-synaptic glutamergic transmission between rat olfactory bulb neurones in culture. Neurosci Lett 299:65–68

Panksepp J, Nelson E Bekkedal M (1997) Brain systems for the mediation of social separation-distress and social reward. Ann NY Acad Sci 807:78–100

Perrett D, Hietanen J, Oram N, Benson P (1992) Organization and functions of cells responsive to faces in the temporal cortex. Philos Trans R Soc Lond B Biol Sci 335:23–30

Pfaus J, Heeb M (1997) Implications of immediate-early gene induction in the brain following sexual stimulation of female and male rodents. Brain Res Bull 44:397–407

Ranote S, Elliott R, Abel, KM, Mitchell R, Deakin JF, Appleby L (2004) The neural basis of maternal responsiveness to infants: an fMRI study. NeuroReport 15:1825–1829

Ridderinkhof KR, van den Wildenbert WP, Segalowitz SJ, Carter CS (2004) Neurocognitive mechanisms of cognitive control: the role of prefrontal cortex in action selection, response inhibition, performance monitoring, and reward-based learning. Brain Cogn 56:129–140

Rogers RD, Ramnani N, Mackay C, Wilson, JL, Jezzard, P, Carter CS, Smith SM (2004) Distinct portions of anterior cingulated cortex and medial prefrontal cortex are activated by reward processing separable phases of decision-making cognition. Biol Psychiat 55:594–602

Silk J, Alberts S, Altmann J (2003) Social bonds of female baboons enhance infant survival. Science 302:1231–1234

Simpson MJA, Gore MA, Janus M, Rayment FD (1989) Prior experience of risk and individual differences in enterprise shown by rhesus monkey infants in the second half of their first year. Primates 30:493–509

Stephan H, Baron G, Frahm HD (1982) Comparison of brain structure volumes in insectivores and primates. II. Accessory olfactory bulb (AOB). J Hirnforsch 23:575–591

Stowers L, Holy TE, Markus M, Dulac C, Koentges G (2002) Electrophysiological characterization of chemosensory neurons from the mouse vomeronasal organ. J Neurosci 16:4625–4637

Suomi SJ, Harlow HF (1975) Effects of differential removal from group on social development of rhesus monkeys. J Child Psychol Psychiat 16:149–164

Surridge A, Mundy N (2002) Trans-specific evolution of opsin alleles and the maintenance of trichromatic colour vision in Callitrichine primates. Mol Ecol 11:2157–2169

Surridge A, Osorio D, Mundy NI (2003) Evolution and selection of trichromatic vision in primates. Trends Ecol Evol 18:198–205

Van Essen D, Anderson C, Felleman D (1992) Information processing in the primate visual system: an integrated systems perspective. Science 255:419–423

Webb D, Cortes-Ortiz L, Zhang J (2004) Genetic evidence for the coexistence of pheromone perception and full trichromatic vision in howler monkey. Mol Biol Evol 21:697–704

Whinnett A, Mundy N (2003) Isolation of novel olfactory receptor genes in marmosets (Callithrix): Insights into pseudogene formation and evidence of functional degeneracy in non-human primates. Gene 304:87–96

Williams J, Catania K, Carter C (1992) Development of partner preferences in female prairie voles (Microtus ochrogaster): the role of social and sexual experience. Horm Behav 117:339–349

Williams J, Insel T, Harbaugh C, Carter C (1994) Oxytocin centrally administered facilitates formation of a partner preference in female prairie voles (Microtus ochragaster). J Neuroendocrinol 6:247–250

Winslow J, Hearn E, Ferguson J, Young L, Matzuk M, Insel T (2000) Infant vocalization, adult aggression, and fear behaviour of an oxytocin null mutant mouse. Horm Behav 37:145–155

Winslow JT, Noble PL, Lyons CK, Sterk SM, Insel TR (2003) Rearing effects of cerebrospinal fluid oxytocin concentration and social buffering in rhesus monkeys. Neuropsychopharmacology 28:910–918
Wrangham R (1980) An ecological model of female-bonded primate groups. Behaviour 75:262–300
Young L, Wang Z, Donaldson R, Rissman E (1998) Estrogen receptor α is essential for induction of oxytocin receptor by estrogen. NeuroReport 9:933–936
Zhang X, Firestein S (2002) The olfactory receptor gene superfamily of the mouse. Nat Neurosci 5:124–133
Zhang J, Webb D (2003) Evolutionary deterioration of the vomeronasal pheromone transduction pathway in catarrhine primates. Proc Natl Acad Sci USA 100:8337–8341

Brain Oxytocin Mediates Beneficial Consequences of Close Social Interactions: From Maternal Love and Sex

Inga D. Neumann[1]

Summary

There is growing interest directed toward understanding positive emotions, and maternal and romantic love are among the most desired and positive social experiences encountered. It is only now that we are beginning to understand not only their neurobiological and neurochemical regulation but also their beneficial health consequences. For example, around parturition, profound adaptations of the maternal brain take place with significant behavioural consequences that ensure the healthy development of the child, or the offspring, including nutrition, protection and maternal emotional care. There is an activation of several neuroendocrine systems, including oxytocin and prolactin, that play important roles as classical hormones in the regulation of parturition, lactogenesis and milk ejection, respectively. Importantly, as signalling molecules of the brain, they were shown to be important promoters of maternal behaviour. Moreover, oxytocin released within the rat brain is correlated with the protection of the offspring, i.e., with the display of maternal aggression. Thus, oxytocin and prolactin are important for meeting the physiological demands of the offspring, but also to satisfy their emotional demands, including protection and close affiliation with the mother. In turn, the maternal brain profits from these adaptations: oxytocin and prolactin exert anxiolytic effects at various brain sites and have been shown to reduce stress responsiveness at neuronal, neuroendocrine and behavioural levels. As a consequence, increased calmness, reduced anxiety levels and blunted hypothalamo-pituitary-adrenal axis and sympathetic responses to numerous stressors have been described in pregnancy and/or lactation, both in human and animal studies. These complex brain adaptations are clearly beneficial for the mother. However, they are vulnerable to stressful life experiences and maladaptations, e.g., lack of adaptive activation of the brain oxytocin and prolactin systems may result in postpartum mood disorders with negative consequences for both maternal health and child development.

Is there a comparable physiological and behavioural situation in males? There is scientific and anecdotal evidence for sedation and calmness after sexual activity. Oxytocin is released within the hypothalamus during mating, where it is crucially involved in the regulation of male sexual behaviour. Evidence will be provided that activation of brain oxytocin, as seen during sexual activity, also mediates beneficial effects in males.

[1] Department of Behavioural and Molecular Neuroendocrinology, University of Regensburg, Germany, e-mail: inga.neumann@biologie.uni-regensburg.de

Pfaff et al.
Hormones and Social Behavior
© Springer-Verlag Berlin Heidelberg 2008

Introduction

For many decades, neurobiologists have focussed on uncovering the neurochemical brain circuitries underlying emotions, in particular of anxiety, fear and aggression. However, there has also been growing interest in understanding positive emotions. In this context, maternal and romantic love are among the most desired and positive experiences encountered in our lives, and we are beginning to understand not only their neurobiological and neurochemical regulation, but also their beneficial health consequences. In this chapter, I will focus on brain neuropeptide systems, in particular on brain oxytocin (OXT) and prolactin (PRL), which are activated, for example, in the maternal brain peripartum and which may mediate the positive effects on various health parameters, including reduced stress vulnerability. Additionally, I will provide initial evidence that, in males, sexual activity and mating represent comparable physiological stimuli activating these neuropeptide circuitries that, in turn, exert long-lasting beneficial effects.

Complex Adaptations of the Maternal Brain Peripartum

Remarkable physiological and behavioural changes have been extensively described in the mammalian maternal brain in the peripartum period. These profound adaptations start during pregnancy as complex and direct consequences of mainly hormonal signals arising from the fetus. They continue around birth and in lactation as a result of close social interactions between mother and offspring, for example during suckling, maternal care and protection. Pup-derived stimuli, for example during the suckling stimulus, in turn, are essential for these neuroendocrine and complex emotional adaptations to continue in the mother until weaning. Several of these maternal physiological adaptations are a primary prerequisite for offspring survival and development, i.e. the provision of sufficient nutrients both in utero and during lactation, and of a stable hormonal and biochemical environment during pregnancy, and a safe birth.

Tellingly however, profound alterations in systems that are not directly linked to reproductive functions, but that may play a supportive role, have also been described. For example, pregnancy- and lactation-associated alterations have been repeatedly demonstrated in several species with respect to maternal stress-coping style. There is a severely attenuated responsiveness of the hypothalamo-pituitary-adrenal (HPA) axis to a broad variety of stressors, with the consequence of lower stress-induced plasma concentrations of glucocorticoids, i.e., cortisol in humans and corticosterone in rodents (de Weerth and Buitelaar 2005; Kammerer et al. 2002; Lightman et al. 2001; Neumann et al. 1998c; Russell et al. 1999; Stattery and Neumann 2007; Stern et al. 1973). Such alterations seem to be essential for the healthy development of the offspring to prevent excessive circulating stress hormone levels, which have been shown to have adverse effects on prenatal development (Weinstock 2001; Welberg and Seckl 2001). Moreover, there is a growing body of evidence suggesting that mechanisms underlying the attenuated stress responses are also important for the mental health of the mother. In this context, several neurobiological mechanisms have been discussed, including the activation of the brain OXT and PRL systems (Fig. 1).

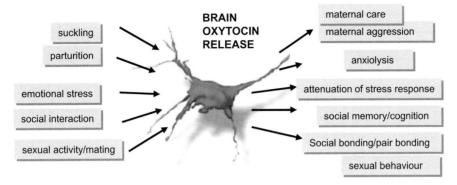

Fig. 1. Stimuli that trigger the release of oxytocin (OXT) within the brain, e.g., within the hypothalamic paraventricular nucleus, include suckling and parturition in females and emotional stress, social interactions and mating also in males. On the right side, consequences of oxytocin actions within the brain in a behavioural context are listed

Activation of Brain OXT and PRL Systems Around Birth

In the context of peripartum adaptations of stress systems, two brain neuropeptides are likely to play a prominent role: OXT and PRL. Whereas the existence of a brain OXT system is well established, there is emerging evidence for a brain PRL system with PRL synthesis in hypothalamic neurons, specifically within the hypothalamic paraventricular nucleus (PVN), and an abundant presence of PRL receptors throughout the brain. As neurohormones, both OXT and PRL are directly related to reproductive functions and become activated before birth, i.e., there is increased hormone storage in the neurohypophysis and in the lactotrophe cell of the adenohypophysis, respectively. When released into the blood stream, they are importantly involved in the delivery process (OXT), lactogenesis (PRL) and milk ejection (OXT).

Importantly, there is also activation of the OXT and PRL systems within the brain in the peripartum period, as witnessed by an increased OXT and PRL gene expression and synthesis within distinct brain regions and an increased expression and binding of their respective receptors. Moreover, OXT is released within the hypothalamic PVN and supraoptic nucleus (SON) and the olfactory bulb during parturition (Kendrick et al. 1988a; Neumann et al. 1993b) and also within the hippocampus and the medio-lateral septum in response to the suckling stimulus (Moos et al. 1984; Neumann et al. 1993b; Neumann and Landgraf 1989; Fig. 1). Recently, using the rather old-fashioned, but more sensitive, push-pull perfusion technique, we have shown that close social contact with the pups and the suckling stimulus also triggers neuronal release of PRL within the PVN (Torner et al. 2004).

Functions of Locally Released OXT and PRL in the Maternal Brain

Several functions of brain OXT have been suggested in a physiological or behavioural context (summarized in Fig. 1). For example, it has been postulated that locally released

OXT within the hypothalamus is involved in the auto-regulation of OXT neuronal activity during the phase of pulsatile release patterns into blood, as seen during the milk ejection reflex or during birth (Kombian et al. 1997; Moos et al. 1984; Neumann et al. 1994, 1996). Moreover, brain OXT seems to play a major role in the neuronal plasticity observed within the hypothalamic SON in the peripartum period (Theodosis 2002). Importantly, various changes in social behaviour have also been attributed to the action of brain OXT in the context of reproductive behaviour. For example, the onset and fine-tuned maintenance of maternal behaviour has been directly linked to the action of OXT (Lonstein and Morrell 2006; Numan and Insel 2003; Pedersen and Boccia 2003; Pedersen and Prange 1979). Moreover, there is compelling evidence of changes in social cognitive functions, including offspring recognition, which have been related to the action of locally released OXT (Dluzen et al. 2000; Kendrick et al. 1988b, 1987, 1997; see below). Therefore, these multiple effects of local OXT provide an excellent example of the synergistic action of a neuropeptide in dependence on the site of release.

Although far less is known about the functions of brain PRL, there is good evidence of a significant involvement of PRL in the regulation of maternal behaviour (Bridges et al. 1984, 1990; Torner et al. 2002). Thus, as seen for OXT, there are also synergistic actions of PRL secreted from lactotroph cells into the bloodstream to promote lactogenesis and of PRL released within distinct brain regions to regulate a respective behavioural profile of the mother. In general, maternal behaviour is regulated in a complex manner, with many neuronal circuits and neurotransmitter systems involved (for review see Lonstein and Morrell 2006; Numan and Insel 2003), and centrally released OXT and PRL seem to be key players in these neuronal systems. Interestingly, breast-feeding women interact more positively with their babies, directing more touching and smiling toward their infants, than do bottle-feeding mothers (Dunn and Richards 1977; for review, see Carter et al. 2001). Therefore, it is likely that the suckling-induced, site-specific release of OXT and PRL contributes to this behavioural effect. As the quality of maternal care is a key component for the healthy emotional development of the offspring, as seen in rodents, primates and also in humans, the central actions of maternal OXT and PRL have far-reaching implications for the future health of the baby and its social competence, as well as the competence of future generations (Francis et al. 1999; Liu et al. 2000).

Brain OXT and Maternal Aggression

Protection of the offspring and enhanced aggressive behaviour toward potential conspecific encounters are features of the complex pattern of maternal behaviour in mammals (Erskine et al. 1978; for review, see Numan and Insel 2003), and there is strong evidence demonstrating a contribution of brain OXT in the display of maternal aggression (Consiglio and Lucion 1996; Elliott et al. 2001; Lubin et al. 2003). Recently, we demonstrated increased OXT release within the central amygdala and within the hypothalamic PVN in rat dams showing a high level of maternal aggression towards a virgin intruder. In both of these regions of the limbic system, local OXT release was found to be directly correlated with the intensity of aggressive behaviour (Bosch et al. 2005). Furthermore, if local OXT actions were blocked by local administration of the selective receptor antagonist, highly aggressive rats showed a reduced number of attacks. In contrast, when synthetic OXT was slowly infused into the PVN of low aggressive dams, they displayed more attacks and lateral threats toward the intruder. These results clearly show that, in the peripartum period, brain OXT mediates, at least in part, the behavioural response to potentially threatening social stimuli, like a conspecific rat placed into the dam's home cage. Thus, locally released OXT promotes the display of relevant aggressive behaviours necessary for the protection of the offspring. Intra-individual differences in the activation of the brain OXT system seem to determine the differences seen in these complex social behaviours.

In contrast to these findings providing robust evidence for OXT as an important regulator of maternal aggression, very little is known about OXT actions on male aggression (but see Winslow et al. 2000). However, OXT is importantly involved in various aspects of social behaviour in males as well (Crawley et al. 2007; Domes et al. 2007; Kirsch et al. 2005; Kosfeld et al. 2005; Winslow et al. 2000).

Beneficial Consequences of Being a Mother

The above-described adaptations of the maternal brain, including activation of the brain OXT and PRL system, are clearly directed towards and beneficial for the offspring, or for the baby, to ensure their survival and healthy development. According to our hypothesis, these adaptations should also be beneficial for the mother, and brain OXT and PRL are importantly involved. For example, lactating dams were reported to show a reduced level of anxiety and emotional stress response (Neumann et al. 2001; Walker et al. 1995; Windle et al. 1997a). The anxiolytic effect of lactation can even be seen in rat dams with a high innate level of anxiety-related behaviour; therefore, being a mother seems to be beneficial for these animals with respect to state anxiety (Neumann 2001). Similarly, in humans, nursing mothers are more likely to describe positive mood states, reduced anxiety levels and increased calmness (Heinrichs et al. 2001; for review, see Carter and Altemus 1997; Carter et al. 2001). It would be interesting to speculate to what extent these emotional adaptations and positive mood effects are prerequisites for mothers to manage the highly demanding multi-tasking of their lives while keeping a balanced and healthy mood.

The peripartum alterations in emotionality, which are dependent upon social stimuli from the offspring, are likely to be related to the changes seen in the neuronal and hormonal responsiveness of the HPA axis. A blunted response to a broad variety of psychological and physical stressors has been found in rats and mice at the end of pregnancy and in lactation (Brunton and Russell 2003; Douglas et al. 2003; Johnstone et al. 2000; Lightman et al. 2001; Neumann 2001; Neumann et al. 1998c; Shanks et al. 1999; Stern et al. 1973; Walker et al. 1995; Windle et al. 1997b). This blunted response is reflected by an attenuated rise in plasma corticotrophin (ACTH) and corticosterone following stressor exposure, despite the elevated plasma glucocorticoid levels found at this time under basal conditions (Neumann et al. 1998a; Russell et al. 2001). Similarly, in pregnant and lactating women, lower cortisol responses to various stressors (Amico et al. 1994; de Weerth and Buitelaar 2005), including treadmill exercise (Altemus et al. 1995), cold stress (Kammerer et al. 2002) and psychological stress (Heinrichs et al.

2001), have been described, indicating similar adaptive mechanisms in the human maternal brain.

Although there is experimental evidence that hypo-responsiveness of the HPA axis in pregnancy prevents excessive levels of circulating glucocorticoids and, thus, negative effects on the fetus in utero (Weinstock 2001; Welberg and Seckl 2001), the positive effects of these adaptations for the offspring are less clear in lactation. In contrast, there are indications for beneficial effects for the mother, which becomes evident if we discuss in more detail the neurobiological mechanisms involved in stress hypo-responsiveness peripartum.

Mechanisms of Blunted Stress Responses Peripartum

Several brain mechanisms contribute to the blunted emotional and neuroendocrine response seen peripartum, as studied in rodent models. These include, for example, a lower level of stress-induced neuronal activation within several forebrain and limbic brain regions (da Costa et al. 2001), which might reflect the process of perception of a given stressor. Moreover, there is a loss of excitatory inputs to the hypothalamic PVN, the main regulatory centre of the HPA axis, in pregnancy and during lactation. For example, the noradrenergic excitatory tone of the PVN is reduced, and there is a lower expression of noradrenergic alpha$_{1A}$-adrenoceptors in the parvo- and magnocellular PVN (Douglas et al. 2005; Toufexis et al. 1998). Also, the excitatory input of the HPA axis exerted by endogenous opioids is reduced at the end of pregnancy (Douglas et al. 1998; Kammerer et al. 2002; Kofman 2002) and is further reversed into a highly significant inhibition during parturition (Wigger et al. 1999). Further, endogenous opioid inhibition of the OXT system disappears at the time of birth and is not seen in virgins (Douglas et al. 1995), which may contribute to differences in regulating stress adaptations peripartum (Wigger and Neumann 2002).

As a consequence of (or in parallel to) these changes, the expression of corticotropin releasing factor (CRF) within the PVN is reduced both in pregnancy (da Costa et al. 2001; Douglas and Russell 1994; Johnstone et al. 2000) and in lactation (Lightman et al. 2001; Walker et al. 2001). Similarly, reduced CRF expression has been described in the central nucleus of the amygdala, a region important for regulating HPA axis activity and emotionality (Davis and Whalen 2001). Moreover, the pituitary sensitivity to CRF is diminished due to reduced CRF receptor binding at pituitary corticotrophs (Neumann et al. 1998b). A potential intracellular mechanism underlying the attenuated CRF system is via the immediate-early gene *nur77* (NGFI-B), which controls CRF gene expression under conditions of stress (Kirschbaum et al. 1999), but hypothalamic NGFI-B expression is lower in pregnancy (Douglas et al. 2003). A generally lowered activity of the CRF system may contribute to the attenuated ACTH and corticosterone responses observed during pregnancy and in lactation. Moreover, a low brain CRF system activity is likely to be related to the reduced anxiety of the dam (Hard and Hansen 1985; Neumann 2003; Toufexis et al. 1998; Windle et al. 1997b) and to the promotion of social behaviours, including maternal behaviour (Pedersen et al. 1991) and maternal aggression (Gammie et al. 2004). CRF has been shown to inhibit both maternal behaviour and aggression. For example, rhesus monkeys that abuse their infants were shown to have higher plasma levels of CRF (Maestripieri et al. 2005).

OXT and PRL Mediate the Beneficial Effects for the Mother

There is substantial evidence that peripartum activation of the brain OXT and PRL systems mediates the beneficial effects of these stress adaptations for the mother in concert with the factors described above. In general, an anxiolytic effect of OXT administered peripherally (McCarthy and Altemus 1997) or centrally (Bale et al. 2001; Ring et al. 2006) has been established. Also, chronic infusion of OXT in virgin rats results in an attenuation of the emotional, neuroendocrine and neuronal responses to an acute stressor (Windle et al. 1997a, 2004). Mice lacking the OXT gene show an increased emotional responsiveness (Amico et al. 2004). Central infusion of a selective OXT receptor antagonist before testing on the elevated plus-maze revealed an anxiolytic effect of endogenous brain OXT in both pregnant and lactating rats (Neumann et al. 2000a), an effect that could be localized within the central amygdala (Neumann 2002). These findings indicate that up-regulation of the activity of the brain OXT system at the end of pregnancy and throughout lactation mediates the lower level of emotionality, including reduced anxiety.

Brain PRL is another important anxiolytic regulator of the brain that, as described above, is up-regulated in the maternal brain. Both female and, to a lesser extent, male rats show a reduced anxiety-related behaviour on the elevated plus-maze following icv PRL treatment (Torner et al. 2001). Also, down-regulation of brain PRL receptors by use of antisense oligodesoxynucleotides directed against the short form of PRL receptors (see Torner and Neumann 2002 for review of the physiology of PRL receptors) in the brain of lactating rats resulted in elevated emotionality, indicating the involvement of brain PRL receptors in the anxiolytic effect (Torner et al. 2001).

In addition to the attenuation of emotional stress responses, both OXT and PRL show common actions in the reduction of hormonal and neuronal stress responses. Thus, chronic intracerebral infusion of OXT (Windle et al. 1997a, 2004) or PRL (Donner et al. 2007) reduced the stress-induced increase in neuronal activity in several brain regions, as revealed using c-fos as a marker, hypothalamic CRF mRNA expression, and hormonal stress responses in virgin rats. Inhibition of brain PRL receptor expression (see above) enhanced HPA axis stress responses in lactating dams.

Indirect evidence suggests that these results can be translated into humans. In lactating mothers, breast-feeding shortly before exposure to a psychological stressor reduced the emotional response and salivary cortisol levels compared with bottle-feeding lactating mothers. As mentioned above, both OXT and PRL are released in several brain regions, including the hypothalamic PVN, in response to the suckling stimulus (Moos et al. 1984; Neumann et al. 1993a; Torner et al. 2004). Therefore, it is likely that such locally released neuropeptides exert inhibitory effects on HPA axis reactivity and state anxiety, possibly via direct or indirect actions on CRF neurons. In conclusion, the high activity of the brain OXT and PRL systems contributes to the blunted stress vulnerability of the mother.

If these physiological adaptations are partially prevented, we believe that mood disorders like postpartum blues or depression are more likely to occur. The dramatic reproduction-related fluctuation in sexual steroid concentration around birth is likely to contribute to an increased vulnerability to mood disturbances and psychopathologies in susceptible individuals, depending on their genetic predisposition and stressful life events. Therefore, attenuation of complex stress circuitries by a high activation of brain OXT and PRL represents a necessary mechanism to protect the maternal brain. Interestingly, postpartum depression is associated (or goes hand in hand) with impaired maternal bonding and sometimes even rejection of the child and with impaired stress management, parameters that are mediated by OXT and PRL.

OXT Effects on Stress Coping in the Male Brain

In comparison to females, relatively little is known about brain OXT actions in males. However, in male rats and mice, comparable effects of OXT on HPA axis responsiveness (Neumann et al. 2000b) and anxiety (Blume et al. 2008; Ring et al. 2006) have been described (Fig. 1). For example, blocking central OXT receptors by infusion of an OXT receptor antagonist increased basal HPA axis activity and responses to swim stress, indicating an inhibitory influence of endogenous OXT also in males (Neumann et al. 2000b). As in females (Bosch et al. 2005; Wigger and Neumann 1998), OXT is released within several regions of the male brain, including the amygdala and the hypothalamic PVN, in response to social stimuli (Ebner et al. 2000; Wotjak et al. 1996) and various non-social stressors (Ebner et al. 2005; Hattori et al. 1992; Wotjak et al. 2001; for review, see Landgraf and Neumann 2004). In addition, locally released OXT regulates the behavioural and neuroendocrine stress response in the male rat (Ebner et al. 2005; Engelmann et al. 2004; Neumann et al. 2006). Furthermore, within the central amygdala, OXT released during stressor exposure promotes a passive stress-coping strategy (Ebner et al. 2005), and effects of OXT on local neuronal activity patterns were also described in males (Huber et al. 2005). Moreover, central manipulation of the OXT system by application of an antagonist or agonist revealed that OXT modulates wakefulness and sleep patterns: under basal, undisturbed conditions, OXT promotes sleep whereas at higher doses OXT delays sleep onset, indicating an acute arousal effect (Lancel et al. 2003). Taken together, these results provide substantial evidence that, also in male rats, brain OXT is significantly involved in the regulation of behavioural and hormonal stress responses.

In humans, intranasal OXT, which has been shown to cross the blood-brain barrier (Born et al. 2002), reduced neuronal responses within the amygdala to threatening, non-social cues and to fearful social stimulation, as revealed by magnetic resonance imaging studies (Kirsch et al. 2005). Thus, OXT seems to be an important modulator of processing social stimuli also in humans, which is further substantiated by the finding of a suppressed anxiety to psychosocial stress (Heinrichs et al. 2003) and of a substantial increase in social trust (Kosfeld et al. 2005) in subjects treated with intranasal OXT.

Positive Effects of Social Interactions in the Male: Involvement of OXT?

Given such effects of OXT in males and since they do not undergo birth or lactation as do females, is there a clearly defined physiological stimulation that triggers a high level of activity of the endogenous brain OXT system in males? In other words, under which physiological circumstances can males benefit from the positive effects of OXT on various aspects of stress coping?

Social support is the most intensively investigated social factor in humans, and there is a growing body of evidence that the intensity of social support is associated with positive effects on various stress-related diseases, including hypertension, cardio-vascular diseases, depression (House et al. 1988; Knox and Uvnas-Moberg 1998; Paykel 2001; Rozanski et al. 1999) and stroke outcome (DeVries et al. 2001). In particular, social support in humans can provide a buffer against stress-induced responses of the HPA axis in humans (for review, see DeVries et al. 2003; Kikusui et al. 2006). For example, the salivary free cortisol response of healthy young men to the Trier Social Stress Test, a psychosocial stressor, was reduced by social support provided by their best friend during the preparation period prior to stressor exposure (Heinrichs et al. 2003; Kirschbaum et al. 1995). Moreover, diseases that respond to cortisol concentrations, like asthma (Buske-Kirschbaum et al. 2003), heal better in socially supported patients.

In animals that show a distinct level of social bonding, like mice, rats, guinea pigs and marmosets, social support by conspecifics was demonstrated to lower plasma glucocorticoid levels, although this has mainly been studied in females (Gonzalez et al. 1982; Sachser et al. 1998; Smith and French 1997).

Furthermore, promoting social interactions of laboratory rodents by group housing lowers their plasma corticosterone concentrations (for review, see DeVries et al. 2007; Kikusui et al. 2006). On the other hand, social stress, an unstable social environment or a subordinate position in the hierarchy results in HPA axis hyper-activity, paralleled by adrenal insufficiency after prolonged stressor exposure (Reber et al. 2006), thymus-atrophy, an increase in pro-inflammatory cytokines, and in impaired recovery from injuries or diseases, such as wounds, stroke, and cardiac arrest (Reber et al. 2007; for review, see DeVries et al. 2007). Moreover, chronic social stress in male laboratory mice, mediated by subordinate colony housing, was shown to induce colonic inflammation and to increase the severity of a pharmacologically induced colitis in mice (Reber et al. 2007). Thus, depending on the circumstances, social factors can buffer the stress response or impair the healthy state of the individual.

Interestingly, effects of social buffering were directly found within the hypothalamic PVN. The stress-induced increase in the immediate early gene product Fos within the PVN was attenuated in rats that were accompanied by a partner rat (Kiyokawa et al. 2004). Similarly, in sheep, the visual presentation of pictures of sheep faces was sufficient to induce social buffering in terms of neuronal responses to stress within the PVN (da Costa et al. 2004). These findings give some indications to presume that social stimuli, either visual, tactile or olfactory, activate the brain OT system, which in turn attenuates stress responsiveness.

Activation of OXT in the Male Brain During Social Stimuli: Effects of Sexual Activity

Although limited, there is evidence of stimulation of the brain OXT system during social interaction in males. For example, OXT release within the septum is triggered in stressful social situations, i.e., defeat by a conspecific male (Ebner et al. 2000). Also, OXT secretion into blood is induced by massage and stroking (Uvnas-Moberg 1997). Moreover, the most intense social behaviour found in males, i.e., sexual behaviour and mating, is accompanied by increased OXT secretion into blood (Carmichael et al. 1987;

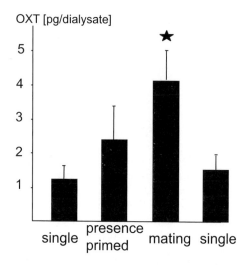

Fig. 2. Oxytocin release within the paraventricular nucleus of the hypothalamus in male Wistar rats, under basal conditions, in the presence of an estrogen-primed female behind a wall and during mating, as revealed by 30-min microdialysis periods. Data from Waldherr and Neumann 2007

Stoneham et al. 1985). Moreover, brain OXT plays an important role in the regulation of male (and female) sexual behaviour (Argiolas and Gessa 1991; Flanagan et al. 1993; McCarthy et al. 1994), and increased Fos-expression was found in OXT neurons within the PVN in response to mating (Witt and Insel 1994). In monogamous species, i.e prairie voles, a mouse-like rodent that forms a lasting pair bond with its mate (Young et al. 1998), release of OXT within relevant brain regions during mating has repeatedly been hypothesized to underlie their monogamous nature, at least in females. OXT actions were found to facilitate pair bonding in female voles whereas vasopressin seemed to play the dominant role in establishing pair bonds in males.

However, central OXT release during mating does not seem to be limited to monogamous species, where mating is a prerequisite for pair bonding. Recently, we demonstrated that the presence of a receptive female rat and successful mating triggered the release of OXT within the hypothalamic PVN, as quantified by microdialysis performed during ongoing behavioural monitoring (Waldherr and Neumann 2007; Fig. 2). Interestingly, local OXT release began to rise in the presence of the primed female behind a perforated wall that allowed olfactory and visual contact but not physical contact and mating (Fig. 2). Because males clearly displayed signs of behavioural arousal under these conditions, it can be concluded that OXT activation is induced by the presence of a receptive female in anticipation of, but without, mating, although this effect was not found to be significant.

OXT Mediates the Anxiolytic Effect of Sexual Activity in Males

Without any doubt, a high level of social interaction is a prerequisite for successful mating. Is there evidence that males benefit from the activation of the central OXT

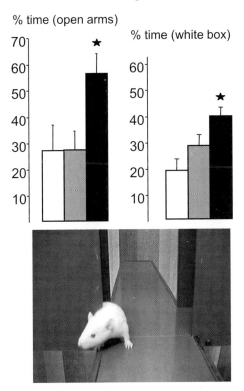

% time (open arms)

% time (white box)

Fig. 3. Effects of sexual activity and mating on anxiety behaviour on the elevated plus-maze, as indicated by the percentage of time spent in the open arms and the percentage of entries performed into the open arms of the maze. Male rats were either single-housed (*white columns*), housed with a non-primed female (*grey columns*) or allowed to mate with a primed female (*black columns*). Behavioural testing was performed four hours after a 30-min mating period as shown in the photograph below. Data from Waldherr and Neumann 2007

system in response to sexual activity? In general, anecdotal and experimental evidence has given rise to the commonly held perception that sedation and calmness are consequences of sexual activity in humans, contributing to a general feeling of well-being. Therefore, it is not surprising that positive consequences of sexual activity have been described in several mammalian species, including humans. For example, greater rates of sexual intercourse have been associated longitudinally with lower risk of mortality (Smith and Ruiz 2002) and lower blood pressure responses (Brody 2006).

We have demonstrated that male rats show a reduced level of anxiety-related behaviour up to four hours after mating with a receptive female but not following olfactory and visual cues (Fig. 3). The anxiolytic effect of sexual activity was already evident after 30 min and could be confirmed both on the elevated plus-maze and in the light-dark box. Importantly, if brain OXT receptors were blocked by icv infusion of a selective OXT receptor antagonist immediately after the 30-min mating period, the anxiolytic effect was abolished. Therefore, it is tempting to conclude that activation of the brain OXT system during sexual activity, i.e., increased release of OXT within the brain and subsequent neuropeptide-receptor interactions in relevant brain regions including the hypothalamus, mediates the anxiolytic effect of mating in males.

In support of our findings, Edinger and Frye (2007) demonstrated reduced anxiety levels in male rats that have experienced a lifetime of sexual stimuli, indicating long-term positive mood effects of repeated sexual activity. These anxiolytic effects were linked to the rise in basal plasma testosterone found in sexually experienced males. Androgens were recently found to have positive effects on mood (Haren et al. 2002), and lower testosterone levels were correlated with the occurrence of anxiety and depression (Aikey et al. 2002; Granger et al. 2003; van Honk et al. 1999).

As discussed above, social support and social bonding exert a variety of positive effects on health and stress susceptibility. As social interactions activate the brain OXT system in males, it is very likely that OXT also mediates positive effects of close social interaction. As mentioned above, social support by the best friend reduced stress-induced HPA axis responses and anxiety levels (Heinrichs et al. 2003). Interestingly, volunteers who were socially supported and also received an intranasal OXT administration showed the lowest hormone levels, whereas OXT alone had little effect. Moreover, the common action of both social support and OXT further increased their calmness and reduced the level of anxiety experienced during the stress test. These results provide further evidence for our hypothesis that endogenous OXT stimulated during social interactions mediates the positive and buffering effects of social support.

Thus, mating and sexual activity represents a physiological stimulus activating OXT release within the brain in males, which could be an important neurobiological mechanism contributing to the positive health effects of sexual activity. In this context, it would be of interest to study whether infant contact regulates the OXT system in paternal circumstances – in parallel with those described above for the mother – and if differences can be found between paternal and non-paternal species.

OXT Mediates the Rewarding Nature of Close Social Interactions: Maternal and Romantic Love

Clearly, social affiliation and sexual behaviour have rewarding effects. Social animals seek affiliation and sexual activity, and these experiences enhance the motivation for seeking it. Thomas Insel (Insel et al. 1997) described the rewarding property of affiliation as "love is addiction," and this statement holds clearly true for both maternal and romantic love. It has been reported in the monogamous prairie vole that establishing social bonds involves neural reward systems, including dopamine and opioid circuitry (Nelson and Panksepp 1998; Young and Wang 2004). Importantly, OXT significantly modulates the activity of these systems and vice versa, e.g., OXT amplifies the mesolimbic dopamine system (Wang and Aragona 2004; Young and Wang 2004) and increases preproenkephaline in the nucleus accumbens, thus activating neural reward systems (Lim et al. 2004). Recently, the existence of a neural circuit has been suggested that integrates OXT and dopamine actions on the consummatory, motivational and rewarding aspects of sexual behaviour (Melis et al. 2007; Succu et al. 2007).

Moreover, evidence exists that endogenous opioids regulate not only stress responsiveness (Douglas et al. 1998) but also OXT neuronal activity, in particular peripartum (Douglas et al. 1995; Wigger and Neumann 2002). Additional support has recently been shown using imaging techniques that the suckling stimulus triggers high activity in mesolimbic reward systems (Febo et al. 2005; Ferris et al. 2005). As suckling activates the OXT system, and given the above-mentioned interactions between OXT, dopamine and endogenous opioids, it is likely that activation of central OXT release both during close maternal-offspring interactions and interactions with the bonding/mating partner, e.g., during sexual behaviour, mediates the rewarding effects of these complex affiliative behaviours.

Another positive effect of a stimulated brain OXT system by close social interactions that necessitates discussion relates to social cognition. Initial studies on OXT in social cognition showed strong dose-dependent effects after peripheral or icv administration of OXT (Popik and van Ree 1991). In females, administration of an OXT antagonist interfered with the animals' ability to establish normal social memory (Engelmann et al. 1998; for review, see Bielsky et al. 2004; Bielsky and Young 2004). Additional support for an involvement of OXT in social cognitive abilities comes from studies using OXT knockout mice, which show clear deficits in social recognition but normal non-social learning and memory abilities (Choleris et al. 2003; Ferguson et al. 2000; Kavaliers et al. 2003; Nishimori et al. 1996). The deficit in social recognition was reversible with OXT administration, clearly demonstrating the importance of this peptide in the processing of social cues and subsequent social recognition. In female OXT knockout mice, the essential role of OXT in social memory has also been demonstrated in the context of the Bruce effect. OXT knockout females failed to remain pregnant if re-exposed to either their mate or a novel male. Only females that were allowed to remain with their mate maintained pregnancy (Temple et al. 2003). This inability to distinguish between the mate and a novel male in females with deficits in the OXT systems further demonstrates the importance of OXT in long-term social memory as well as short-term social recognition.

Other examples of OXT being essential for social memory and recognition come from experiments performed in ewes and in monogamous prairie voles. In ewes, lamb recognition and bonding immediately after birth could clearly be related to the intracerebral release of OXT, for example within the olfactory bulb, during parturition (Kendrick et al. 1988b), where OXT modulates GABA, noradrenaline and acetylcholine neurotransmission, and, consequently, mitral cell activity (Levy et al. 1995). Thus, OXT seems to be the common signal for the development of selective offspring recognition.

In the monogamous prairie vole, social recognition of the mate is clearly a prerequisite for monogamous behaviour and the ability to form a selective pair-bond. Similar to the offspring bonding in ewes, OXT plays a critical role in the social bonding in female prairie voles, as does vasopressin in the male prairie voles (Insel and Hulihan 1995). Thus, mating-induced stimulation of OXT release within distinct brain regions seems to be a promoting factor for social cognition and pair-bond formation. Importantly, the distribution of OXT receptors differs greatly between the monogamous and promiscuous species (the montane vole), with a high OXT receptor density found in the nucleus accumbens of female and a high vasopressin receptor density found in the ventral pallidum of male prairie voles (Insel and Shapiro 1992). These brain regions are important components of the reward system, further indicating a functional and behaviourally relevant relation between close social interactions, as seen during mating or during suckling, intracerebral OXT release and activation of reward systems beneficial for mental health.

In related studies, OXT has been shown to increase social skills in humans. As described above, OXT makes humans more trusting (Kosfeld et al. 2005), which is clearly a necessary emotion to have when forming and maintaining social bonds. Furthermore, OXT has been shown to increase the ability to gauge the mental state of others using social cues from facial expressions (Domes et al. 2007), which provides further indication of the likelihood of a similar role of OXT in social recognition in humans.

References

Aikey JL, Nyby JG, Anmuth DM, James PJ (2002) Testosterone rapidly reduces anxiety in male house mice (Mus musculus). Horm Behav 42:448–460

Altemus M, Deuster PA, Galliven E, Carter CS, Gold PW (1995) Suppression of hypothalmic-pituitary-adrenal axis responses to stress in lactating women. J Clin Endocrinol Metab 80:2954–2959

Amico JA, Johnston JM, Vagnucci AH (1994) Suckling-induced attenuation of plasma cortisol concentrations in postpartum lactating women. Endocr Res 20:79–87

Amico JA, Mantella RC, Vollmer RR, Li X (2004) Anxiety and stress responses in female oxytocin deficient mice. J Neuroendocrinol 16:319–324

Argiolas A, Gessa GL (1991) Central functions of oxytocin. Neurosci Biobehav Rev 15:217–231

Bale TL, Davis AM, Auger AP, Dorsa DM, McCarthy MM (2001) CNS region-specific oxytocin receptor expression: importance in regulation of anxiety and sex behavior. J Neurosci 21:2546–2552

Bielsky IF, Young LJ (2004) Oxytocin, vasopressin, and social recognition in mammals. Peptides 25:1565–1574

Bielsky IF, Hu SB, Szegda KL, Westphal H, Young LJ (2004) Profound impairment in social recognition and reduction in anxiety-like behavior in vasopressin V1a receptor knockout mice. Neuropsychopharmacology 29:483–493

Blume A, Bosch OJ, Miklos S, Torner L, Wales L, Waldherr M, Neumann ID (2008) Oxytocin reduces anxiety via ERK 1/2 activation: local effect within the rat hypothalamic paraventricular nucleus. Eur J Neurosci 27(8):1947–1956

Born J, Lange T, Kern W, McGregor GP, Bickel U, Fehm HL (2002) Sniffing neuropeptides: a transnasal approach to the human brain. Nature Neurosci 5:514–516

Bosch OJ, Meddle SL, Beiderbeck DI, Douglas AJ, Neumann ID (2005) Brain oxytocin correlates with maternal aggression: link to anxiety. J Neurosci 25:6807–6815

Bridges RS, Dibiase R, Loundes DD, Doherty PC (1984) Prolactin stimulation of maternal behavior in female rats. Science 227:782–784

Bridges RS, Numan M, Ronsheim PM, Mann PE, Lupini CE (1990) Central prolactin infusions stimulate maternal behavior in steroid-treated, nulliparous female rats. Proc Natl Acad Sci USA 87:8003–8007

Brody S (2006) Blood pressure reactivity to stress is better for people who recently had penile-vaginal intercourse than for people who had other or no sexual activity. Biol Psychol 71:214–222

Brunton PJ, Russell JA (2003) Hypothalamic-pituitary-adrenal responses to centrally administered orexin-A are suppressed in pregnant rats. J Neuroendocrinol 15:633–637

Buske-Kirschbaum A, von Auer K, Krieger S, Weis S, Rauh W, Hellhammer D (2003) Blunted cortisol responses to psychosocial stress in asthmatic children: a general feature of atopic disease? Psychosom Med 65:806–810

Carmichael MS, Humbert R, Dixen J, Palmisano G, Greenleaf W, Davidson JM (1987) Plasma oxytocin increases in the human sexual response. J Clin Endocrinol Metab 64:27–31

Carter CS, Altemus M (1997) Integrative functions of lactational hormones in social behavior and stress management. Ann NY Acad Sci 807:164–174

Carter CS, Altemus M, Chrousos GP (2001) Neuroendocrine and emotional changes in the post-partum period. Prog Brain Res 133:241–249

Choleris E, Gustafsson J-A, Korach KS, Muglia LJ, Pfaff DW, Ogawa S (2003) An estrogen-dependent four-gene micronet regulating social recognition: a study with oxytocin and estrogen receptor-α and -β knockout mice. Proc Natl Acad Sci USA 100:6192–6197

Consiglio AR, Lucion AB (1996) Lesion of hypothalamic paraventricular nucleus and maternal aggressive behavior in female rats. Physiol Behav 59:591–596

Crawley JN, Chen T, Puri A, Washburn R, Sullivan TL, Hill JM, Young NB, Nadler JJ, Moy SS, Young LJ, Caldwell HK, Young WS (2007) Social approach behaviors in oxytocin knockout mice: comparison of two independent lines tested in different laboratory environments. Neuropeptides 41:145–163

da Costa AP, Ma X, Ingram CD, Lightman SL, Aguilera G (2001) Hypothalamic and amygdaloid corticotropin-releasing hormone (CRH) and CRH receptor-1 mRNA expression in the stress-hyporesponsive late pregnant and early lactating rat. Brain Res Mol Brain Res 91:119–130

da Costa AP, Leigh AE, Man MS, Kendrick KM (2004) Face pictures reduce behavioural, autonomic, endocrine and neural indices of stress and fear in sheep. Proc Biol Sci 271:2077–2084

Davis M, Whalen PJ (2001) The amygdala: vigilance and emotion. Mol Psychiat 6:13–34

de Weerth C, Buitelaar JK (2005) Physiological stress reactivity in human pregnancy – a review. Neurosci Biobehav Rev 29:295–312

DeVries AC, Joh HD, Bernard O, Hattori K, Hurn PD, Traystman RJ, Alkayed NJ (2001) Social stress exacerbates stroke outcome by suppressing Bcl-2 expression. Proc Natl Acad Sci USA 98:11824–11828

DeVries AC, Glasper ER, Detillion CE (2003) Social modulation of stress responses. Physiol Behav 79:399–407

DeVries AC, Craft TK, Glasper ER, Neigh GN, Alexander JK (2007) 2006 Curt P. Richter award winner: Social influences on stress responses and health. Psychoneuroendocrinology 32:587–603

Dluzen DE, Muraoka S, Engelmann M, Ebner K, Landgraf R (2000) Oxytocin induces preservation of social recognition in male rats by activating alpha-adrenoceptors of the olfactory bulb. Eur J Neurosci 12:760–766

Domes G, Heinrichs M, Glascher J, Buchel C, Braus DF, Herpertz SC (2007) Oxytocin Attenuates Amygdala Responses to Emotional Faces Regardless of Valence. Biol Psychiatry

Donner N, Bredewold R, Maloumby R, Neumann ID (2007) Chronic intracerebral prolactin attenuates neuronal stress circuitries in virgin rats. Eur J Neurosci 25:1804–1814

Douglas AJ, Russell JA (1994) Corticotrophin-releasing hormone, proenkephalin A and oxytocin mRNA's in the paraventricular nucleus during pregnancy and parturition in the rat. Gene Ther 1(Suppl 1):S85

Douglas AJ, Neumann I, Meeren HK, Leng G, Johnstone LE, Munro G, Russell JA (1995) Central endogenous opioid inhibition of supraoptic oxytocin neurons in pregnant rats. J Neurosci 15:5049–5057

Douglas AJ, Johnstone HA, Wigger A, Landgraf R, Russell JA, Neumann ID (1998) The role of endogenous opioids in neurohypophysial and hypothalamo-pituitary-adrenal axis hormone secretory responses to stress in pregnant rats. J Endocrinol 158:285–293

Douglas AJ, Brunton PJ, Bosch OJ, Russell JA, Neumann ID (2003) Neuroendocrine responses to stress in mice: hyporesponsiveness in pregnancy and parturition. Endocrinology 144:5268–5276

Douglas AJ, Meddle SL, Toschi N, Bosch OJ, Neumann ID (2005) Reduced activity of the noradrenergic system in the paraventricular nucleus at the end of pregnancy: implications for stress hyporesponsiveness. J Neuroendocrinol 17:40–48

Dunn J, Richards MP (1977) Observations on the developing relationship between mother and baby in the neonatal period. In: Scaefeer HR (ed) Studies in mother-infant interaction New York: Academic Press New York, pp 427–455

Ebner K, Wotjak CT, Landgraf R, Engelmann M (2000) A single social defeat experience selectively stimulates the release of oxytocin, but not vasopressin, within the septal brain area of male rats. Brain Res 872:87–92

Ebner K, Bosch OJ, Kromer SA, Singewald N, Neumann ID (2005) Release of oxytocin in the rat central amygdala modulates stress-coping behavior and the release of excitatory amino acids. Neuropsychopharmacology 30:223–230

Edinger KL, Frye CA (2007) Sexual experience of male rats influences anxiety-like behavior and androgen levels. Physiol Behav 92:443–453

Elliott JC, Lubin DA, Walker CH, Johns JM (2001) Acute cocaine alters oxytocin levels in the medial preoptic area and amygdala in lactating rat dams: implications for cocaine-induced changes in maternal behavior and maternal aggression. Neuropeptides 35:127–134

Engelmann M, Ebner K, Wotjak CT, Landgraf R (1998) Endogenous oxytocin is involved in short-term olfactory memory in female rats. Behav Brain Res 90:89–94

Engelmann M, Landgraf R, Wotjak CT (2004) The hypothalamic-neurohypophysial system regulates the hypothalamic-pituitary-adrenal axis under stress: an old concept revisited. Front Neuroendocrinol 25:132–149

Erskine MS, Barfield RJ, Goldman BD (1978) Intraspecific fighting during late pregnancy and lactation in rats and effects of litter removal. Behav Biol 23:206–218

Febo M, Numan M, Ferris CF (2005) Functional magnetic resonance imaging shows oxytocin activates brain regions associated with mother-pup bonding during suckling. J Neurosci 25:11637–11644

Ferguson JN, Young LJ, Hearn EF, Matzuk MM, Insel TR, Winslow JT (2000) Social amnesia in mice lacking the oxytocin gene. Nat Genet 25:284–288

Ferris CF, Kulkarni P, Sullivan JM Jr., Harder JA, Messenger TL, Febo M (2005) Pup suckling is more rewarding than cocaine: evidence from functional magnetic resonance imaging and three-dimensional computational analysis. J Neurosci 25:149–156

Flanagan LM, Pfaus JG, Pfaff DW, McEwen BS (1993) Induction of FOS immunoreactivity in oxytocin neurons after sexual activity in female rats. Neuroendocrinology 58:352–358

Francis DD, Caldji C, Champagne F, Plotsky PM, Meaney MJ (1999) The role of corticotropin-releasing factor–norepinephrine systems in mediating the effects of early experience on the development of behavioral and endocrine responses to stress. Biol Psychiat 46:1153–1166

Gammie SC, Negron A, Newman SM, Rhodes JS (2004) Corticotropin-releasing factor inhibits maternal aggression in mice. Behav Neurosci 118:805–814

Gonzalez CA, Coe CL, Levine S (1982) Cortisol responses under different housing conditions in female squirrel monkeys. Psychoneuroendocrinology 7:209–216

Granger DA, Shirtcliff EA, Zahn-Waxler C, Usher B, Klimes-Dougan B, Hastings P (2003) Salivary testosterone diurnal variation and psychopathology in adolescent males and females: individual differences and developmental effects. Dev Psychopathol 15:431–449

Hard E, Hansen S (1985) Reduced fearfulness in the lactating rat. Physiol Behav 35:641–643

Haren MT, Morley JE, Chapman IM, O'Loughlin PD, Wittert GA (2002) Defining 'relative' androgen deficiency in aging men: how should testosterone be measured and what are the relationships between androgen levels and physical, sexual and emotional health? Climacteric 5:15–25

Hattori T, Sundberg DK, Morris M (1992) Central and systemic oxytocin release: a study of the paraventricular nucleus by in vivo microdialysis. Brain Res Bull 28:257–263

Heinrichs M, Meinlschmidt G, Neumann I, Wagner S, Kirschbaum C, Ehlert U, Hellhammer DH (2001) Effects of suckling on hypothalamic-pituitary-adrenal axis responses to psychosocial stress in postpartum lactating women. J Clin Endocrinol Metab 86:4798–4804

Heinrichs M, Baumgartner T, Kirschbaum C, Ehlert U (2003) Social support and oxytocin interact to suppress cortisol and subjective responses to psychosocial stress. Biol Psychiat 54:1389–1398

House JS, Landis KR, Umberson D (1988) Social relationships and health. Science 241:540–545

Huber D, Veinante P, Stoop R (2005) Vasopressin and oxytocin excite distinct neuronal populations in the central amygdala. Science 308:245–248

Insel TR, Hulihan TJ (1995) A gender-specific mechanism for pair bonding: oxytocin and partner preference formation in monogamous voles. Behav Neurosci 109:782–789

Insel TR, Shapiro LE (1992) Oxytocin receptor distribution reflects social organization in monogamous and polygamous voles. Proc Natl Acad Sci USA 89:5981–5985

Insel TR, Young L, Wang Z (1997) Molecular aspects of monogamy. Ann NY Acad Sci 807:302–316

Johnstone HA, Wigger A, Douglas AJ, Neumann ID, Landgraf R, Seckl JR, Russell JA (2000) Attenuation of hypothalamic-pituitary-adrenal axis stress responses in late pregnancy: changes in feedforward and feedback mechanisms. J Neuroendocrinol 12:811–822

Kammerer M, Adams D, Castelberg Bv B, Glover V (2002) Pregnant women become insensitive to cold stress. BMC Pregnancy Childbirth 2:8

Kavaliers M, Colwell DD, Choleris E, Agmo A, Muglia LJ, Ogawa S, Pfaff DW (2003) Impaired discrimination of and aversion to parasitized male odors by female oxytocin knockout mice. Genes Brain Behav 2:220–230

Kendrick KM, Keverne EB, Baldwin BA (1987) Intracerebroventricular oxytocin stimulates maternal behaviour in the sheep. Neuroendocrinology 46:56–61

Kendrick KM, Keverne EB, Chapman C, Baldwin BA (1988a) Intracranial dialysis measurement of oxytocin, monoamine and uric acid release from the olfactory bulb and substantia nigra of sheep during parturition, suckling, separation from lambs and eating. Brain Res 439:1–10

Kendrick KM, Keverne EB, Chapman C, Baldwin BA (1988b) Microdialysis measurement of oxytocin, aspartate, gamma-aminobutyric acid and glutamate release from the olfactory bulb of the sheep during vaginocervical stimulation. Brain Res 442:171–174

Kendrick KM, Da Costa AP, Broad KD, Ohkura S, Guevara R, Levy F, Keverne EB (1997) Neural control of maternal behaviour and olfactory recognition of offspring. Brain Res Bull 44:383–395

Kikusui T, Winslow JT, Mori Y (2006) Social buffering: relief from stress and anxiety. Phil Trans R Soc B 361:2215–2228

Kirsch P, Esslinger C, Chen Q, Mier D, Lis S, Siddhanti S, Gruppe H, Mattay VS, Gallhofer B, Meyer-Lindenberg A (2005) Oxytocin modulates neural circuitry for social cognition and fear in humans. J Neurosci 25:11489–11493

Kirschbaum C, Klauer T, Filipp SH, Hellhammer DH (1995) Sex-specific effects of social support on cortisol and subjective responses to acute psychological stress. Psychosom Med 57:23–31

Kirschbaum C, Kudielka BM, Gaab J, Schommer NC, Hellhammer DH (1999) Impact of gender, menstrual cycle phase, and oral contraceptives on the activity of the hypothalamus-pituitary-adrenal axis. Psychosom Med 61:154–162

Kiyokawa Y, Kikusui T, Takeuchi Y, Mori Y (2004) Partner's stress status influences social buffering effects in rats. Behav Neurosci 118:798–804

Knox SS, Uvnas-Moberg K (1998) Social isolation and cardiovascular disease: an atherosclerotic pathway? Psychoneuroendocrinology 23:877–890

Kofman O (2002) The role of prenatal stress in the etiology of developmental behavioural disorders. Neurosci Biobehav Rev 26:457–470

Kombian SB, Mouginot D, Pittman QJ (1997) Dendritically released peptides act as retrograde modulators of afferent excitation in the supraoptic nucleus in vitro. Neuron 19:903–912

Kosfeld M, Heinrichs M, Zak PJ, Fischbacher U, Fehr E (2005) Oxytocin increases trust in humans. Nature 435:673–676

Lancel M, Kromer S, Neumann ID (2003) Intracerebral oxytocin modulates sleep-wake behaviour in male rats. Regul Pept 114:145–152

Landgraf R, Neumann ID (2004) Vasopressin and oxytocin release within the brain: a dynamic concept of multiple and variable modes of neuropeptide communication. Front Neuroendocrinol 25:150–176

Levy F, Kendrick KM, Goode JA, Guevara-Guzman R, Keverne EB (1995) Oxytocin and vasopressin release in the olfactory bulb of parturient ewes: changes with maternal experience and effects on acetylcholine, gamma-aminobutyric acid, glutamate and noradrenaline release. Brain Res 669:197–206

Lightman SL, Windle RJ, Wood SA, Kershaw YM, Shanks N, Ingram CD (2001) Peripartum plasticity within the hypothalamo-pituitary-adrenal axis. Prog Brain Res 133:111–129

Lim MM, Murphy AZ, Young LJ (2004) Ventral striatopallidal oxytocin and vasopressin V1a receptors in the monogamous prairie vole (Microtus ochrogaster). J Comp Neurol 468:555–570

Liu D, Diorio J, Day JC, Francis DD, Meaney MJ (2000) Maternal care, hippocampal synaptogenesis and cognitive development in rats. Nature Neurosci 3:799–806

Lonstein JS, Morrell JI (2006) Neuropharmacology and neuroendocrinology of maternal behavior and motivation. In: Blaustein JD (ed) Handbook of neurochemistry and molecular biology. New York: Kluwer Press pp 195–245

Lubin DA, Elliott JC, Black MC, Johns JM (2003) An oxytocin antagonist infused into the central nucleus of the amygdala increases maternal aggressive behavior. Behav Neurosci 117:195–201

Maestripieri D, Lindell SG, Ayala A, Gold PW, Higley JD (2005) Neurobiological characteristics of rhesus macaque abusive mothers and their relation to social and maternal behavior. Neurosci Biobehav Rev 29:51–57

McCarthy MM, Altemus M (1997) Central nervous system actions of oxytocin and modulation of behavior in humans. Mol Med Today 3:269–275

McCarthy MM, Kleopoulos SP, Mobbs CV, Pfaff DW (1994) Infusion of antisense oligodeoxynucleotides to the oxytocin receptor in the ventromedial hypothalamus reduces estrogen-induced sexual receptivity and oxytocin receptor binding in the female rat. Neuroendocrinology 59:432–440

Melis MR, Melis T, Cocco C, Succu S, Sanna F, Pillolla G, Boi A, Ferri GL, Argiolas A (2007) Oxytocin injected into the ventral tegmental area induces penile erection and increases extracellular dopamine in the nucleus accumbens and paraventricular nucleus of the hypothalamus of male rats. Eur J Neurosci 26:1026–1035

Moos F, Freund-Mercier MJ, Guerne Y, Guerne JM, Stoeckel ME, Richard P (1984) Release of oxytocin and vasopressin by magnocellular nuclei in vitro: specific facilitatory effect of oxytocin on its own release. J Endocrinol 102:63–72

Nelson EE, Panksepp J (1998) Brain substrates of infant-mother attachment: contributions of opioids, oxytocin, and norepinephrine. Neurosci Biobehav Rev 22:437–452

Neumann ID (2001) Alterations in behavioral and neuroendocrine stress coping strategies in pregnant, parturient and lactating rats. Prog Brain Res 133:143–152

Neumann ID (2002) Involvement of the brain oxytocin system in stress coping: interactions with the hypothalamo-pituitary-adrenal axis. Prog Brain Res 139:147–162

Neumann ID (2003) Brain mechanisms underlying emotional alterations in the peripartum period in rats. Depress Anxiety 17:111–121

Neumann ID, Landgraf R (1989) Septal and hippocampal release of oxytocin, but not vasopressin, in the conscious lactating rat during suckling. J Neuroendocrinol 1:305–308

Neumann I, Ludwig M, Engelmann M, Pittman QJ, Landgraf R (1993a) Simultaneous microdialysis in blood and brain: oxytocin and vasopressin release in response to central and peripheral osmotic stimulation and suckling in the rat. Neuroendocrinology 58:637–645

Neumann I, Russell JA, Landgraf R (1993b) Oxytocin and vasopressin release within the supraoptic and paraventricular nuclei of pregnant, parturient and lactating rats: a microdialysis study. Neuroscience 53:65–75

Neumann I, Koehler E, Landgraf R, Summy-Long J (1994) An oxytocin receptor antagonist infused into the supraoptic nucleus attenuates intranuclear and peripheral release of oxytocin during suckling in conscious rats. Endocrinology 134:141–148

Neumann I, Douglas AJ, Pittman QJ, Russell JA, Landgraf R (1996) Oxytocin released within the supraoptic nucleus of the rat brain by positive feedback action is involved in parturition-related events. J Neuroendocrinol 8:227–233

Neumann ID, Johnstone H, Hatzinger M, Landgraf R, Russell JA, Douglas A (1998a) Neuroendocrine adaptations of the hypothalamo-pituitary-adrenal (HPA) axis throughout pregnancy. J Physiol 508:289–300

Neumann ID, Johnstone HA, Hatzinger M, Liebsch G, Shipston M, Russell JA, Landgraf R, Douglas AJ (1998b) Attenuated neuroendocrine responses to emotional and physical stressors in pregnant rats involve adenohypophysial changes. J Physiol 508(Pt 1):289–300

Neumann ID, Wigger A, Liebsch G, Holsboer F, Landgraf R (1998c) Increased basal activity of the hypothalamo-pituitary-adrenal axis during pregnancy in rats bred for high anxiety-related behaviour. Psychoneuroendocrinology 23:449–463

Neumann ID, Torner L, Wigger A (2000a) Brain oxytocin: differential inhibition of neuroendocrine stress responses and anxiety-related behaviour in virgin, pregnant and lactating rats. Neuroscience 95:567–575

Neumann ID, Wigger A, Torner L, Holsboer F, Landgraf R (2000b) Brain oxytocin inhibits basal and stress-induced activity of the hypothalamo-pituitary-adrenal axis in male and female rats: partial action within the paraventricular nucleus. J Neuroendocrinol 12:235–243

Neumann ID, Toschi N, Ohl F, Torner L, Kromer SA (2001) Maternal defence as an emotional stressor in female rats: correlation of neuroendocrine and behavioural parameters and involvement of brain oxytocin. Eur J Neurosci 13:1016–1024

Neumann ID, Torner L, Toschi N, Veenema AH (2006) Oxytocin actions within the supraoptic and paraventricular nuclei: differential effects on peripheral and intranuclear vasopressin release. Am J Physiol Regul Integr Comp Physiol 291:R29–R36

Nishimori K, Young LJ, Guo Q, Wang Z, Insel TR, Matzuk MM (1996) Oxytocin is required for nursing but is not essential for parturition or reproductive behavior. Proc Natl Acad Sci USA 93:11699–11704

Numan M, Insel TR (2003) The neurobiology of parental behaviour. In: Ball GF, Balthazart J, Nelson RJ (eds) Hormones, brain, and behavior series New York, Springer

Paykel ES (2001) Stress and affective disorders in humans. Semin Clin Neuropsychiatry 6:4–11

Pedersen CA, Boccia ML (2003) Oxytocin antagonism alters rat dams' oral grooming and upright posturing over pups. Physiol Behav 80:233–241

Pedersen CA, Prange AJ, Jr. (1979) Induction of maternal behavior in virgin rats after intracerebroventricular administration of oxytocin. Proc Natl Acad Sci USA 76:6661–6665

Pedersen CA, Caldwell JD, McGuire M, Evans DL (1991) Corticotropin-releasing hormone inhibits maternal behavior and induces pup-killing. Life Sci 48:1537–1546

Popik P, van Ree JM (1991) Oxytocin but not vasopressin facilitates social recognition following injection into the medial preoptic area of the rat brain. Eur Neuropsychopharmacol 1:555–560

Reber SO, Obermeier F, Straub HR, Falk W, Neumann ID (2006) Chronic intermittent psychosocial stress (social defeat/overcrowding) in mice increases the severity of an acute DSS-induced colitis and impairs regeneration. Endocrinology 147:4968–4976

Reber SO, Birkeneder L, Veenema AH, Obermeier F, Falk W, Straub RH, Neumann ID (2007) Adrenal insufficiency and colonic inflammation after a novel chronic psycho-social stress paradigm in mice: implications and mechanisms. Endocrinology 148:670–682

Ring RH, Malberg JE, Potestio L, Ping J, Boikess S, Luo B, Schechter LE, Rizzo S, Rahman Z, Rosenzweig-Lipson S (2006) Anxiolytic-like activity of oxytocin in male mice: behavioral and autonomic evidence, therapeutic implications. Psychopharmacology (Berl) 185:218–225

Rozanski A, Blumenthal JA, Kaplan J (1999) Impact of psychological factors on the pathogenesis of cardiovascular disease and implications for therapy. Circulation 99:2192–2217

Russell JA, Johnstone H, Douglas AJ, Landgraf R, Wigger A, Shipston M, Seckl JR, Neumann ID (1999) Neuroendocrine stress mechanisms regulating ACTH and oxytocin in pregnancy. In: Yamashita H (ed) Control mechanisms of stress and emotions: neuroendocrine-based studies. Amsterdam, Elsevier pp 33–51

Russell JA, Douglas AJ, Ingram CD (2001) Brain preparations for maternity–adaptive changes in behavioral and neuroendocrine systems during pregnancy and lactation. An overview. Prog Brain Res 133:1–38

Sachser N, Durschlag M, Hirzel D (1998) Social relationships and the management of stress. Psychoneuroendocrinology 23:891–904

Shanks N, Windle RJ, Perks P, Wood S, Ingram CD, Lightman SL (1999) The hypothalamic-pituitary-adrenal axis response to endotoxin is attenuated during lactation. J Neuroendocrinol 11:857–865

Slattery DA, Neumann ID (2007) No stress please! Mechanisms of stress hyporesponsiveness of the maternal brain. J Physiol 586:377–385

Smith TE, French JA (1997) Social and reproductive conditions modulate urinary cortisol excretion in black tufted-ear marmosets (Callithrix kuhli). Am J Primatol 42:253–267

Smith TW, Ruiz JM (2002) Psychosocial influences on the development and course of coronary heart disease: current status and implications for research and practice. J Consult Clin Psychol 70:548–568

Stern JM, Goldman L, Levine S (1973) Pituitary-adrenal responsiveness during lactation in rats. Neuroendocrinology 12:179–191

Stoneham MD, Everitt BJ, Hansen S, Lightman SL, Todd K (1985) Oxytocin and sexual behaviour in the male rat and rabbit. J Endocrinol 107:97–106

Succu S, Sanna F, Melis T, Boi A, Argiolas A, Melis MR (2007) Stimulation of dopamine receptors in the paraventricular nucleus of the hypothalamus of male rats induces penile erection and increases extra-cellular dopamine in the nucleus accumbens: Involvement of central oxytocin. Neuropharmacology 52:1034–1043

Temple JL, Young WSI, Wersinger SR (2003) Disruption of the genes for either oxytocin or the vasopressin 1B receptor alters male-induced pregnancy block (the Bruce effect). In: Society for Neuroscience, New Orleans 404.13

Theodosis DT (2002) Oxytocin-secreting neurons: A physiological model of morphological neuronal and glial plasticity in the adult hypothalamus. Front Neuroendocrinol 23:101–135

Torner L, Neumann ID (2002) The brain prolactin system: involvement in stress response adaptations in lactation. Stress 5:249–257

Torner L, Toschi N, Nava G, Clapp C, Neumann ID (2002) Increased hypothalamic expression of prolactin in lactation: involvement in behavioural and neuroendocrine stress responses. Eur J Neurosci 15:1381–1389

Torner L, Toschi N, Pohlinger A, Landgraf R, Neumann ID (2001) Anxiolytic and anti-stress effects of brain prolactin: improved efficacy of antisense targeting of the prolactin receptor by molecular modeling. J Neurosci 21:3207–3214

Torner L, Maloumby R, Nava G, Aranda J, Clapp C, Neumann ID (2004) In vivo release and gene upregulation of brain prolactin in response to physiological stimuli. Eur J Neurosci 19:1601–1608

Toufexis DJ, Thrivikraman KV, Plotsky PM, Morilak DA, Huang N, Walker CD (1998) Reduced noradrenergic tone to the hypothalamic paraventricular nucleus contributes to the stress hyporesponsiveness of lactation. J Neuroendocrinol 10:417–427

Uvnas-Moberg K (1997) Physiological and endocrine effects of social contact. In: Carter S, Lederhendler I, Kirkpatrick B (eds) The integrative neurobiology of affiliation. Cambridge (MA): MIT Press, pp 245–262

van Honk J, Tuiten A, Verbaten R, van den Hout M, Koppeschaar H, Thijssen J, de Haan E (1999) Correlations among salivary testosterone, mood, and selective attention to threat in humans. Horm Behav 36:17–24

Waldherr M, Neumann ID (2007) From the Cover: Centrally released oxytocin mediates mating-induced anxiolysis in male rats. Proc Natl Acad Sci USA 104:16681–16684

Walker CD, Trottier G, Rochford J, Lavallee D (1995) Dissociation between behavioral and hormonal responses to the forced swim stress in lactating rats. J Neuroendocrinol 7:615–622

Walker CD, Toufexis DJ, Burlet A (2001) Hypothalamic and limbic expression of CRF and vasopressin during lactation: implications for the control of ACTH secretion and stress hyporesponsiveness. Prog Brain Res 133:99–110

Wang Z, Aragona BJ (2004) Neurochemical regulation of pair bonding in male prairie voles. Physiol Behav 83:319–328

Weinstock M (2001) Alterations induced by gestational stress in brain morphology and behaviour of the offspring. Prog Neurobiol 65:427–451

Welberg LA, Seckl JR (2001) Prenatal stress, glucocorticoids and the programming of the brain. J Neuroendocrinol 13:113–128

Wigger A, Neumann ID (1998) Endogenous opioids suppress the stress-induced release of oxytocin in the paraventricular nucleus of the pregnant rat. Eur J Neurosci 10(suppl. 10):167.118

Wigger A, Neumann ID (2002) Endogenous opioid regulation of stress-induced oxytocin release within the hypothalamic paraventricular nucleus is reversed in late pregnancy: a microdialysis study. Neuroscience 112:121–129

Wigger A, Lorscher P, Oehler I, Keck ME, Naruo T, Neumann ID (1999) Nonresponsiveness of the rat hypothalamo-pituitary-adrenocortical axis to parturition-related events: inhibitory action of endogenous opioids. Endocrinology 140:2843–2849

Windle RJ, Shanks N, Lightman SL, Ingram CD (1997a) Central oxytocin administration reduces stress-induced corticosterone release and anxiety behavior in rats. Endocrinology 138:2829–2834

Windle RJ, Wood S, Shanks N, Perks P, Conde GL, da Costa AP, Ingram CD, Lightman SL (1997b) Endocrine and behavioural responses to noise stress: comparison of virgin and lactating female rats during non-disrupted maternal activity. J Neuroendocrinol 9:407–414

Windle RJ, Kershaw YM, Shanks N, Wood SA, Lightman SL, Ingram CD (2004) Oxytocin attenuates stress-induced c-fos mRNA expression in specific forebrain regions associated with modulation of hypothalamo-pituitary-adrenal activity. J Neurosci 24:2974–2982

Winslow JT, Hearn EF, Ferguson J, Young LJ, Matzuk MM, Insel TR (2000) Infant vocalization, adult aggression, and fear behavior of an oxytocin null mutant mouse. Horm Behav 37:145–155

Witt DM, Insel TR (1994) Increased Fos expression in oxytocin neurons following masculine sexual behavior. J Neuroendocrinol 6:13–18

Wotjak CT, Kubota M, Liebsch G, Montkowski A, Holsboer F, Neumann I, Landgraf R (1996) Release of vasopressin within the rat paraventricular nucleus in response to emotional stress: a novel mechanism of regulating adrenocorticotropic hormone secretion? J Neurosci 16:7725–7732

Wotjak CT, Naruo T, Muraoka S, Simchen R, Landgraf R, Engelmann M (2001) Swim stress stimulates the expression of vasopressin and oxytocin in magnocellular neurons of the hypothalamic paraventricular nucleus. Eur J Neurosci 13:2273–2281

Young LJ, Wang Z (2004) The neurobiology of pair bonding. Nature Neurosci 7:1048–1054

Young LJ, Wang Z, Insel TR (1998) Neural bases of monogamy. Trends Neurosci 21:71–75

Hormones, Brain Plasticity and Reproductive Functions

Dionysia T. Theodosis[1]

Summary

The magnocellular oxytocin system of the hypothalamus illustrates remarkably well activity-dependent structural plasticity in the adult brain. Its neurons secrete the neurohormone oxytocin, which plays a key role in the initiation of parturition and maintenance of lactation. The somata and dendrites of oxytocin neurons accumulate in the supraoptic and paraventricular nuclei of the hypothalamus whereas their axons project to the neurohypophysis. There, oxytocin is secreted into the bloodstream from neurosecretory terminals upon electrical and biosynthetic activation of the neurons driven by afferent stimulation from the periphery. Oxytocin is released centrally as well, including within the hypothalamic nuclei, where it facilitates the electrical, biosynthetic and secretory activities of its own neurons. During conditions that stimulate peripheral and central oxytocin release, like parturition and lactation, there is a significant reduction in ensheathing of oxytocin neurons and their synapses by fine processes of astrocytes. As a consequence, the geometry and diffusion properties of the extracellular space surrounding the cells are significantly modified. In addition, there is a concomitant formation of new functional synapses on oxytocin neurons, which, in the main, are inhibitory. The anatomical changes are rapid, occuring within an hour, and reversible with arrest of stimulation. In vivo and in vitro evidence shows that oxytocin, in synergy with estrogen, mediates this neuronal, glial and synaptic remodeling. It is mediated specifically by oxytocin receptors, requires de novo protein synthesis, ongoing neuronal activity and expression of cell adhesion molecules that are permissive for plasticity. Similar neuro-glial changes occur in other hypothalamic nuclei whose neurons intervene in estrogen-dependent reproductive behaviors, like ovarian cyclicity and puberty. The functional consequences of such structural plasticity are important since the plasticity modifies neurotransmission, gliotransmission, neurohormone secretion and, ultimately, behaviors associated with reproduction.

Introduction

Parturition and lactation are neuroendocrine events vital for reproduction in mammals, and, therefore, of utmost import to the survival of the species. Like all physiological phenomena, their regulation involves numerous and diverse molecules that

---

[1] Inserm Research Center U862, Bordeaux F33077, France; University Victor Segalen-Bordeaux 2, Bordeaux F33077, France, e-mail: dionysia.theodosis@bordeaux.inserm.fr

Pfaff et al.
Hormones and Social Behavior
© Springer-Verlag Berlin Heidelberg 2008

intervene in signaling, genomic and biosynthetic mechanisms. Of these, the non-apeptide oxytocin (OT) is particularly important. OT is synthetized in magnocellular neurons that accumulate in well-delineated regions of the hypothalamus, the paired supraoptic (SON) and paraventricular (PVN) nuclei. In these structures, oxytocinergic neurons occur intermingled with their close relatives, neurons secreting vasopressin (VP), a neurohormone important in cardiovascular and osmotic regulation. After synthesis, the hormones, packaged in secretory granules, follow the regulated secretory pathway to be released from axon terminals in the posterior lobe of the pituitary or neurohypophysis (for a recent review, see Burbach et al. 2001). Synthesis and release of OT, like VP, and ultimately circulating levels of the neurohormones, are in large part determined by the electrical activity of the neurons, which in turn is regulated by afferent inputs. The latter utilize neurotransmitters common to all central systems, including GABA, glutamate, the monoamines and acetylcholine (reviewed in Poulain and Wakerley 1982; Armstrong and Stern 1998). In addition, OT is released in many areas of the central and peripheral nervous systems, where it participates in different neurovegetative and limbic functions (see Landgraf and Neumann 2004). It is secreted in the SON and PVN. mainly via a somato-dendritic exocytotic mechanism, and exerts a positive feedback action, ultimately facilitating the electrical and secretory activities of its own system (reviewed in Ludwig and Pittman 2003).

It is now generally acknowledged that many adult neurons, as well as the synapses controlling their activities, are not static anatomical entities since they can undergo dynamic structural transformations that alter their morphologies and interrelationships. This alteration occurs under normal physiological conditions of heightened neuronal activity and highlights the brain's remarkable capacity for restructuring to meet particular functional requirements. Together with morphological changes in neurons and synapses, there is remodeling of the other major cellular elements in the nervous system, glia and, in particular, astrocytes. This neuronal-glial plasticity not only has direct consequences on the respective functions of each type of cell but also may affect neuronal and glial behavior by modifying the immediate extracellular environment, with consequences on synaptic and volume transmission.

The OT system is an excellent model illustrating this kind of activity-dependent structural plasticity. Whenever it is strongly or persistently stimulated, as at parturition and lactation, its neurons respond by significantly increased electrophysiological and secretory activities (Poulain and Wakerley 1982; Armstrong and Stern 1998; Burbach et al. 2001). At the same time, their overall morphology is modified since they progressively hypertrophy, their dendrites change in size and branching and their axons in the neurohypophysis enlarge and ramify. In the hypothalamus, there is a concomitant remodeling of their afferent inputs as well as of their associated astrocytes. Several recent reviews describe this physiological structural plasticity in detail (see, for example, Theodosis 2002; Miyata and Hatton 2002; Theodosis et al. 2008), and only its most salient features will be presented here. I will then briefly show that this kind of neuronal-glial plasticity is not limited to the hypothalamo-neurohypophysial system (HNS) since it occurs in other central systems, including in hypothalamic neuroendocrine centers involved in reproductive functions like ovarian cyclicity and puberty (reviewed in Theodosis et al. 2008). In the latter, plasticity takes place in concert with fluctuations in circulating levels of sexual steroids. I will then discuss the functional consequences of such plasticity at the cellular and systems levels. Finally, I shall present molecular mechanisms that may shed some light on how such plasticity takes place in the adult nervous system, whose structure, until now, has been considered to be relatively unchangeable, except in response to aging, trauma or degeneration.

Morphological Plasticity of the OT System

Like most other central neurons, oxytocinergic neurons are normally ensheathed by processes of astrocytes, the most abundant glial cells in the magnocellular nuclei. Astrocytes in the SON and PVN have a variable, complex morphology (Bonfanti et al. 1993; Bobak and Salm 1996; Israel et al. 2003b), consisting of relatively small cell bodies, several thick processes extending into the neuronal network, and numerous thin processes, at times consisting merely of two membranes enclosing little cytoplasm. It is these lamellipodia that ensheath the somata, dendrites and axons of the neurons, as well as their synapses driving the activity. As has been illustrated in the hippocampus, their tips probably surround several synapses (Halassa et al. 2007), thereby creating glial microdomains enabling neuron-glia interactions in a restricted microenvironment (Grosche et al. 1999). Astrocytes respond to physiological stimuli by increases in intracellular calcium (Perea and Araque 2005), which consequently affect glial structure and function via different intracellular signaling mechanisms and gene activation.

Numerous observations obtained over the past two decades have made it clear that neurons, synapses and astrocytes of the HNS undergo significant morphological transformations under different physiological conditions. In particular, as clearly seen with electron microscopy coupled to morphometric analyses of immunoidentified profiles, this system's OT somata and dendrites, as well as their neighboring astrocytic processes, are surprisingly dynamic, continually changing their morphology in relation to neuronal activity. OT neurons usually occur in tightly packed clusters, yet, under basal conditions of neurosecretion, they remain separated by astrocytic processes. In contrast, during parturition, lactation, chronic dehydration, or in response to elevated ambient levels of OT, there is a significant reduction in astrocytic coverage of all portions of OT neurons. Thus, in the rat SON under basal conditions, astrocytic processes cover about 90% of any OT soma, a proportion that is reduced to 70% during lactation or chronic dehydration (Chapman et al. 1986; Theodosis et al. 1986a; Theodosis and Poulain 1987). This reduction in glial coverage leaves soma and dendritic surfaces directly and extensively juxtaposed. Astrocytic coverage of synapses contacting OT neurons is also significantly reduced (Oliet et al. 2001). It is important to note that this plasticity is not limited to one particular hypothalamic center but occurs throughout the hypothalamus, in all nuclei containing OT neurons (Theodosis and Poulain 1989). In contrast, in response to most stimuli for VP secretion, including severe chronic salt loading (Chapman et al. 1986), astrocytic coverage of VP neurons is not altered and remains around 90%. While VP neurons display some juxtapositions, their incidence and extent are low and show no variation with changing conditions of VP secretion (Chapman et al. 1986; Theodosis et al. 1986a).

Activity-dependent restructuring is visible not only in the magnocellular nuclei in the hypothalamus but also in the neurohypophysis (reviewed in Hatton et al. 1984; Theodosis and MacVicar 1996; Miyata and Hatton 2002). The gland is composed essentially of axons of SON and PVN neurons and astrocyte-like glial cells, the pituicytes.

The gland is highly vascularized and its capillaries are fenestrated, which permits passage of the secreted neurohormones into the circulation. Under basal conditions of neurosecretion, about 40% of the perivascular basal lamina is covered by neurosecretory terminals and about 60% by pituicyte processes. During stimulated conditions, as in the neurohypophyses of parturient and lactating animals (Tweedle and Hatton 1987; Luckman and Bicknell 1991) or when the glands are exposed in vitro to media that enhance secretion (Perlmutter et al. 1984; Smithson et al. 1990; Monlezun et al. 2005), pituicyte processes retract from the basal lamina and these proportions are reversed. Moreover, there is multiplication of terminals (Monlezun et al. 2005), and the end result is a significantly enlarged neurovascular contact zone. In addition, under stimulated conditions, throughout the gland, there is a reduction in the extent to which neurosecretory axons are engulfed or ensheated by pituicytes (Tweedle and Hatton 1982).

The structural transformations in the hypothalamic nuclei and neurohypophysis occur rapidly. This is evident in vivo, where ultrastructural changes can be detected within a few hours of the onset of parturition (Montagnese et al. 1987). It is even more apparent in vitro, in acute slices of adult hypothalamus that include the SON treated with OT (Langle et al. 2003; Theodosis et al. 2006) and in hemi-neurohypophyses exposed to hypertonic media or beta-adrenergic stimulation (Perlmutter et al. 1984; Monlezun et al. 2005). In both preparations, changes can be detected within one hour of treatment. When ambient levels of OT are again reduced (for example, after weaning the young, or in slices exposed to normal media), astrocytic processes reappear between neuronal profiles. Similarly, the extent of neurovascular contact in the neurohypophysis returns to baseline, non-stimulated levels upon cessation of stimulation of neurohypophysial secretion (Tweedle and Hatton 1987; Monlezun et al. 2005).

In the magnocellular nuclei, variations in astrocytic coverage of neuronal somata and dendrites are invariably accompanied by synapse turnover (reviewed in Theodosis 2002; Theodosis et al. 2005). This is represented by a changing number of boutons making synaptic contact onto more than one postsynaptic element simultaneously ("multiple" synapses) and boutons making single synaptic contacts on OT somata and dendrites (Theodosis et al. 1986c; Gies and Theodosis, 1994; El Majdoubi et al. 1997). Moreover, analyses of immunoidentified elements have allowed identification of the circuits undergoing plasticity as inhibitory (GABAergic) and excitatory (glutamatergic and noradrenergic ; reviewed in Theodosis et al. 2005). The most important increases affect GABAergic inputs, so that in the SON of lactating rats, about 50% of all axo-somatic and axo-dendritic synapses are GABAergic, compared to about 35% under basal conditions (El Majdoubi et al. 1997). Once stimulation is over, synaptic numbers revert to control levels. This synaptic remodeling can be reproduced in vitro in acute hypothalamic slices of adult SON. Electron microscopy and patch clamp electrophysiology of such preparations showed without ambiguity that synapse formation is extremely rapid, occurring within an hour, and is reversible within hours as well and results in the formation of inhibitory synapses that are functional (Theodosis et al. 2006).

How neuronal surfaces become extensively juxtaposed remains to be determined. The suggestion that juxtaposed neuronal surfaces are due simply to glial retraction is debatable. On the other hand, it is highly unlikely that astrocytic processes are passively squeezed away by hypertrophied neuronal profiles. For example, this mechanism does not explain the significant reduction in astrocytic ensheathing of dendrites or the numerous juxtaposed elements in tissues where hypertrophy of neuronal elements has yet to take place (Langle et al. 2003). It is noteworthy that VP neurons significantly hypertrophy during chronic dehydration, yet their surfaces do not become increasingly juxtaposed (Chapman et al. 1986). A more likely scenario is that neuronal juxtapositions result from both active retraction and elongation of glial processes over neuronal surfaces whose morphology is constantly changing. In the neurohypophysis, glial process retraction from the perivascular zone could explain reduction in glio-vascular contact associated with stimulation,whereas the return to baseline conditions could be associated with a reinsertion of pituicyte processes between the neurosecretory terminals. The modified expression of several cytoskeletal proteins (Nothias et al. 1996; Hawrylak et al. 1999; Miyata et al. 1999) probably reflects this remodeling. In comparison to other systems (Bailey and Kandel 1993), one expects that these cell transformations are accompanied by differential gene expression and de novo protein synthesis. In the SON, new macromolecular synthesis is essential since there is no glial or neuronal remodeling when protein synthesis is blocked by agents like anisomycin (Langle et al. 2003).

Neuronal-glial Plasticity in Other Neuroendocrine Centers

Rapid, activity-dependent morphological changes similar to those visible in the magnocellular nuclei are detectable in other areas of the basal hypothalamus. In the rat arcuate nucleus, for example, which includes neurons secreting reproductive hormones like gonadotropin releasing hormone (GnRH), the proportion of neuronal somatic surface covered by astrocytic processes fluctuates with changing sexual steroid levels, being high when plasma estrogen is elevated (afternoon of proestrus and morning of estrus) and low 24 hours later at metestrus, when estrogen levels have diminished (reviewed in Garcia-Segura et al. 1994). Administration of estradiol to ovariectomized animals mimics the effects of the estrous cycle and shows clearly that the astro-neuronal changes are rapid, occurring within 2 hours of steroid injection. Similar phenomena have been described in the infundibulum and preoptic area of primates, like the Rhesus and African green monkey (Witkin et al. 1991; Garcia-Segura et al. 1994).

Synaptic changes accompany astrocytic remodeling in these areas of the hypothalamus, as they do in the magnocellular nuclei. In adult females, there is a natural phasic synaptic remodeling that is linked to variations of the ovarian cycle and is reflected in a changing number of inhibitory GABAergic synapses on somata of arcuate neurons (see Garcia-Segura et al. 1994a). A negative correlation between the level of glial ensheathment and number of synaptic inputs in relation to fluctuations in steroid levels has also been detected in primates (Witkin et al. 1991; Garcia-Segura et al. 1994a). In sheep, seasonal variations in glial ensheathment of GnRH neurons, together with changes in the number of synaptic inputs to GnRH neurons, occur in the preoptic area. Thus, the number of synapses decreases between the breeding and non-breeding seasons in conjunction with a decreased pulsatile GnRH secretion that leads to anestrous (Viguié et al. 2001), a decline accompanied by a significantly increased coverage of the neurons by astrocytic processes. Interestingly, in the rodent arcuate, rewiring of inhibitory inputs also occurs on POMC neurons, in response to enhanced circulating levels of the gut hormone ghrelin, which intervenes in the control of energy balance and growth hormone release (Pinto et al. 2004). It is not unlikely that these latter synaptic changes are accompanied by astrocytic changes similar to those seen in response to estrogen, but this remains to be demonstrated.

The axons of GnRH neurons project to the external layer of the median eminence where, as in the neurohypophysis, they release the hormone from neurosecretory terminals in close proximity to fenestrated capillaries. In this neurohemal structure, it is fluctuations in sexual steroid levels that lead to axo-glial changes similar to those of the stimulated neurohypophysis. They result in retraction of end feet of tanycytes (modified ependymoglial cells) from the perivascular zone and exposure of GnRH terminals to fenestrated capillaries (King and Rubin 1995; De Serrano et al. 2004). In neurohemal structures, therefore, glial rearrangements ultimately permit direct access of neurosecretory axons to perivascular zones.

Consequences of Neuronal-glial Plasticity at the Cellular Level

In addition to supportive and nutritive functions (Magistretti et al. 1999), astrocytic processes, by their mere presence, act as a physical barrier to restrict spillover and diffusion of neuroactive substances in the extracellular space surrounding neurons and synapses. Therefore, a major consequence of astrocytic remodeling during stimulated conditions of neuronal activity is to reduce the extent to which astrocytic processes fill the extracellular space surrounding all neuronal elements, including synapses. As recent studies have demonstrated, this retraction has several important consequences on neuronal functions.

First, the ionic homeostasis of the extracellular space will be modified. A major function of astrocytic processes is to remove ions that can potentially influence neuronal activity. When absent during enhanced neuronal activity, there will be accumulation of ions like $K+$, which can facilitate further neuronal excitability. Such increases have been recorded in the SON (Coles and Poulain 1991) and neurohypophysis (Leng and Shibuki 1986) of lactating animals.

Secondly, the matrix (ECM) of all extracellular spaces is composed of many glycoproteins secreted by astrocytes, including cell adhesion molecules, proteoglycans and tenascins. While several of these molecules may act as permissive molecular factors to allow glial and neuronal remodeling (Theodosis et al. 2004a), they can also intervene more directly in neuron-glia interactions. They are large, complex, often charged molecules that can hinder access to receptors and transporters. In addition, they can interact homo- and heterophilically, between each other and/or with other ECM components, interactions that can affect neuronal activity (see for example, Dityatev and Schachner, 2003). Where astrocytic processes are withdrawn, therefore, the expression of such molecules will be absent or reduced (Theodosis et al. 1999), which will modify further intercellular communication and dynamic cell interactions.

Thirdly, since astrocytic processes possess many neurotransmitter receptors, transporters and ion channels (Danbolt 2001; Verkhratsky et al. 1998), they can sense activity in neighboring neurons. Indeed, as shown by numerous recent studies, astrocytes intervene actively in neuronal communication (Araque et al. 1999) and are considered integral parts of the synapse, which is now termed "tripartite" and seen to consist of pre- and post-synaptic neuronal elements and a glial component (Haydon 2001). In this context, then, a modified ensheathment of synapses will have important consequences on neurotransmission, especially that due to the excitatory amino acid, glutamate. This is because astrocytic processes in the vicinity of glutamatergic synapses, because of their high content of glutamate transporters, limit glutamate spillover and are therefore critical for the maintenance of point-to-point synaptic transmission (Oliet et al. 2001). As clearly shown by the SON of lactating animals, a reduction of astrocytic coverage will enhance levels of ambient glutamate (Oliet et al. 2001). Glutamate then stimulates inhibitory metabotropic receptors at presynaptic sites of glutamate and even neighboring GABA synapses and results in homo- and heterosynaptic depression of neurotransmitter release (see Oliet et al. 2004). A reduced synaptic efficacy at glutamatergic synapses will also give rise to a decrease in background synaptic noise, which renders the neuron more electrically compact, increasing input resistance and the gain of the input-output neuronal response (Oliet et al. 2004). Such changes may be critical for tuning the responsiveness of neurons to pertinent synaptic information. In addition, astrocytes can potentiate inhibitory neurotransmission by activating presynaptic GABA-B receptors, an effect that is also potentiated by glutamate (Kang et al. 1998).

Fourth, the extracellular space is a kind of communication channel for molecules implicated in extrasynaptic or volume transmission (reviewed in Sykova 2004). A physical lack of astrocytic processes, therefore, could potentially facilitate diffusion of neurotransmitters like glutamate, GABA, and catecholamines to sites distant from their release (Piet et al. 2004), which could then allow crosstalk between neighboring synapses and neurons. In the same vein, facilitated diffusion of neureptides like OT and VP could contribute to their autocrine and paracrine actions (Moos et al. 1998; Ludwig and Pittman 2003).

Fifth, retraction of astrocytic processes will have further direct effects on neuronal function by affecting gliotransmission. It is now generally admitted that astrocytes themselves release different signalling molecules, or gliotransmitters, such as glutamate (Kang et al. 1998), D-serine (Wolosker et al. 1999; Panatier et al. 2006), taurine (Hussy 2002), and ATP (Gordon et al. 2005; Neumann 2003; Fields and Burnstock 2006) and these can mediate astrocyte-neuron cross-talk (Oliet and Mothet 2006) and affect further neuronal excitability (Volterra and Meldolesi 2005). Thus, glutamate (Kang et al. 1998) and D-serine (Miller 2004; Panatier et al. 2006), acting as gliotransmitters, activate NMDA receptors. The degree of astrocytic coverage of neurons will then govern the level of glycine site occupancy of these receptors, thereby affecting their availability for activation. Besides the direct effects on glutamatergic transmission, this means that the activity dependence of long-term synaptic changes, whose direction and magnitude depend on the number of NMDA receptors activated during afferent input stimulation, is also affected. This effect is clearly illustrated in the SON. Its astrocytes are enriched in D-serine, the endogenous coagonist of NMDA receptors in this hypothalamic area (Panatier et al. 2006), where the levels of D-serine and therefore the occupancy of NMDA receptors are controlled by astrocytic coverage. In this nucleus, then, NMDA-dependent phenomena like LTP and LTD are modified by its glial remodeling so that, on withdrawal of astrocytic processes, the number of activated NMDA receptors is reduced and the activity dependence of long-term synaptic changes is shifted towards higher activity values.

Finally, besides direct effects, astrocytic withdrawal can have indirect consequences on neuronal function by favoring synapse formation. As noted earlier, changes in astrocytic coverage in hypothalamic neuroendocrine centers like the SON and arcuate

decreasing the number of inhibitory GABAergic inputs impinging on the neurons. In the median eminence, as in the neurohypophysis, concurrent retraction of glial processes and tanycyte end feet from the perivascular area exposes GnRH terminals directly to the portal capillaries (King and Rubin 1995; De Serrano et al. 2004), thereby facilitating diffusion of GnRH into the general circulation.

Cell Mechanisms Underlying Astro-neuronal Plasticity

Permissive Molecular Factors

The structural plasticity described in this review connotes interactions that will bring into play cell surface and ECM molecules, as well as soluble factors, many of which have been identified by molecular neurobiology in developing systems undergoing similar glial and neuronal transformations. In the developing brain, the effects of these molecules result from mutual interactions and via activation of intracellular signal transduction mechanisms through diverse cell surface receptors, ultimately determining the architecture of nervous tissue. It is not too surprising, then, that adult neural systems capable of remodeling continue to express many of these "juvenile" molecules. The list includes cell adhesion molecules like the cadherins, neurexins and those like NCAM that belong to the immunoglobulin superfamily. Complex ECM glycoproteins, like the chondroitin sulphate proteoglycans and tenascins, as well as their receptors, also contribute (Theodosis et al. 2004a; Kleene and Schachner 2004; Waites et al. 2005; Dalva et al. 2007). There are many excellent reviews describing these molecules and their contributions to cell interactions, especially in the context of axon outgrowth and synaptic plasticity (see, for example, Levinson and El-Husseini 2005; Dityatev and Schachner 2003). We will focus here on NCAM, and in particular, its highly sialylated isoform, PSA-NCAM, since we have strong evidence that this cell surface molecule does intervene in astro-neuronal remodeling.

While PSA-NCAM is abundant in developing tissues, most adult tissues contain NCAM with little PSA. However, PSA-NCAM continues to be strongly expressed in adult systems endowed with the capacity for morphological plasticity (Bonfanti et al. 1992; Seki and Arai 1993; Bonfanti 2006). Thus, in the HNS, PSA-NCAM is made by astrocytes and neurons throughout life (Theodosis et al. 1991; Kiss et al. 1993; Theodosis et al. 1999). In some systems, like the hippocampus, PSA-NCAM expression is linked to synaptic activity (Kiss and Muller 2001), but in the HNS (Pierre et al. 2001), its expression is constitutive and not markedly affected by neuronal activity. Nevertheless, it is a prerequisite for all dynamic phases of plasticity. Thus, specific enzymatic removal of PSA from NCAM in the SON in situ inhibited glial and neuronal remodeling associated with lactation and chronic dehydration; there was no effect if PSA was removed once morphological changes in the nuclei had already taken place (Theodosis et al. 1999). Likewise, PSA removal from cell surfaces in the neurohypophysis prevented stimulation-related induction and reversal of axonal and glial changes but had no effect once remodeling had occurred (Monlezun et al. 2005). A similar strong, quite constant expression characterizes PSA-NCAM in the GnRH system of rodents (Bonfanti et al. 1992; Hoyk et al. 2001), sheep (Viguié et al. 2001) and primates (Perera et al. 1994), and in this system as well, removal of PSA inhibits the onset of astrocytic and synaptic changes associated with reproductive status (Hoyk et al. 2001). How PSA intervenes to permit morphological changes remains undetermined, but a possible mechanism is that large quantities of the carbohydrate on cell surfaces attenuate adhesion via physical impedance or charge repulsion (Rutishauser and Landmesser 1996). Cells can then detach from their neighbors or from the extracellular matrix and undergo changes in their conformation.

We consider that a molecule like NCAM to be permissive for morphological plasticity because its expression, while not tightly linked to neuronal activity in the neuroendocrine centers, appears obligatory for their morphological plasticity. This was clearly evident from enzyme perturbation experiments (Theodosis et al. 1999; Hoyk et al. 2001; Monlezun et al. 2005). Nonetheless, there can be compensatory replacement by other molecules, since remodeling occurs in lactating and salt-loaded mice genetically deficient in NCAM (Theodosis et al. 2004b), which reflects a redundancy in the molecular systems permitting such plasticity. Similar phenomena have been described in other neuronal systems in which NCAM is highly expressed and which continue to undergo plasticity in NCAM -/- mutants (Durbec and Cremer 2001). In a sense, the specific identity of molecules that are permissive for remodeling may not be important provided that they activate the same intracellular mechanism. On the other hand, the response of neurons and astrocytes implicated in remodeling would be invariant and independent of the identity of the factor, provided the proper stimulus intervenes.

Signaling Molecules

If molecules like PSA-NCAM act as primers, providing a permissive environment for remodeling, then there must be molecules whose expression is particular to each potentially plastic system that act as specific stimuli, triggering cascades of intracellular events that result in glial and neuronal transformations. Such molecules include those expressed at the onset of enhanced activity to bring on remodeling as well as molecules, not necessarily identical to the former, that signal the system to revert to its original condition. There are many candidates for such functions, including neuropeptides, neurotransmitters, steroids and trophic factors that are released by neighboring elements. Nevertheless, we still have little knowledge of how these signaling pathways consequently operate, through genomic and non-genomic pathways, to influence the morphology of the brain's cells and its synaptic wiring.

In the OT system, parturition and lactation, the conditions in which plasticity is most striking, are characterized by enhanced peripheral release of OT and by increased secretion within the hypothalamic nuclei. Central OT has a positive feedback action on the activity of its own system (Jourdain et al. 1998; Israel et al. 2003a; de Kock et al. 2003). It can also induce its morphological plasticity, since intracerebroventricular infusion of the peptide, presumably mimicking this central release, induced neuronal-glial and synaptic changes in the SON similar to those detected during lactation (Theodosis et al. 1986b). These effects can be reproduced in vitro, in acute slices of the adult hypothalamus, a preparation that allows pharmacological manipulation. We were thus able to determine that the neuropeptide acts specifically via its receptors since its action was mimicked by close analogues and inhibited with specific OT receptor antagonists (Langle et al. 2003). Addition of even structurally similar peptides like VP had no effect.

The receptor-mediated action of the neuropeptide may explain why morphological changes in the HNS are specific to its OT system. In the hypothalamic magnocellular nuclei, OT receptors occur on OT but not on VP neurons (Barberis and Tribollet 1996); they are present on astrocytes as well (Guenot-Di Scala and Strosser 1992).

Nevertheless, OT does not act alone but in synergy with sexual steroids, especially estrogens (Montagnese et al. 1990; Langle et al. 2003; Theodosis et al. 2006). In view of the rapidity of the effects of the steroid (Langle et al. 2003; Theodosis et al. 2006), it is probable that it acts via a plasmalemmal mechanism (Revankar et al. 2005), mobilizing intracellular Ca^{2+} and ultimately inducing remodeling. Such a mechanism is likely when one considers the extremely rapid beneficial effects of the steroid on the electrical activity of OT neurons (Israel and Poulain 2000), their gene expression (Crowley and Amico 1993) and central and peripheral release (Yamaguchi et al. 1979; Wang et al. 1995). It is noteworthy that estrogens affect OT gene regulation if treatment is accompanied by a progesterone withdrawal protocol (Amico et al. 1995), as in the endocrine conditions characterizing the end of gestation (Bridges 1984) when remodeling occurs under physiological conditions. Nevertheless, although OT, with or without steroids, appears essential for remodeling in the magnocellular nuclei, there are other candidates for such signaling and OT may act in a secondary fashion, by facilitating their expression.

Of these, glutamate is an excellent candidate since it can serve as a bi-directional signal to transfer information between activated neurons and adjacent astrocytes. In the cerebellum, activation of AMPA receptors on Bergmann glia is required for the maintenance of neuron-glia interrelationships (Iino et al. 2001). It is to be expected, then, that changes in glutamate transmission may lead to rapid and concerted modifications in the morphology of neurons and their astrocytes. In the SON, exposure to a combination of metabotropic and ionotropic glutamate receptor antagonists prevented OT/estrogen-mediated remodeling (Langle et al. 2003). Likewise, such a treatment inhibits the appearance of new GABA synapses (Trailin, Israel and Theodosis, unpublished observations). This finding strongly suggests that glutamate itself may be a more immediate signaling agent than OT. In the preoptic area of the hypothalamus, a mediator of astro-neuronal communication via glutamate appears to be prostaglandin-estrogen2 (PGE2). PGE2 induces astrocytic release of glutamate, which in turn activates glutamate receptors on adjacent neurons, an effect that can have important consequences on neuronal morphology and dendritic spine formation (Amateu and McCarthy, 2002).

Another neurotransmitter that may signal glial-neuronal changes is nitric oxide (NO). Electron microscopic observations of the external layer of the median eminence indicate that vascular endothelial cells use a signaling pathway mediated by NO to regulate neuronal-glial plasticity (De Serrano et al. 2004). Thus, activation of endogenous NO release induced a rapid structural remodeling resulting in the freeing of GnRH terminals from ensheathing astrocytic processes.

Other excellent signaling candidates are the purines, especially in the neurohypophysis. Neurohypophysial pituicytes possess purinergic receptors (Loesch and Burnstock 2001; Rosso et al. 2002), ATP can be released from neurosecretory granules in the terminals (Sperlagh et al. 1999), and adenosine, secondary to the metabolism of ATP, induces pituicyte stellation (Miyata et al. 1999; Rosso et al. 2002). Activated Rho A GTPase activation is a key event in coupling purine receptor activation and stellation (Rosso et al. 2002). In line with these results are preliminary observations of the SON in the acute slice preparation, where adenosine can substitute for OT in inducing glial and neuronal changes similar to those visible under physiological conditions (Trailin, Oliet, Poulain and Theodosis, unpublished observations).

Finally, there is abundant evidence indicating that gonadal steroids on their own signal the onset of morphological changes. As noted earlier, estrogen can substitute for OT, at least in vitro, to induce neuronal-glial (Langle et al. 2003) and synaptic (Theodosis et al. 2006) changes in the SON. In the arcuate nucleus, administration of one single dose of 17ß-estradiol resulting in plasma levels similar to those at proestrus induced a change in synaptic numbers and astrocytic transformations similar to those detected at proestrus (Garcia-Segura et al. 1994). GnRH neurons themselves do not express estrogen receptors, so the effects of the steroid must be mediated through effects on presynaptic axons and/or astrocytes (Witkin et al. 1991). Indeed, in this area of the hypothalamus, not only are astrocytes targets for estrogen action, they themselves release factors that could affect neuron-glia interactions. Thus, gonadal steroids facilitate astrocytic expression of growth factors of the epidermal growth factor family and their tyrosine kinase receptors, thereby contributing to neuron-glia signaling intervening at the initiation of puberty (Ojeda and Ma 1999). Moreover, median eminence astrocytes and tanycytes release factors like PGE2 that contribute to estrogen-induced synaptic remodeling in the arcuate nucleus and to GnRH terminal remodeling in the external layer of the median eminence (Ojeda and Ma 1999; Garcia-Segura and McCarthy 2004).

References

Aldskogius H, Liu L, Svensson M (1999) Glial responses to synaptic damage and plasticity. J Neurosci Res 58:33–41

Amateu SK, McCarthy MM (2002) A novel mechanism of dendritic spine plasticity involving estradiol induction by prostaglandin-E2. J Neurosci 22:8586–8596

Amico JA, Crowley RS, Insel TR, Thomas A, O'Keefe JA (1995) Effect of gonadal steroids upon hypothalamic oxytocin expression. Adv Exp Med Biol 395:23–36

Araque A, Parpura V, Sanzgiri RP, Haydon PG (1999) Tripartite synapses: glia, the unacknowledged partner. Trends Neurosci 22:208–215

Armstrong WE, Stern JE (1998) Phenotypic and state-dependent expression of the electrical and morphological properties of oxytocin and vasopressin neurones. Prog Brain Res 119:101–113

Bailey CH, Kandel ER (1993) Structural changes accompanying memory storage. Annu Rev Physiol 55:397–426

Barberis C, Tribollet E (1996) Vasopressin and oxytocin receptors in the central nervous system. Crit Rev Neurobiol 10:119–154

Bobak JB, Salm AK (1996) Plasticity of astrocytes of the ventral glial limitans subjacent to the supraoptic nucleus. J Comp Neurol 376:188–197

Bonfanti L (2006) PSA-NCAM in mammalian structural plasticity and neurogenesis. Prog Neurobiol 80:129–164

Bonfanti L, Olive S, Poulain DA, Theodosis DT (1992) Mapping of the distribution of polysialylated neural cell adhesion molecule throughout the central nervous system of the adult rat: an immunohistochemical study. Neuroscience 49:419–436

Bonfanti L, Poulain DA, Theodosis DT (1993) Radial glia-like cells in the supraoptic nucleus of the adult rat. J Neuroendocrinol 5:1–6

Bridges RS (1984) A quantitative analysis of the roles of dosage, sequence, and duration of estradiol and progesterone exposure in the regulation of maternal behavior in the rat. Endocrinology 114:930–940

Burbach JPH, Luckman SM, Murphy D, Gainer H (2001) Gene regulation in the magnocellular hypothalamo-neurohypophysial system. Physiol Rev 81:1197–1267

Chapman DB, Theodosis DT, Montagnese C, Poulain DA, Morris JF (1986) Osmotic stimulation causes structural plasticity of neurone-glia relationships of the oxytocin but not vasopressin secreting neurones in the hypothalamic supraoptic nucleus. Neuroscience 17:679–686

Coles JA, Poulain DA (1991) Extracellular K+ in the supraoptic nucleus of the rat during reflex bursting activity by oxytocin neurones. J Physiol 439:383–409

Crowley RS, Amico JA (1993) Gonadal steroid modulation of oxytocin and vasopressin gene expression in the hypothalamus of the osmotically stimulated rat. Endocrinology 133:2711–2718

Daftary SS, Boudaba C, Szabo K, Tasker JG (1998) Noradrenergic excitation of magnocellular neurons in the rat hypothalamic paraventricular nucleus via intranuclear glutamatergic circuits. J Neurosci 18:10619–10628

Dalva MB, McClelland AC, Kayser MS (2007) Cell adhesion molecules: signaling functions at the synapse. Nature Rev Neurosci 8:206–220

Danbolt NC (2001) Glutamate uptake. Prog Neurobiol 65:1–105

Day TA, Ferguson AV, Renaud LP (1984) Facilitatory influence of noradrenergic afferents on the excitability of rat paraventricular nucleus neurosecretory cells. J Physiol 355:237–249

de Kock CPJ, Wierda KDB, Bosman LWJ, Min R, Koksma JJ, Mansvelder HD, Verhage M, Brussaard AB (2003) Somatodendritic secretion in oxytocin neurons is upregulated during the female reproductive cycle. J Neurosci 23:2726–2734

De Serrano S, Estrella C, Loyens A, Cornea A, Ojeda SR, Beauvillain JC, Prevot V (2004) Vascular endothelial cells promote acute plasticity in ependymoglial cells of the neuroendocrine brain. J Neurosci 24:10353–10363

Dityatev A, Schachner M (2003) Extracellular matrix molecules and synaptic plasticity. Nature Rev Neurosci 4:456–468

Durbec P, Cremer H (2001) Revisiting the function of PSA-NCAM in the nervous system. Mol Neurobiol 24:53–64

El Majdoubi M, Poulain DA, Theodosis DT (1997) Lactation-induced plasticity in the supraoptic nucleus augments axodendritic and axosomatic gabaergic and glutamatergic synapses: an ultrastructural analysis using the disector method. Neuroscience 80:1137–1147

Fenelon VS, Theodosis DT, Poulain DA (1994) Fos synthesis in identified magnocellular neurons varies with phenotype, stimulus, location in the hypothalamus and reproductive state. Brain Res 662:165–177

Fields RD, Burnstock G (2006) Purinergic signalling in neuron-glia interactions. Nature Rev Neurosci 7:423–436

Garcia-Segura LM, McCarthy MM (2004) Minireview: role of glia in neuroendocrine function. Endocrinology 145:1082–1086

Garcia-Segura LM, Chowen JA, Parducz A, Naftolin F (1994) Gonadal hormones as promoters of structural synaptic plasticity: cellular mechanisms. Prog Neurobiol 44:279–307

Gies U, Theodosis DT (1994) Synaptic plasticity in the rat supraoptic nucleus during lactation involves GABA innervation and oxytocin neurons: a quantitative immunocytochemical analysis. J Neurosci 14:2861–2869

Gordon GR, Baimoukhametova DV, Hewitt SA, Rajapaksha WR, Fisher TE, Bains JS (2005) Norepinephrine triggers release of glial ATP to increase postsynaptic efficacy. Nature Neurosci 8:1078–1086

Grosche J, Matyash V, Möller T, Verkhratsky A, Reichenbach A, Kettenmann H (1999) Microdomains for neuron-glia interaction: parallel fiber signaling to Bergmann glial cells. Nature Neurosci 2:139–143

Guenot-Di Scala D, Strosser M-T (1992) Oxytocin receptors on cultured astroglial cells. Kinetic and pharmacological characterization of oxytocin-binding sites on intact hypothalamic and hippocampic cells from foetal rat brain. Biochem J 284:491–497

Halassa MM, Fellin T, Takano H, Dong J-H, Haydon PG (2007) Synaptic islands defined by the territory of a single astrocyte. J Neurosci 27:6473–6477

Hatton GI, Perlmutter LS, Salm AK, Tweedle CD (1984) Dynamic neuronal-glial interactions in hypothalamus and pituitary: implications for control of hormone synthesis and release. Peptides 5:121–138

Hawrylak N, Boone D, Salm AK (1999) The surface of glial fibrillary acidic protein immunopositive astrocytic processes in the rat supraoptic nucleus is reversibly altered by dehydration and rehydration. Neurosci Lett 277:57–60

Haydon PG (2001) Glia: listening and talking to the synapse. Nature Rev Neurosci 2:185–193

Hirrlinger J, Hülsmann S, Kirchhoff F (2004) Astroglial processes show spontaneous motility at active synaptic terminals in situ. Eur J Neurosci 20:2235–2239

Hoyk Zs, Parducz A, Theodosis DT (2001) The highly sialylated isoform of the neural cell adhesion molecule is required for estradiol-induced morphological synaptic plasticity in the adult arcuate nucleus. Eur J Neurosci 13:649–656

Hussy N (2002) Glial cells in the hypothalamo-neurohypophysial system: key elements of the regulation of neuronal activity and secretory activity. Prog Brain Res 139:113–139

Iino M, Goto K, Kakegawa W, Okado H, Sudo M, Ishiuchi S, Miwa A, Takayasu Y, Saito I, Tsuzuki K, Ozawa S (2001) Glia-synapse interaction through Ca^{2+}-permeable AMPA receptors in Bergmann glia. Science 292:926–929

Israel J-M, Poulain DA (2000) 17 beta-oestradiol modulates in vitro electrical properties and responses to kainate of oxytocin neurones in lactating rats. J Physiol 524:457–470

Israel J-M, Le Masson G, Theodosis DT, Poulain DA (2003a) Glutamate afferent input governs periodicity and synchronisation of bursting electrical activity in oxytocin neurons. Eur J Neurosci 17:2619–2629

Israel J-M, Schipke CG, Ohlemeyer C, Theodosis DT, Kettenmann H (2003b) GABA-A receptor-expressing astrocytes in the supraoptic nucleus lack glutamate uptake and receptor currents. Glia 44:102–110

Jourdain P, Israel J-M, Dupouy B, Oliet SHR, Allard M, Vitiello S, Theodosis DT, Poulain DA (1998) Evidence for a hypothalamic oxytocin-sensitive pattern-generating network governing oxytocin neurons in vitro. J Neurosci 18:6641–6649

Kang J, Jiang L, Goldman SA, Nedergaard M (1998) Astrocyte-mediated potentiation of inhibitory synaptic transmission. Nature Neurosci 1:683–692

King JC, Rubin BS (1995) Dynamic alterations in luteinizing hormone-releasing hormone (LHRH) neuronal cell bodies and terminals of adult rats. Cell Mol Neurobiol 15:89–106

Kiss JZ, Wang C, Rougon G (1993) Nerve-dependent expression of high polysialic acid neural cell adhesion molecule in neurohypophysial astrocytes of adult rats. Neuroscience 53:213–222

Kiss JZ, Muller D (2001) Contribution of the neural cell adhesion molecule to neuronal and synaptic plasticity. Rev Neurosci 12:297–310

Kleene R, Schachner M (2004) Glycans and neural cell interactions. Nature Rev Neurosci 5:195–208

Landgraf R, Neumann ID (2004) Neuropeptide release within the brain: a dynamic concept of multiple and variable modes of communication. Front Neuroendocrinol 25:150–176

Langle SL, Poulain DA, Theodosis DT (2003) Induction of rapid, activity-dependent neuronal-glial remodeling in the adult hypothalamus in vitro. Eur J Neurosci 18:206–214

Leng G, Shibuki K (1986) Extracellular potassium changes in the rat neurohypophysis during activation of the magnocellular neurosecretory system. J Physiol 392:97–111

Levinson JN, El-Husseini A (2005) Building excitatory and inhibitory synapses: balancing neuroligin partnerships. Neuron 48:171–174

Lightman SL, Young III WS (1989) Lactation inhibits stress mediated secretion of corticosterone and oxytocin and hypothalamic accumulation of CRF and enkephalin messenger ribonucleic acids. Endocrinology 124:2358–2364

Loesch A, Burnstock G (2001) Immunoreactivity to P2X6 receptors in the rat hypothalamo-neurohypophysial system: an ultrastructural study with extravidin and colloidal gold-silver labelling. Neuroscience 106:621–631

Luckman SM, Bicknell RJ (1991) Morphological plasticity that occurs in the neurohypophysis following activation of the magnocellular neurosecretory system can be mimicked in vitro by beta-adrenergic stimulation. Neuroscience 39:701–709

Ludwig M, Pittman QJ (2003) Talking back: dendritic neurotransmitter release. Trends Neurosci 26:255–261

Magistretti P, Pellerin L, Rothman DL, Shulman RG (1999) Energy on demand. Science 283:496–497

Michaloudi HC, El Majdoubi M, Poulain DA, Papadopoulos GC, Theodosis DT (1997) The noradrenergic innervation of identified hypothalamic somata and its contribution to lactation-induced synaptic plasticity. J Neuroendocrinol 9:17–23

Miller RF (2004) D-Serine as a glial modulator of nerve cells. Glia 47:275–283

Mitchell SJ, Silver RA (2000) Glutamate spillover suppresses inhibition by activating presynaptic mGluRs. Nature 404:498–502

Miyata S, Hatton GI (2002) Activity-related, dynamic neuron-glia interactions in the hypothalamo-neurohypophysial system. Microsc Res Tech 56:143–157

Miyata S, Furuya K, Nakai S, Bun H, Kiyohara T (1999) Morphological plasticity and rearrangement of cytoskeletons in pituicytes cultured from adult rat neurohypophyses. Neurosci Res 33:299–306

Monlezun S, Ouali S, Poulain DA, Theodosis DT (2005) Polysialic acid is required for active phases of morphological plasticity of neurosecretory axons and their glia. Mol Cell Neurosci 29:516–524

Montagnese C, Poulain DA, Vincent JD, Theodosis DT (1987) Structural plasticity in the rat supraoptic nucleus during gestation, post-partum lactation and suckling-induced pseudogestation and lactation. J Endocrinol 115:97–105

Montagnese C, Poulain DA, Theodosis DT (1990) Influence of ovarian steroids on the ultrastructural plasticity of the adult supraoptic nucleus induced by central administration of oxytocin. J Neuroendocrinol 2:225–231

Moos FC (1995) GABA-induced facilitation of the periodic bursting activity of oxytocin neurones in suckled rats. J Physiol 488:103–114

Moos F, Gouzènes L, Brown D, Dayanithi G, Sabatier N, Boissin L, Rabie A, Richard P (1998) New aspects of firing pattern autocontrol in oxytocin and vasopressin neurones. Adv Exp Med Biol 449:153–162

Newman EA (2003) Glial cell inhibition of neurons by release of ATP. J Neurosci 23:1659–1666

Nothias F, Fischer I, Murray M, Simone M, Vincent JD (1996) Expression of a phosphorylated isoform of MAP1B is maintained in adult central nervous system areas that retain capacity for structural plasticity. J Comp Neurol 368:317–334

Ojeda SR, Ma YJ (1999) Glial-neuronal interactions in the neuroendocrine control of mammalian puberty: facilitatory effects of gonadal steroids. J Neurobiol 40:528–540

Oliet SHR, Mothet J-P (2006) Molecular determinants of D-serine-mediated gliotransmission: from release to function. Glia 54:726–737

Oliet SHR, Piet R, Poulain DA (2001) Control of glutamate clearance and synaptic efficacy by glial coverage of neurons. Science 292:923–926

Oliet SHR, Piet R, Poulain DA, Theodosis DT (2004) Glial modulation of synaptic transmission: insights from the hypothalamic supraoptic nucleus. Glia 47:258–267

Panatier A, Theodosis DT, Mothet J-P, Touquet B, Pollegioni L, Poulain DA, Oliet SHR (2006) Glial control of NMDA receptor activity contributes to synaptic memory. Cell 125:775–784

Parker SL, Crowley WR (1993) Stimulation of oxytocin release in the lactating rat by a central interaction of alpha-1-adrenergic and alpha-amino-3-hydroxy-5-methylisoxazole-4-propionic acid-sensitive excitatory amino acid mechanisms. Endocrinology 133:2855–2860

Perea G, Araque A (2005) Properties of synaptically evoked astrocyte calcium signal reveal synaptic information processing by astrocytes. J Neurosci 25:2192–2203

Perera AD, Lagenaur CF, Plant TM (1994) Postnatal expression of polysialic acid-neural cell adhesion molecule (PSA-NCAM) in the hypothalamus of the male rhesus monkey (Macaca mulatta). Endocrinology 133:2729–2735

Perlmutter LS, Hatton GI, Tweedle CD (1984) Plasticity in the in vitro neurohypophysis: effects of osmotic changes on pituicytes. Neuroscience 12:503–511

Pierre K, Bonhomme R, Dupouy B, Poulain DA, Theodosis DT (2001) The polysialylated Neural Cell Adhesion Molecule (PSA-NCAM) reaches cell surfaces of hypothalamic neurons and astrocytes via the constitutive pathway. Neuroscience 103:133–142

Piet R, Bonhomme R, Theodosis DT, Poulain DA, Oliet SHR (2003) Modulation of GABAergic transmission by endogenous glutamate in the rat supraoptic nucleus. Eur J Neurosci 17:1777–1785

Piet R, Vargova L, Sykova E, Poulain DA, Oliet SHR (2004) Physiological contribution of the astrocytic environment of neurons to intersynaptic crosstalk. Proc Natl Acad Sci USA 101:2151–2155

Pinto S, Roseberry AG, Liu H, Diano S, Shanabrough M, Cai X, Friedman JM, Horvath TL (2004) Rapid rewiring of arcuate nucleus feeding circuits by leptin. Science 304:110–115

Poulain DA, Wakerley JB (1982) Electrophysiology of hypothalamic magnocellular neurones secreting oxytocin and vasopressin. Neuroscience 7:773–808

Revankar CM, Cimino DF, Sklar LA, Arterburn JB, Prossnitz ER (2005) A transmembrane intracellular estrogen receptor mediates rapid cell signaling. Science 307:1625–1630

Rosso L, Peteri-Brunbäck B, Vouret-Craviari V, Deroanne C, Troadec J-D, Thirion S, Van Obberghen-Schilling E, Mienville J-M (2002) Rho A inhibition is a key step in pituicyte stellation induced by A1-type adenosine receptor activation. Glia 38:351–362

Rutishauser U, Landmesser LT (1996) Polysialic acid in the vertebrate nervous system: a promoter of plasticity in cell-cell interactions. Trends Neurosci 19:422–427

Seki T, Arai Y (1993) Distribution and possible roles of the highly polysialylated neural cell adhesion molecule (NCAM-H) in the developing and adult central nervous system. Neurosci Res 17:265–290

Smithson KG, Suarez I, Hatton GI (1990) Beta-adrenergic stimulation decreases glial and increases neural contact with the basal lamina in rat neurointermediate lobes incubated in vitro. J Neuroendocrinol 2:693–699

Sperlagh B, Mergl Zs, Juranyi Zs, Vizi ES, Makara GB (1999) Local regulation of vasopressin and oxytocin secretion by extracellular ATP in the isolated posterior lobe of the rat hypophysis. J Endocrinol 160:343–350

Sykova E (2004) Extrasynaptic volume transmission and diffusion parameters of the extracellular space. Neuroscience 129:861–876

Theodosis DT (2002) Oxytocin-secreting neurons: a physiological model of morphological neuronal and glial plasticity in the adult hypothalamus. Front Neuroendocrinol 23:101–135

Theodosis DT, MacVicar BA (1996) Neuron-glia interactions in the hypothalamus and pituitary. Tr Neurosci 19:363–367

Theodosis DT, Poulain DA (1987) Oxytocin-secreting neurones : a physiological model for structural plasticity in the adult mammalian brain. Trends Neurosci 10:426–430

Theodosis DT, Poulain DA (1989) Neuronal-glial and synaptic plasticity in the adult rat paraventricular nucleus. Brain Res 484:361–366

Theodosis DT, Chapman DB, Montagnese C, Poulain DA, Morris JF (1986a) Structural plasticity in the hypothalamic supraoptic nucleus at lactation affects oxytocin- but not vasopressin-secreting neurones. Neuroscience 17:661–678

Theodosis DT, Montagnese C, Rodriguez F, Vincent JD, Poulain DA (1986b) Oxytocin induces morphological plasticity in the adult hypothalamo-neurohypophysial system. Nature 322:738–740

Theodosis DT, Paut L, Tappaz ML (1986c) Immunocytochemical analysis of the GABAergic innervation of oxytocin- and vasopressin-secreting neurones in the rat supraoptic nucleus. Neuroscience 19:207–222

Theodosis DT, Rougon G, Poulain DA (1991) Retention of embryonic features by an adult neuronal system capable of plasticity: Polysialylated N-CAM in the hypothalamo-neurohypophysial system. Proc Natl Acad Sci USA 88:5494–5498

Theodosis DT, Bonhomme R, Vitiello S, Rougon G, and Poulain DA (1999) Cell surface expression of polysialic acid on NCAM is a prerequisite for activity-dependent morphological neuronal and glial plasticity. J Neurosci 19:10228–10236

Theodosis DT, Piet R, Poulain DA, Oliet SHR (2004a) Neuronal,glial and synaptic remodeling in the adult hypothalamus: functional consequences and role of cell surface and extracellular matrix adhesion molecules. Neurochem Int 45:491–501

Theodosis DT, Schachner M, Neumann ID (2004b) Oxytocin neuron activation in NCAM-deficient mice: anatomical and functional consequences. Eur J Neurosci 20:3270–3280

Theodosis DT, Trailin A, Poulain DA (2005) Remodeling of astrocytes, a prerequisite for synapse turnover in th adult brain? Insights from the oxytocin system of the hypothalamus. Am J Physiol Regul Integr Comp Physiol 290:R1175–R1182

Theodosis DT, Koksma JJ, Trailin A, Langle SL, Piet R, Lodder JC, Timmerman J, Mansvelder H, Poulain DA, Oliet SHR, Brussaard AB (2006) Oxytocin and estrogen promote rapid synapse formation of functional GABA synapses in the adult supraoptic nucleus. Mol Cell Neurosci 31:785–794

Theodosis DT, Poulain DA, Oliet SHR (2008) Physiological glial-neuronal plasticity in the adult brain. Physiol Rev, in press

Tweedle CD, Hatton GI (1982) Magnocellular neuropeptidergic terminals in neurohypophysis: rapid glial release of enclosed axons during parturition. Brain Res Bull 8:205–209

Tweedle CD, Hatton GI (1987) Morphological adaptability at neurosecretory axonal endings on the neurovascular contact zone of the rat neurohypophysis. Neuroscience 20:241–246

Verkhratsky A, Orkand RK, Kettenmann H (1998) Glial calcium: homeostasis and signaling function. Physiol Rev 78:99–141

Viguié C, Jansen HT, Glass JD, Watanabe M, Billings HJ, Coolen L, Lehman MN, Karsch FJ (2001) Potential for polysialylated form of neural cell adhesio molecule-mediated neuroplasticity within the gonadotropin-releasing hormone neurosecretory system of the ewe. Endocrinology 142:1317–1324

Voisin DL, Herbison AE, Poulain DA (1995) Central inhibitory effects of muscimol and bicuculline on the milk ejection reflex in the anaesthetized rat. J Physiol 483:211–224

Volterra A, Meldolesi J (2005) Astrocytes, from brain glue to communication elements: the revolution continues. Nature Rev Neurosci 6:626–640

Waites CL, Craig AM, Garner CC (2005) Mechanisms of vertebrate synaptogenesis. Annu Rev Neurosci ARI:251–274

Wang H, Ward AR, Morris JF (1995) Oestradiol acutely stimulates exocytosis of oxytocin and vasopressin from dendrites and somata of hypothalamic magnocellular neurons. Neuroscience 68:1179–1188

Witkin JW, Ferin M, Popilskis SJ, Silverman A-J (1991) Effects of gonadal steroids on the ultrastructure of GnRH neurons in the rhesus monkey: synaptic input and glial apposition. Endocrinology 129:1083–1092

Wolosker H, Sheth KN, Takahashi M, Mothet J-P, Brady ROJr, Ferris CD, Snyder SH (1999) Purification of serine racemase: biosynthesis of the neuromodulator D-serine. Proc Natl Acad Sci USA 96:721–725

Yamaguchi K, Akaishi T, Negoro H (1979) Effects of estrogen treatment on plasma oxytocin and vasopressin in ovariectomised rats. Endocrinol Jpn 26:197–205

Neuroendocrine Mechanisms Underlying the Intergenerational Transmission of Maternal Behavior and Infant Abuse in Rhesus Macaques

Dario Maestripieri[1]

Summary

Parenting style in rhesus macaques (*Macaca mulatta*) can vary dramatically among individuals along the two orthogonal dimensions of maternal protectiveness and maternal rejection. High rates of maternal rejection can be accompanied by infant abuse. We investigated the effects of exposure to variable parenting styles on offspring behavioral and neuroendocrine development to identify the possible mechanisms underlying the intergenerational transmission of maternal behavior and infant abuse. Forty-three non-crossfostered male and female infants and 16 crossfostered female infants were followed through their first three years of life or until they reproduced for the first time. Half of the infants were reared by abusive mothers and half by nonabusive controls. Cerebral spinal fluid (CSF) concentrations of the serotonin metabolite, 5-HIAA, were measured at six-month intervals. Abused infants were rejected more by their mothers than controls, and infants exposed to higher rates of maternal rejection had significantly lower CSF 5-HIAA in the first three years of life. When the crossfostered females gave birth for the first time, their rates of maternal rejection matched those of their foster mothers and were negatively correlated with CSF 5-HIAA. Approximately half of the females reared by the abusive mothers exhibited abusive parenting, whereas none of the females reared by controls did. The abused females who became abusive mothers had lower CSF 5-HIAA than the abused females who did not. These findings provide evidence that maternal rejection and infant abuse are transmitted across generations and suggest that experience-induced, long-term alterations in brain serotonergic function may play an important role in the intergenerational transmission of normal and abnormal parenting.

Introduction

Studies of macaques and other Old World monkeys have shown that most variability in parenting style occurs along the two orthogonal dimensions of maternal protectiveness and rejection (Tanaka 1989; Schino et al. 1995; Fairbanks 1996; Maestripieri 1998a). The maternal protectiveness dimension includes variation in the extent to which the mother physically restrains her infant, initiates proximity and contact, and cradles

[1] Department of Comparative Human Development, The University of Chicago, Chicago, IL 60637, e-mail: dario@uchicago.edu

Pfaff et al.
Hormones and Social Behavior
© Springer-Verlag Berlin Heidelberg 2008

and grooms her infant. The maternal rejection dimension includes the extent to which the mother limits the timing and duration of contact, suckling, or carrying. Although maternal behavior changes as a function of infant age and the mother's own age and experience, individual differences in parenting style are generally consistent over time and across infants (Hinde and Spencer-Booth 1971; Fairbanks 1996).

Studies of macaques and vervet monkeys have shown that exposure to a particular parenting style in infancy can have long-term effects on the offspring's behavior. For example, infants reared by highly rejecting mothers generally develop independence at an earlier age than infants reared by mothers with low rejection levels (Simpson 1985; Simpson and Simpson 1985; Simpson et al. 1989; Simpson and Datta 1990). In contrast, infants reared by more protective mothers appear to be delayed in the acquisition of their independence and are relatively fearful and cautious when faced with challenging situations (Fairbanks and McGuire 1987, 1988, 1993; Vochteloo et al. 1993). Effects of parenting style on offspring behavior can extend into adulthood (Fairbanks and McGuire 1988, 1993; Schino et al. 2001; Bardi et al. 2005; Bardi and Huffman 2006; Maestripieri et al. 2006b). These effects have also been demonstrated with experimental manipulations of maternal behavior (Vochteloo et al. 1993) and with infant crossfostering studies (Maestripieri 2005,b; Maestripieri et al. 2006b). Parenting style has also been shown to affect the offspring's parenting behavior in adulthood, as there are often significant similarities in maternal rejection between mothers and daughters (Fairbanks 1989; Berman 1990; Maestripieri 2005a; Maestripieri et al. 2007). The mechanisms underlying the intergenerational transmission of parenting style in monkeys, however, are still poorly understood.

Brain Serotonin and Naturally Occurring Variation in Primate Maternal Behavior

In the past decade, we have conducted a series of studies investigating the neurobiological and neuroendocrine mechanisms underlying the cross-generational effects of naturally occurring variation in parenting style, including infant abuse, in rhesus macaques. The project was conducted with a population of approximately 1,500 rhesus macaques living at the Field Station of the Yerkes National Primate Research Center in Lawrenceville, GA. Previous studies had shown that 5 to 10% of adult females in this population abuse their offspring and that abusive parenting runs in families, being present in some matrilines for more than six to seven generations and completely absent in others (Maestripieri et al. 1997; Maestripieri 1998b; Maestripieri and Carroll 1998a,b). At the Yerkes Field Station, the rhesus macaques are housed in large outdoor corrals, where they live in social groups of naturalistic size and composition. In our research project, the individuals are studied in their own social groups, where they have the opportunity to express naturally occurring variation in behavioral tendencies. The monkeys are trained for capture and handling, so that procedures involving experimental testing and collection of biological samples are generally brief and the subjects are immediately returned to their groups for observation.

The project involved the longitudinal study of 16 females that were crossfostered at birth between abusive and nonabusive mothers, along with 43 males and females that were born and raised by their biological mothers, half of which were abusive and half nonabusive. In addition to studying the social development and behavioral reactivity to stress of offspring exposed to variable maternal behavior in infancy, we assessed the development of hypothalamic-pituitary-adrenal (HPA) function and the functionality of brain monoamine systems, such as serotonin, dopamine, and norepinephrine, by measuring the plasma concentrations of ACTH and cortisol in a variety of experimental conditions, and by measuring the CSF concentrations of serotonin, dopamine, and norepinephrine metabolites (5-HIAA, HVA, and MHPG, respectively) at six-month intervals (see Maestripieri et al. 2006a, for details of the experimental procedures). A subset of infants and their mothers was also genotyped for the polymorphism in the serotonin transporter gene (Lesch et al. 1996), which has been shown to modulate the effects of early experience on adult behavior and psychopathology in both humans and rhesus macaques. In particular, individuals with the short (s) allele of this gene are more likely to develop anxiety disorders and dysregulation of the HPA axis as a result of early adverse experience than individuals with the long (l) allele (Lesch et al. 1996; Bennett et al. 2002; Caspi et al. 2002, 2003; Barr et al. 2004a,b). Analyses of the hormonal data are still in progress; therefore, the rest of this chapter will focus on the behavioral and brain monoamine data, with particular emphasis on serotonin.

We found that abusive mothers were significantly more likely to carry the s allele of the serotonin transporter gene than nonabusive mothers; however, there was no significant difference in the prevalence of the l and s alleles between the offspring of abusive and nonabusive mothers. Individual differences in the CSF concentrations of 5-HIAA in the offspring measured at 6, 12, 18, 24, 30, and 36 months of age were highly stable over time (see also Higley et al. 1992). Infants that were heterozygous (l/s genotype) or homozygous for the long or the short allele (l/l and s/s genotype) of the serotonin transporter gene did not differ significantly from each other in their CSF concentrations of 5-HIAA. Moreover, we found no significant variation in CSF concentrations of 5-HIAA in relation to infant abuse experienced in the first three months of life (abuse is concentrated in the first month and generally ends by the end of the third month; Maestripieri et al. 2006b). Therefore, we focused our analysis of offspring development on the effects of exposure to variable parenting style in infancy.

We found stable individual differences in many measures of maternal behavior in the first six postpartum months and, similar to previous studies, we found that these measures clustered around two factors, or parenting style dimensions: protectiveness and rejection. We obtained composite measures of these two dimensions and classified all mothers in our sample as being high or low in protectiveness and high or low in rejection depending on whether their scores were above or below the median value for the composite measures.

The individuals exposed to high rates of maternal rejection in infancy had significantly lower CSF concentrations of 5-HIAA across their first three years of life than the individuals exposed to low rates of maternal rejection (Maestripieri et al. 2006a). Data were analyzed separately for crossfostered and non-crossfostered individuals, and a similar relation between maternal rejection and CSF 5-HIAA was found in both groups, suggesting that this association was not due to genetic similarities between mothers and offspring. In contrast, there were no differences in CSF 5-HIAA between offspring reared by high and low protectiveness mothers. Long-term effects of early experience on the development of the brain serotonergic system have also been reported in other studies of rhesus macaques (Kraemer et al. 1989; Higley et al. 1992; Shannon et al. 2005) as well as rodents (e.g., Ladd et al. 1996; Gardner et al. 2005).

Exposure to variable maternal behavior early in life had little impact on the off-spring's social interactions with other group members prior to puberty. In fact, the general affiliative and aggressive tendencies of crossfostered females in their first two years of life were more similar to those of their biological mothers than to those of their foster mothers (Maestripieri 2003b). There was, however, a significant negative correlation between CSF 5-HIAA and rates of scratching (Maestripieri et al. 2006b), suggesting that individuals with low CSF 5-HIAA were more anxious than those with high 5-HIAA (see Schino et al. 1991; Maestripieri et al. 1992, for the relation between scratching and anxiety). Differences in anxiety associated with serotonergic function may have contributed to some of the effects of exposure of variable parenting style that we observed after our female subjects reached puberty and gave birth for the first time.

Although there were no similarities between the maternal protectiveness scores of mothers and daughters, the maternal rejection rates of daughters closely resembled those of their mothers (Maestripieri et al. 2007). The resemblance was particularly strong for the crossfostered females and their foster mothers. This finding is con-sistent with a previously reported intergenerational correlation of maternal rejection rates in another population of rhesus macaques (Berman 1990) and suggests that this correlation is the result of early experience and not of genetic similarities between mothers and daughters. Although learning through direct experience with one's own mother and/or observations of maternal interactions with siblings may play a role in the intergenerational transmission of maternal rejection in macaques (Berman 1990), biological mechanisms are also important.

In our study, we found that the crossfostered females' CSF concentrations of 5-HIAA were negatively correlated with their rates of maternal rejection, such that the individuals with lower CSF 5-HIAA exhibited higher rates of rejection with their infants (Maestripieri et al. 2007). Therefore, exposure to variable rates of maternal rejection in infancy may affect the development of the brain serotonergic system, and variation in serotonergic function, in turn, may contribute to the expression of maternal rejection with one's own offspring later in life. Interestingly, a preliminary study by Lindell et al. (1997) found that the CSF 5-HIAA concentrations of rhesus macaque mothers were significantly correlated with those of their nine-month-old infants, but this study did not assess whether these correlations had a genetic or environmental nature. Evidence of both genetic and environmental effects on CSF concentrations of 5-HIAA and other monoamine metabolites was provided by Rogers et al. (2004) in a study of a large pedigreed population of baboons.

In addition to demonstrating the intergenerational transmission of maternal re-jection rates, we found evidence for the intergenerational transmission of infant abuse. Specifically, about half of the females who were abused by their mothers early in life, whether crossfostered or non-crossfostered (all crossfostered females reared by abu-sive mothers were also abused by them), exhibited abusive parenting toward their first-born offspring, whereas none of the females reared by nonabusive mothers did (including those born to abusive mothers; Maestripieri 2005a). Moreover, the abused females, both crossfostered and non-crossfostered, who became abusive mothers had lower CSF 5-HIAA concentrations than the abused females who did not become abu-sive mothers (Maestripieri et al. 2006a). This finding suggests that experience-induced, long-term alterations in serotonergic function in females reared by abusive mothers contribute to the manifestation of abusive parenting in adulthood. It is possible that experience-induced reduction in serotonergic function results in elevated anxiety and impaired impulse control and that high anxiety and impulsivity increase the probability of occurrence of abusive parenting (e.g., Troisi and D'Amato 1991, 1994), perhaps in conjunction with social learning resulting from direct experience of abuse early in life or observation of abusive parenting displayed by one's own mother with siblings. The intergenerational transmission of infant abuse, however, is likely to be a complex process with multiple determinants and influences. The finding that abusive mothers were more likely to carry the *s* allele of the serotonin transporter gene suggests that genetic variation in brain serotonergic function may play a role in the manifestation of abusive parenting and its transmission across generations. To understand the complex relationship between serotonin and abusive parenting, one must understand the relation between serotonin and maternal rejection as well as the relationship between maternal rejection and abuse.

Serotonin and Maternal Behavior

The brain serotonergic system is believed to play an important role in impulse control and in reducing the probability that risky, dangerous or aggressive behaviors will be expressed in response to internal pressures or external stimuli (e.g., Gollan and Coccaro 2005). Consistent with a large body of human research (e.g., Linnoila and Virkkunnen 1992), studies of rhesus macaques and vervet monkeys have shown that, in adult males, low levels of CSF 5-HIAA are associated with high impulsivity, risk-taking behavior and a propensity to engage in severe forms of aggression (see Higley 2003, for a review). In young males, low levels of CSF 5-HIAA are associated with earlier age of emigration from the natal group (e.g., Mehlman et al. 1995) and with the attainment of high dominance rank in adulthood (Fairbanks et al. 2004). Similar to the adult males, adult monkey females with low CSF 5-HIAA have been reported to be more likely to be wounded, to engage in violent aggression, and to be lower ranking than females with high CSF 5-HIAA (see Higley 2003 for review; but see Cleveland et al. 2004). Adult females with low CSF 5-HIAA also appear to be less socially oriented, spending more time alone, grooming less, and having fewer conspecifics in close proximity (Cleveland et al. 2004; rhesus macaque abusive mothers fit this behavioral profile quite well; see Maestripieri 1998b). Westergaard et al. (2003) also reported that the infants born to adult rhesus females with low CSF 5-HIAA concentrations are more likely to die within a year after birth than infants born to females with high CSF 5-HIAA concentrations.

Early studies of serotonin and maternal behavior in monkeys reported that mothers with low CSF 5-HIAA were more protective and restrictive, and that their infants spent more time in contact with them, than mothers with high CSF 5-HIAA (Lindell et al. 1997; Fairbanks et al. 1998). Cleveland et al. (2004) found no relationship between CSF 5-HIAA and maternal behavior in the first few post-partum days, but on post-partum days 15 and 20, females with low CSF 5-HIAA broke contact and left their infants less frequently than females with high CSF 5-HIAA. A preliminary study in our laboratory reported a positive correlation between CSF 5-HIAA concentrations measured during pregnancy and maternal rejection behaviors in the first post-partum month in multiparous females (Maestripieri et al. 2005). Our more recent work involving multiple measurements of CSF 5-HIAA during development, however, reported a negative correlation between CSF 5-HIAA and maternal rejection among first-time mothers (Maestripieri et al. 2007). Taken together, these studies support the notion that variation in serotonergic function can contribute to the expression of differences in maternal behavior, although the relationship between serotonin and primate maternal behavior is not yet fully understood.

Although serotonin might affect maternal motivation through its actions on oxytocin or prolactin release, serotonin and other monoamines are generally viewed as having aspecific effects on emotionality, motivation, or memory rather than specific effects on parentally motivated behaviors (Insel and Winslow 1998; Numan and Insel 2003). Research with rodents has established a strong link between anxiety/impulsivity and maternal aggression (e.g., Lonstein and Gammie 2002), but the emotional substrate of rodent maternal behavior is not well established (but see Weller et al. 2003).

Emotions, however, play a fundamental role in the regulation of maternal behavior in nonhuman primates and humans (Dix 1991; Pryce 1992; Maestripieri 1999). Emotions can be powerful elicitors of maternal behavior and play a crucial role in mediating the impact of the surrounding environment on the mother-infant dyad. For example, Pryce (1992) argued that two emotional systems, the attraction/arousal system and the anxiety system, play a central role in the regulation of primate maternal behavior. The attraction-arousal system involves the activation of positive emotions (e.g., excitement or joy) that elicit nurturing maternal behavior, whereas the anxiety system involves the activation of negative emotions (e.g., anxiety and fear) that elicit protective or rejecting maternal behaviors. Whereas the postpartum period is associated with lower reactivity to stress in rodents (Tu et al. 2006; but see Deschamps et al. 2003), pregnancy and the postpartum period in nonhuman primates and humans are characterized by high emotional instability and reactivity. For example, high cortisol levels and high arousability in the early postpartum period have been associated with greater sensitivity to infant cues and greater maternal responsiveness in humans (Fleming et al. 1987, 1997; see also Maestripieri et al. 2008, for rhesus macaques). Interestingly, etiological theories of postpartum psychosis based on estrogen's interaction with serotonin systems have been proposed (Fink and Sumner 1996). For example, it has been shown that variation in the SERT genotype affects susceptibility to bipolar affective puerperal psychosis (Coyle et al. 2000).

Motherhood is a psychologically stressful condition in human and nonhuman primates. In rhesus macaques, the first few months of an infant's life result in a number of anxiety-eliciting situations for the mother (Maestripieri 1993a). There are marked individual differences in anxiety among rhesus mothers, and such differences translate into differences in maternal style (Maestripieri 1993b). Maternal anxiety has also been implicated in the etiology of infant abuse (Troisi and D'Amato 1984, 1991, 1994). Although the role of emotionality, and particularly of impulsivity, in primate maternal behavior is still poorly understood, it is possible that impulsivity affects how primate mothers interact with their infants, and that high impulsivity is expressed as high rejection rates as well as, as other studies suggest, greater maternal protectiveness. Our recent findings suggest that variation in impulsivity and maternal rejection originates, at least in part, from early experience and that there may be causal relationships between these two variables, such that high rates of maternal rejection result in low serotonergic function, which in turn results in high rates of maternal rejection later in life.

Maternal rejection also has a complex relation with infant abuse, perhaps not dissimilar from the relationship between child neglect and abuse in humans. Although abusive parenting in monkeys is probably maladaptive (Maestripieri 1998b), maternal rejection is a behavior that belongs to the normal maternal repertoire and is used by mothers to limit the amount of time spent by infants in bodily and nipple contact, thus encouraging the infant's social and nutritional independence (e.g., Simpson and Simpson 1985). Abusive parenting in rhesus macaques co-occurs with high rates of maternal rejection. Abusive mothers begin rejecting their infants shortly after birth (rejection normally begins after three to four weeks) and continue to do so at much higher rates than nonabusive mothers (Maestripieri 1998b; McCormack et al. 2006). Although we found no direct effects of infant abuse on CSF 5-HIAA, the observed significant effects of maternal rejection on CSF 5-HIAA were likely driven by abused infants, who were exposed to much higher levels of rejection than nonabused infants. Rejection occurs more frequently than abuse and, although it does not cause physical harm to the infants, it may be even more psychologically traumatic than abuse. Interestingly, human studies have found that child neglect tends to have stronger and more consistent effects on brain structure and function in maltreatment victims than physical abuse does, although both are transmitted across generations (e.g., Glaser 2000; DeBellis 2005). Although social learning probably plays an important role in the intergenerational transmission of both maternal rejection and abuse in monkeys, our results suggest that rejection is more likely than abuse to cause long-term alterations in neuroendocrine and emotional functioning and that these alterations may contribute to the expression of both rejecting and abusive parenting later in life.

Acknowledgements. The research reviewed in this chapter was supported by NIH and involved the participation of many collaborators and assistants, including Richelle Fulks, Anne Graff, Dee Higley, Stephen Lindell, Kai McCormack, Nancy Megna, Timothy Newman, and Mar Sanchez.

References

Bardi M, Huffman MA (2006) Maternal behavior and maternal stress are associated with infant behavioral development in macaques. Dev Psychobiol 48:1–9

Bardi M, Bode AE, Ramirez SM, Brent LY (2005) Maternal care and the development of the stress response. Am J Primatol 66:263–278

Barr CS, Newman TK, Shannon C, Parker C, Dvoskin RL, Becker ML, Schwandt M, Champoux M, Lesch KP, Goldman D, Suomi SJ, Higley JD (2004a) Rearing condition and rh5-HTTLPR interact to influence LHPA-axis response to stress in infant macaques. Biol Psychiat 55:733–738

Barr CS, Newman TK, Lindell S, Shannon C, Champoux M, Lesch KP, Suomi SJ, Higley JD (2004b) Interaction between serotonin transporter gene variation and rearing condition in alcohol preference and consumption in female primates. Arch Gen Psychiat 61:1146–1152

Bennett AJ, Lesch KP, Heils A, Long JC, Lorenz JG, Shoaf SE, Champoux M, Suomi SJ, Linnoila MV, Higley JD (2002) Early experience and serotonin transporter gene variation interact to influence primate CNS function. Mol Psychiat 7:118–122

Berman CM (1984) Variation in mother-infant relationships: traditional and nontraditional factors. In: Small MF (ed) Female primates: studies by women primatologists. Alan Liss, New York, pp 17–36

Berman CM (1990) Intergenerational transmission of maternal rejection rates among free-ranging rhesus monkeys. Anim Behav 39:329–337

Caspi A, McClay J, Moffitt TE, Mill J, Martin J, Craig IW, Taylor A, Poulton R (2002) Role of genotype in the cycle of violence in maltreated children. Science 297:851–854

Caspi A, Sugden K, Moffitt TE, Taylor A, Craig IW, Harrington H, McClay J, Mill J, Martin J, Braithwaite A, Poulton R (2003) Influence of life stress on depression: Moderation by a polymorphism in the 5-HTT gene. Science 301:386–389

Champoux M, Coe CL, Schanberg SM, Kuhn CM, Suomi SJ (1989) Hormonal effects of early rearing conditions in the infant rhesus monkey. Am J Primatol 19:111–117

Cleveland A, Westergaard GC, Trenkle MK, Higley JD (2004) Physiological predictors of reproductive outcome and mother-infant behaviors in captive rhesus macaque females (*Macaca mulatta*). Neuropsychopharmacology 29:901–910

Coyle N, Jones I, Robertson E, Lendon C, Craddock N (2000) Variation at the serotonin transporter gene influences susceptibility to bipolar affective puerperal psychosis. Lancet 356:1490–1491

DeBellis MD (2005) The psychobiology of neglect. Child Maltreatment 10:150–172

Deschamps S, Woodside B, Walker CD (2003) Pups' presence eliminates the stress hyporesponsiveness of early lactating females to a psychological stress representing a threat to the pups. J Neuroendocrinol 15:486–497

Dix T (1991) The affective organization of parenting: Adaptive and maladaptive processes. Psych Bull 110:3–25

Fairbanks LA (1989) Early experience and cross-generational continuity of mother-infant contact in vervet monkeys. Dev Psychobiol 22:669–681

Fairbanks LA (1996) Individual differences in maternal styles: causes and consequences for mothers and offspring. Adv Study Behav 25:579–611

Fairbanks LA (2003) Parenting. In: Maestripieri D (ed) Primate psychology. Harvard University Press, Cambridge, MA, pp 144–170

Fairbanks LA, McGuire MT (1987) Mother-infant relationships in vervet monkeys: response to new adult males. Intl J Primatol 8:351–366

Fairbanks LA, McGuire MT (1988) Long-term effects of early mothering behavior on responsiveness to the environment in vervet monkeys. Dev Psychobiol 21:711–724

Fairbanks LA, McGuire MT (1993) Maternal protectiveness and response to the unfamiliar in vervet monkeys. Am J Primatol 30:119–129

Fairbanks LA, Melega WP, McGuire MT (1998) CSF 5-HIAA is associated with individual differences in maternal protectiveness in vervet monkeys. Am J Primatol 45:179–180 (abstract)

Fairbanks LA, Jorgensen MJ, Huff A, Blau K, Hung Y, Mann JJ (2004) Adolescent impulsivity predicts adult dominance attainment in male vervet monkeys. Am J Primatol 64:1–17

Fink G, Sumner BEH (1996) Estrogen and mental state. Nature 383:306

Fleming AS, Steiner M, Anderson V (1987) Hormonal and attitudinal correlates of maternal behavior during the early postpartum period in first-time mothers. J Reprod Inf Psychol 5:193–205

Fleming AS, Steiner M, Corter C (1997) Cortisol, hedonics, and maternal responsiveness in human mothers. Horm Behav 32:85–98

Gardner KL, Thrivikraman KV, Lightman SL, Plotsky PM, Lowry CA (2005) Early life experience alters behavior during defeat: focus on serotonergic systems. Neuroscience 136:181–191

Glaser D (2000) Child abuse and neglect and the brain: A review. J Child Psychol Psychiat 41:97–116

Gollan JK, Lee R, Coccaro EF (2005) Developmental psychopathology and neurobiology of aggression. Dev Psychopathol 17:1151–1171

Higley JD (2003) Aggression. In: Maestripieri D (ed) Primate psychology. Harvard University Press, Cambridge, MA, pp 17–40

Higley JD, Suomi SJ, Linnoila M (1992) A longitudinal study of CSF monoamine metabolite and plasma cortisol concentrations in young rhesus monkeys: Effects of early experience, age, sex and stress on continuity of interindividual differences. Biol Psychiat 32:127–145

Hinde RA, Spencer-Booth Y (1971) Towards understanding individual Ddifferences in rhesus mother-infant interaction. Anim Behav 19:165–173

Insel TR, Winslow JT (1998) Serotonin and neuropeptides in affiliative behaviors. Biol Psychiat 44:207–219

Kraemer GW, Ebert MH, Schmidt DE, McKinney WT (1989) A longitudinal study of the effect of different social rearing conditions on cerebrospinal fluid norepinephrine and biogenic amine metabolites in rhesus monkeys. Neuropsychopharmacol 2:175–189

Ladd CO, Owens MJ, Nemeroff CB (1996) Persistent changes in corticotropin-releasing factor neuronal systems induced by maternal deprivation. Endocrinology 137:1212–1218

Lesch KP, Bengel D, Heils A, Sabol SZ, Greenberg BD, Petri S, Benjamin J, Muller C, Hamer D, Murphy D (1996) Association of anxiety-related traits with a polymorphism in the serotonin transporter gene regulatory region. Science 274:1527–1531

Lindell SG, Higley JD, Shannon C, Linnoila M (1997) Low levels of CSF 5-HIAA in female rhesus macaques predict mother-infant interaction patterns and mother's CSF 5-HIAA correlates with infant's CSF 5-HIAA. Am J Primatol 42:129 (abstract)

Linnoila VM, Virkkunen M (1992) Aggression, suicidality, and serotonin. J Clin Psychiat 53:46–51

Lonstein JS, Gammie SC (2002) Sensory, hormonal, and neural control of maternal aggression in laboratory rodents. Neurosci Biobehav Rev 26:869–888

Maestripieri D (1993a) Maternal anxiety in rhesus macaques (Macaca mulatta). I. Measurement of anxiety and identification of anxiety-eliciting situations. Ethology 95:19–31

Maestripieri D (1993b) Maternal anxiety in rhesus macaques (Macaca mulatta). II. Emotional bases of individual differences in mothering style. Ethology 95:32–42

Maestripieri D (1998a) Social and demographic influences on mothering style in pigtail macaques. Ethology 104:379–385

Maestripieri D (1998b) Parenting styles of abusive mothers in group-living rhesus macaques. Anim Behav 55:1–11

Maestripieri D (1999) The biology of human parenting: Insights from nonhuman primates. Neurosci Biobehav Rev 23:411–422

Maestripieri D (2003a) Attachment. In: Maestripieri D (ed) Primate psychology. Harvard University Press, Cambridge, MA, pp 108–143

Maestripieri D (2003b) Similarities in affiliation and aggression between cross-fostered rhesus macaque females and their biological mothers. Dev Psychobiol 43:321–327

Maestripieri D (2005a) Early experience affects the intergenerational transmission of infant abuse in rhesus monkeys. Proc Natl Acad Sci USA 102:9726–9729

Maestripieri D (2005b) Effects of early experience on female behavioural and reproductive development in rhesus macaques. Proc R Soc Lond B 272:1243–1248

Maestripieri D, Carroll KA (1998a) Child abuse and neglect: Usefulness of the animal data. Psych Bull 123:211–223

Maestripieri D, Carroll KA (1998b) Risk factors for infant abuse and neglect in group-living rhesus monkeys. Psych Sci 9:65–67

Maestripieri D, Schino G, Aureli F, Troisi A (1992) A modest proposal: displacement activities as an indicator of emotions in primates. Anim Behav 44:967–979

Maestripieri D, Wallen K, Carroll KA (1997) Infant abuse runs in families of group-living pigtail macaques. Child Ab Negl 21:465–471

Maestripieri D, Lindell SG, Ayala A, Gold PW, Higley JD (2005) Neurobiological characteristics of rhesus macaque abusive mothers and their relation to social and maternal behavior. Neurosci Biobehav Rev 29:51–57

Maestripieri D, Higley JD, Lindell SG, Newman TK, McCormack K, Sanchez MM (2006a) Early maternal rejection affects the development of monoaminergic systems and adult abusive parenting in rhesus macaques. Behav Neurosci 120:1017–1024

Maestripieri D, McCormack K, Lindell SG, Higley JD, Sanchez MM (2006b) Influence of parenting style on the offspring's behavior and CSF monoamine metabolites levels in crossfostered and noncrossfostered female rhesus macaques. Behav Brain Res 175:90–95

Maestripieri D, Lindell SG, Higley JD (2007) Intergenerational transmission of maternal behavior in rhesus monkeys and its underlying mechanisms. Dev Psychobiol 49:165–171

Maestripieri D, Hoffman CL, Fulks R, Gerald MS (2008) Plasma cortisol responses to stress in lactating and nonlactating female rhesus macaques. Horm Behav, 53:170–176

McCormack KM, Sanchez MM, Bardi M, Maestripieri D (2006) Maternal care patterns and behavioral development of rhesus macaque abused infants in the first 6 months of life. Dev Psychobiol 48:537–550

Mehlman PT, Higley JD, Faucher I, Lilly AA, Taub DM, Vickers J, Suomi SJ, Linnoila M (1995) Correlation of CSF 5-HIAA concentration with sociality and the timing of emigration in free-ranging primates Am J Psychiat 152:907–913

Numan M, Insel TR (2003) The neurobiology of parental behavior. Springer, New York

Pryce CR (1992) A comparative systems model of the regulation of maternal motivation in mammals. Anim Behav 43:417–441

Rogers J, Martin LJ, Comuzzie AG, Mann JJ, Manuck SB, Leland M, Kaplan JR (2004) Genetics of monoamine metabolites in baboons: overlapping sets of genes influence levels of 5-hydroxyindolacetic acid, 3-hydroxy-4-methoxyphenylglycol, and homovanillic acid. Biol Psychiat 55:739–744

Schino G, Troisi A, Perretta G, Monaco V (1991) Measuring anxiety in nonhuman primates: Effect of lorazepam on macaque scratching. Pharm Biochem Behav 38:889–891

Schino G, D'Amato FR, Troisi A (1995) Mother-infant relationships in Japanese macaques: Sources of interindividual variation. Anim Behav 49:151–158

Schino G, Speranza L, Troisi A (2001) Early maternal rejection and later social anxiety in juvenile and adult Japanese macaques. Dev Psychobiol 38:186–190

Shannon C, Schwandt ML, Champoux M, Shoaf SE, Suomi SJ, Linnoila M, Higley JD (2005) Maternal absence and stability of individual differences in CSF5-HIAA concentrations in rhesus monkey infants. Am J Psychiat 162:1658–1664

Simpson MJA (1985) Effects of early experience on the behaviour of yearling rhesus monkeys (*Macaca mulatta*) in the presence of a strange object: classification and correlation approaches. Primates 26:57–72

Simpson AE, Simpson MJA (1985) Short-term consequences of different breeding histories for captive rhesus macaque mothers and young. Behav Ecol Sociobiol 18:83–89

Simpson MJA, Datta SB (1990) Predicting infant enterprise from early relationships in rhesus macaques. Behaviour 116:42–63

Simpson MJA, Gore MA, Janus M, Rayment FDG (1989) Prior experience of risk and individual differences in enterprise shown by rhesus monkey infants in the second half of their first year. Primates 30:493–509

Tanaka I (1989) Variability in the development of mother-infant relationships among free-ranging Japanese macaques. Primates 30:477–491

Troisi A, D'Amato FR (1984) Ambivalence in monkey mothering: infant abuse combined with maternal possessiveness. J Nerv Ment Dis 172:105–108

Troisi A, D'Amato FR (1991) Anxiety in the pathogenesis of primate infant abuse: A pharmacological study. Psychopharmacology 103:571–572

Troisi A, D'Amato FR (1994) Mechanisms of primate infant abuse: the maternal anxiety hypothesis. In: Parmigiani S, vom Saal F (eds) Infanticide and parental care. Harwood, London, pp 199–210

Tu MT, Lupien SJ, Walker C-D (2006) Measuring stress in postpartum mothers: Perspectives from studies in human and animal populations. Stress 8: 19–34

Vochteloo JD, Timmermans PJA, Duijghuisen JAH, Vossen JMH (1993) Effects of reducing the mother's radius of action on the development of mother-infant relationships in longtailed macaques. Anim Behav 45:603–612

Weller A, Leguisamo AC, Towns L, Ramboz S, Bagiella E, Hofer M, Hen R, Brunner D (2003) Maternal effects in infant and adult phenotypes of 5HT(1A) and 5HT(1B) receptor knockout mice. Dev Psychobiol 42:194–205

Westergaard GC, Cleveland A, Trenkle MK, Lussier ID, Higley JD (2003) CSF 5-HIAA concentrations as an early screening tool for predicting significant life history outcomes in female specific-pathogen-free (SPF) rhesus macaques (*Macaca mulatta*) maintained in captive breeding groups. J Med Primatol 32:95–104

Brain Corticosteroid Receptor Function in Response to Psychosocial Stressors

E.R de Kloet[1], *N.A. Datson*[1], *Y. Revsin*[1], *D.L. Champagne*[1], and *M.S. Oitzl*[1]

Summary

A fundamental question in the neuroendocrinology of stress and adaptation is how stress mediators that are crucial for resilience and health can change into harmful signals enhancing vulnerability to disease. To address this question, we focus in the rodent on corticosterone as the end product of the hypothalamic-pituitary-adrenal (HPA) axis, which coordinates the behavioural and physiological response to stressors. The action of corticosterone is mediated by mineralocorticoid (MR) and glucocorticoid receptors (GR) that are abundantly expressed in neurons of the limbic hippocampus, amygdala and prefrontal cortex. The receptors are transcription factors regulating gene transcription but recently – much to our surprise – these nuclear receptors also were discovered to mediate rapid, non-genomic action on glutamate transmission. MR participates in initial stress reactions important for appraisal and coping processes, whereas management of the later adaptive phase primarily depends on GR. Gene variants of MR and GR have been identified. Moreover, the expression of MR and GR shows enduring epigenetic changes in response to early life experience. Both gene variants and the altered expression of MR and GR have lasting consequences for stress responsiveness, cognitive performance and emotional arousal in later life. In conclusion, an imbalance in stress mediators caused by genetic factors and early life experience is a characteristic feature of a phenotype vulnerable for later life stressors. This concept calls for recovery of the MR/GR balance as a therapeutic strategy to promote the resilience that is still present in the diseased brain.

Introduction

The contributions to this volume concentrate on the molecular and neural biology of hormone actions relevant to social and sexual behavior and on the therapeutic perspectives for treatment of patients impaired in these behaviors. A substantial number of the presentations focused on the neurohypophyseal hormones, vasopressin and oxytocin. These neuropeptides have been known for several decades to coordinate body and brain functions in social behaviors, reproduction, adaptation, and autonomic and neuroendocrine regulations. Hence, oxytocin promotes patterns of affiliative, sexual and maternal behavior and, while doing so, attenuates fear-motivated behavior.

---

[1] Division of Medical Pharmacology, Leiden/Amsterdam Center for Drug Research and Leiden University Medical Center, Leiden, The Netherlands, e-mail: e.kloet@lacdr.leidenuniv.nl

Pfaff et al.
Hormones and Social Behavior
© Springer-Verlag Berlin Heidelberg 2008

Vasopressin is, in some instances, its counterpart, promoting aggression and territorial behaviors and enhancing fear-motivated behavior rather than being amnestic, as oxytocin is under such conditions (de Wied 1997).

A particularly interesting experimental animal model for the study of neurohypophyseal hormone action on behavior is the male canary. During the breeding season, sexually mature males produce a magnificient, stable stereotyped song pattern that serves to impress rivals, mark territory and attract females. Song nuclei in the brain [nucleus robustus archistriatalis (RA) and hyperstriatum vertrale, pars caudalis (HVc)] undergo a profound volume change and neurogenesis to accommodate the enhanced function of trachea and syrinx during singing (Nottebohm 2005). Vasotocin, the equivalent of mammalian vasopressin, is expressed in the brain and innervates the song nuclei (Kiss et al. 1987). For identification of vasotocin receptors, a radioiodinated vasotocin analogue, $[^{125}I]d(CH_2)_5[Tyr(Me)^2, Thr^4, Orn^8, Tyr-NH_2^9]$vasotocin ($[^{125}I]$-OTA) was used. Such labelled vasotocin receptors are abundantly expressed in the capsular regions of the robustus archistriatalis (Voorhuis et al. 1988, 1990). In our final experiments, we showed that administration of this vasotocin advanced song learning (Voorhuis et al. 1991). The lesson we learned from these experiments is that the canary can outdo rivals not only by singing better but also by singing earlier in the breeding season.

At first glance these experiments with neurohypophyseal hormones seem to bear little relevance to the topic of stress and stress hormones. However, vasopressin and oxytocin affect fear-motivated behaviors, and vasopressin is a co-secretagogue of the corticotrophin-releasing hormone released during stress that activates the hypothalamic-pituitary-adrenal (HPA) axis. Corticosteroids (CORT) secreted from the adrenal have profound effects on adaptation to stress and, therefore, also on the behaviors modulated by oxytocin and vasopressin.

This chapter is focused on the role of CORT in the neurobiology underlying adaptive behaviors and provides an argument for targeting the stress system with drugs to correct stress-related dysregulations causal to disease. To do this, we will briefly discuss the following five topics: 1) the principle of CORT action and receptors, 2) the function of these receptors in behavioral adaptation, 3) the mechanism from the perspective of its responsive gene patterns and pathways, 4) diabetes as a disease model characterized by aberrant actions of CORT that can be corrected by a CORT antagonist, and 5) genetics and early experience that interact and may lead to re-programming stress responsiveness and brain plasticity.

The Stress Response

Any stressor – either real or imagined – that threatens to disturb homeostasis triggers a physiological and behavioral response aimed at promoting adaptation. The stress response is coordinated in body and brain by humoral and nervous systems, of which the HPA axis and the sympathetic nervous system (adrenaline) are the primary mediators. The most potent stressful condition is psychosocial in nature, that is, when there is insufficient information and poor predictability of upcoming events leading to poor control over the situation, uncertainty and feelings of fear and anxiety. Briefly, the individual cannot cope with the stress or a situation that becomes more severe in times of socially compromising situations (Levine 2005).

We will focus in this contribution on the role of the HPA axis, notably its end products cortisol (human) and corticosterone (human, rodents), collectively called CORT here. Naturally, CORT does not act alone but operates in the context of the humoral and nervous signals that mediate the stress response (McEwen 2007). CORT dampens the initial stress (defense) reactions to the stressor and prevents them from overshooting (Sapolsky et al. 2000). This action has a diversity as wide as the variety of stressors. For example, after tissue damage, CORT limits inflammatory reactions, suppresses the immune response during infection and curtails neurochemical reactions in specific circuits mediating the processing of psychosocial stressors.

However, the very same CORT can actually also boost the initial stress reaction, a concept that recently earned its molecular underpinning with the discovery of membrane receptors for the hormone in the hippocampus that enhanced excitatory neurotransmission (Karst et al. 2005; Joëls et al. 2007, 2008). CORT promotes motivation, arousal and cognitive performance. The energy needed for these reactions is also provided by CORT, which promotes the availability of substrates for energy metabolism and coordinates, for that purpose, appetite, nutrient choice and food intake with energy disposition to the challenged tissues (Peters et al. 2007). In fact, the physiological role of CORT is essential for health and well being. A healthy, resilient organism is characterized by a rapid activation of the CORT as long as it is also turned off efficiently. In fact, the secretory pattern has been used widely as a marker for health and disease of the organism.

CORT is secreted under basal conditions in approximately hourly pulses that are produced within minutes and usually last about 20 minutes (Young et al. 2004). CORT pulses are increased in amplitude during the activity period, which is nighttime in rodents. Deconvolution analysis is required to construct these pulsatile patterns. During stress-related disease and aging, the patterns become disordered, a sign that the HPA axis pulsatility has become dysregulated (Young et al. 2004). A disease condition such as human depression is characterized by an increase in the frequency and amplitude of the pulses, particularly during the resting period, which is otherwise a period of small amplitudes (Veldhuis et al. 2005). The pulse generator is located in the suprachiasmatic nucleus and in the adrenal, but its nature and mechanism are not known. Nor do we know how tissue responsiveness is altered with the exposure to variable pulsatile patterns.

CORT secretory bursts can be triggered by a stressor any time. Like basal patterns, the stress-induced CORT pattern also serves as a biomarker for breakdown of adaptation and stress-related disease. Such patterns become manifest as either excessive and prolonged or inadequate CORT responses. Feedback regulation is disturbed, which can be assessed by the effect of potent synthetic glucocorticoids that target the pituitary corticotrophs because of their poor penetration in the brain. Escape from dexamethasone suppression, enhanced by CRH (DEX-CRH test), is therefore a hallmark for the hyperactive HPA axis and, at times, hypercorticism during depression. In contrast, post-traumatic stress disorder usually is characterized by enhanced dexamethasone suppression and an apparent underexposure to CORT (Yehuda 2006; de Kloet et al. 2007). These tests, however, have a history of two to three decades. There is an urgent need, therefore, for better biomarkers of a dysregulated stress system during stress-related disorders.

The Principle of CORT Action and Receptors

The HPA axis coordinates behavior and experience with the secretion and action of CORT. In its basal pulsatile pattern, this function relates to the coordination and synchronization of daily- and sleep-related events. During the stress response, the HPA axis and CORT mediate the ability to cope. For this purpose, CORT targets in the brain precisely those circuits that have perceived the initial trigger of the stress response; its action can be divided in two domains: fast and slow. These actions are mediated by two types of corticosteroid receptors: mineralocorticoid receptors (MR) and glucocorticoid receptors (GR; de Kloet et al. 1998, 2005).

MR and GR are nuclear receptors operating as transcription factors. The nuclear MR binds CORT with a very high affinity and is abundantly expressed in limbic structures involved in mood, affect and memory processes. Nuclear GR has a ten-fold lower affinity and is expressed widely in neurons and glial cells, with highest expression in centers involved in regulating the stress response. Thus, in limbic structures, such as the neuronal circuits of hippocampus (CA1-2 and dentate gyrus), the amygdala nuclei and areas of the prefrontal cortex, MR and GR are co-localized and expressed in large amounts (de Kloet et al. 1998).

Because of the difference in affinity, the hourly pulses maintain occupancy of MR in the nucleus, whereas the lower affinity GR follows in nuclear translocation the pulsatile changes in plasma level of the hormone under basal conditions and after stress (Conway-Campbell et al. 2007). Their action mechanisms in transactivation and transrepression show profound differences: both receptors interact as dimers with the transcription machinery, but GR rather than MR monomers can modulate the action of other transcription factors that are activated by the initial stressor. Transrepression therefore underlies the dampening of the stress reaction by CORT. MR and GR recruit distinctly different co-regulator patterns, and their properties are differently affected by sumoylation and proteasomal activity (Meijer et al. 2006; Tirard et al. 2007).

CORT exerts a strong influence on monoaminergic neurons, which is characterized by enhancing the turnover and release of the amines during stress on the one hand and dampening their post-synaptic action on the other. The latter actions are mostly mediated by GR; under solely MR activation the aminergic activity is low and stable. In CA, hippocampal neurons CORT also potently affects the Ca^{2+}-current amplitude, also in a U-shaped dose dependency (Joëls and de Kloet 1994; Joëls 1997, 2006). Ca^{2+} currents are low with predominant MR activation; as a consequence, the frequency accommodation and AHP amplitude, which strongly depend on Ca^{2+}-influx, will be small with predominant MR activation, which guarantees maintenance of basal firing activity in the hippocampus. By contrast, GR (in addition to MR) activation not only increases Ca^{2+}-influx but also compromises Ca^{2+} extrusion, resulting, under physiological conditions, in strong frequency accommodation and large AHP amplitudes, thus attenuating the transmission of prolonged excitatory input (Joëls and de Kloet 1989; Karst and Joëls 2007).

Recently, Henk Karst and Marian Joëls (Karst et al. 2005; Joëls et al. 2007, 2008) discovered that the very same nuclear MR controlling gene expression also resides in the membrane of the hippocampal CA1 neurons. In the slice, the miniature excitatory post-synaptic currents (EPSC) frequency profoundly increased in parallel with the presence of CORT, an effect that was abolished in mutants with brain-specific MR knockouts.

This increase in mEPSC frequency reflects enhanced probability of glutamate release, which indeed was also observed after microdialysis. In subsequent experiments, Joëls and colleagues identified the primary site of this non-genomic corticosterone action as pre-synaptic through the ERK pathway known to control mEPSC-dependent glutamate release (Olijslager et al. 2008). Postsynaptic corticosterone rapidly suppresses the I_k potassium current. Therefore, activation of membrane MR results pre- and postsynaptic collectively in a rapidly enhanced excitability. This increased excitability requires stress levels of CORT, since the affinity of this putative membrane MR for CORT is ten-fold lower than its high-affinity nuclear MR variant.

Function in behavioral adaptation

MR and GR exert complementary actions in the initial phase of the stress reaction and in the management of the later adaptive phase (Fig. 1).

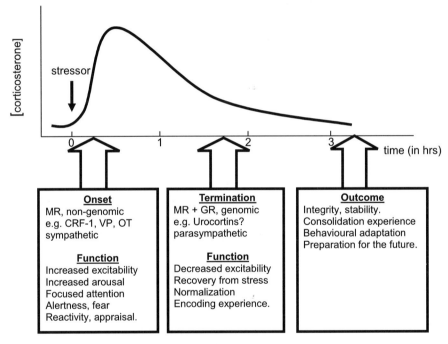

Fig. 1. A stressor triggers an HPA response leading to rising CORT levels. In limbic structures, rising CORT can cause non-genomic actions that amplify the action of the initial stress mediators, e.g., the CRH and sympathetic nervous activity, which is modulated by vasopressin and oxytocin, underlying enhanced arousal, alertness, behavioral reactivity and appraisal processes. At the same time, gene-mediated pathways are activated that are aimed at dampening the initial stress reactions by transrepression to prevent them from overshooting. Other actions through transactivation cause structural and functional changes aimed at promoting recovery, replenishment of depleted energy resources and encoding of the experience. Collectively the outcome of the fast non-genomic and slow genomic actions is storage of the coping response in the memory, behavioral adaptation and thus preparation for the future (see also Joëls et al. 2007, 2008)

The Fast Initial Phase

Based on the discovery of the membrane MR, an entirely new concept is evolving on the rapid-amplifying action of CORT in the stress response (Joëls et al. 2006). Briefly, the low-affinity, MR-mediated mechanism would respond to the rising CORT levels in the initial phase of the stress response and could amplify ongoing excitatory activity, which is also facilitated through the CRH-1, vasopressin (V1a and V1b), angiotensin I receptors and the sympathetic nervous system. The membrane MRs are probably the substrates for a rapid feedforward mode driving violent and fear-motivated behavior, and probably also various types of schedule-induced behaviors occurring in anticipation of an upcoming event (Bohus and de Kloet 1981; Kruk et al. 2004; Mikics et al. 2005). This MR would be involved in appraisal processes, attention and vigilance to allow acquisition of a behaviorally adaptive response (Oitzl and de Kloet 1992; Zorawski and Killcross 2002).

The Slow and Recovery Phase

Through the slower nuclear MR- and GR-mediated actions, complementary actions are being exerted in recovery from the stressor. MR is important for the maintenance of neuronal integrity and stability in the face of the stress response. This fact can be easily demonstrated after adrenalectomy, which leads to enhanced apoptosis in the hippocampal dentate gyrus, which can be restored by substitutions with CORT (Stienstra et al. 1998; Nair et al. 2004). In mouse mutants with a site-specific knockout of MR, viability of neurons is also compromised (Gass et al. 2000). In the brain, GR prevents the initial stress reaction from overshooting, brings the target cell back to baseline and facilitates recovery through promotion of energy metabolism. In cooperation with the amine and neuropeptide signal, GR facilitates encoding of the experience.

The fast and slow phases of the stress response are crucial for the processes underlying memory storage. Experience, problem solving, coping style and response patterns are stored in memory for future use. It is well established that CORT promotes memory consolidation through GR-mediated actions. Strong emotions that are also promoted by CORT are remembered best. At the same time, behavioral responses that are of no more relevance are extinguished by CORT (Bohus and de Kloet 1981; Oitzl and de Kloet 1992; Zorawski and Killcross 2002). Moreover, incoming information not relevant to the situation is suppressed (Pu et al. 2007). These actions are predominantly GR dependent, but require the concomitant action of MR and other stress signals, such as CRH, vasopressin and the catecholamines. Whether the MR-mediated actions in retrieval are mediated by membrane or nuclear MR remains to be established.

The role of MR and GR in information processing and behavior was disentangled in the previous century by systemic and intracerebral administration of agonists and antagonists for either receptor (de Kloet et al. 1993, 1999). These studies were of great conceptual value. However, some of the drugs are not as selective for corticosteroid receptors and are metabolized differently than in humans. For instance, the glucocorticoid antagonist RU38486 (mifepristone) needs to be administered in 10^6 higher dose systemically than in the brain, whereas the steroid also has potent anti-progestin activities. Likewise, the MR antagonist spironolactone is required in mg amounts when given systemically to rodents. Both synthetic ligands are rapidly degraded. The blood-brain barrier forms another obstacle for steroid ligands, like the glucocorticoid agonist dexamethasone, which is a substrate for P-glycoprotein extrusion pumps (Meijer et al. 1998; Karssen et al. 2005).

The generation of transgenic mice with site-specific conditional overexpression or knockout of MR and GR was a great leap forward. Next, viral transfer allowing brain-site localized overexpression or knockdown was introduced to rapidly modulate MR and/or GR gene expression (Ferguson and Sapolsky 2007). Homozygous GR knockout mice were used to illustrate that MR- and GR-mediated effects are different but interact and proceed in a coordinated manner and are linked in time to the particular stage of information processing. These mice displayed the expected impairment in GR-related, long-term memory processes. Interestingly, they also failed to display MR-dependent search strategies, suggesting a role for MR-GR heterodimerization (Oitzl et al. 1997).

In a next step, mice with a point mutation at A458T in the GR were generated, i.e., in exon 4, the amino acid sequence of the second zinc finger in the DNA-binding domain of the GR was exchanged from alanine 458 to threonine. This prevented GR homodimerization and DNA binding ($GR^{dim/dim}$), whereas protein–protein interactions can still take place (Reichardt et al. 1998). The $GR^{dim/dim}$ mice were 100% viable as opposed to the first line of GR knockout mice (5% viability). The specific elimination of GR homodimerization is causal to a selective impairment of spatial memory in the water maze (Fig. 2). This defect cannot be rescued by corticosterone (Oitzl et al. 2001). Importantly, MR-related behavior is left intact, as indicated by, e.g., similar exploration

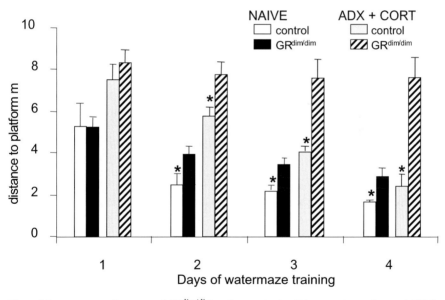

Fig. 2. Water maze performance of $GR^{dim/dim}$ and control mice. Distances in cm (mean ± SEM) to reach the submerged platform were longer in $GR^{dim/dim}$. Removal of the adrenals (ADX) induced a deficit in performance in both groups (not shown). Corticosterone administration (CORT 250 µg/kg i.p) before the daily training trials improved the performance of ADX controls but not $GR^{dim/dim}$ mice. *$p < 0.05$ between groups during spatial training trials. (Adapted from Oitzl et al. 2001)

patterns in the novel environments of open field, light/dark box and during the first exposure to the swimming pool. Thus, the unique experimental model of GR$^{dim/dim}$ mice suggests that DNA binding and transactivation of the GR homodimer are required for CORT effects on spatial memory in the face of unaltered functioning of the MR.

A recurrent and controversial issue in stress research is the rather general belief that *acute* stress and CORT can impair memory retrieval (de Quervain et al. 1998). Retrieval of spatial memory is disturbed if stress and CORT are administered one hour prior to the session, and so is the retrieval of other conditioned behaviors if the treatments continue beyond the context of the learning, consolidation and retention session. However, from a physiological perspective, prior exposure to a stressor competes with the display of learned information, which is at that time considered irrelevant. Actually, it has been shown on the cellular level that, in the context of high-frequency stimulation, CORT facilitates long-term potentiation (LTP; Wiegert et al. 2006; Pu et al. 2007) but suppresses LTP if given one hour before. This finding supports the notion that, instead of CORT-induced impairment of retrieval, CORT facilitates the elimination of a no more relevant response. This distinction is more than merely semantics: CORT-induced impairment demonstrates a healthy, behaviorally adaptive system rather than a defect (de Kloet et al. 1999; Joëls et al. 2006). This finding may have clinical implications if unwanted intrusive memories need to be eliminated, as is the case in post-traumatic stress disorder (de Kloet et al. 2007).

Under conditions of chronic stress, the physiology of the brain changes dramatically: cell survival, proliferation and neurogenesis are compromised in the dentate gyrus, including changes in morphology and synaptic organization of the CA3, CA1 and dentate gyrus (Joëls et al. 2007, 2008). Chronic stress procedures differ largely, but the consensus is that the most powerful designs are based on lack of predictability and controllability. Studies usually report stress-related deficits in hippocampus-dependent spatial learning and memory tasks (McEwen 1999; McLaughlin et al. 2007). In contrast, it enhanced fear conditioning to the context, most probably as a result of stress-induced sensitization of amygdala function (Sandi et al. 2001). During chronic CORT administration to C57BL/6 mice, it appeared that progressive activation of GR induced strong emotional arousal at the expense of cognitive performance (Brinks et al. 2007).

Individual differences in stress reactivity for the cognitive outcome of stress also have been taken into account (Grootendorst et al. 2001a,b; Touyarot et al. 2004). Depending on the genetic background and the activity of the HPA axis, chronic stress either facilitated spatial learning in apolipoprotein E-knockout mice or impaired it in C57BL/6 mice (Grootendorst et al. 2001a,b). There are striking changes in learning strategies (Fig. 3). Superior performance is achieved by a spatially guided, persistent strategy, whereas chronically stressed C57BL/6 mice show concentric and random learning strategies. It is conceivable that, in face of a shift in MR/GR balance, MR-mediated behavior is altered and consequently this altered behavior is consolidated by GR.

There is a paradox, however, since CORT can be increased not only by chronic adverse conditions but also by exercise, food deprivation and enriched environments, but the outcome is opposite. While chronic stress suppresses plasticity (Joëls et al. 2007, 2008), spatial learning increases plasticity processes in the hippocampus (Dupret et al. 2007) and context-dependent increases in CORT facilitate memory (Joëls et al. 2006). Constraining GR activation by continuous intracerebral infusion of a GR antagonist improves spatial learning in rats (Oitzl et al. 1998). GR antagonism will restore

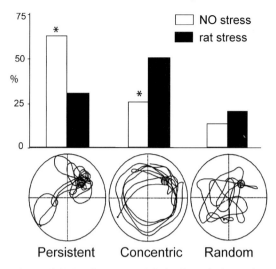

Fig. 3. Search strategies used during free swim trials (at the end of spatial training, on day 3) by naïve and rat-stressed C57BL/6J mice (percentage of mice using either a persistent, concentric or random strategy). Mice were exposed to rats for one to three hrs per day over two weeks. One week thereafter, three days of water maze training followed. On day 3, naïve mice took 12 ± 5 sec and rat-stressed mice took 31 ± 7 sec to reach the platform. Rat-stressed mice switched the strategies from a persistent, hippocampus-dependent strategy to a non-spatial, concentric strategy. *$p < 0.05$. (Adapted from Grootendorst et al. 2001a)

cognitive effects induced by chronic stress and high CORT (see below), a finding that supports its beneficial effect on hippocampal CA1 synaptic plasticity (Krugers et al. 2006).

Translation of MR and GR responses from the cellular level (mainly hippocampus) to behavioral functions is a tempting and fruitful approach. In the behavioral realm, the membrane- and gene-mediated CORT actions are extremely interesting because of their conditional nature, which implies that CORT can change the infrastructure of the target cell via MR and GR. How this change affects neuronal function is dependent on the specific nature of the stimulus. Hence, the context in which CORT is acting is crucial for the result. Thus, knowledge of the source, duration, intensity and timing of the stressor, as well as its predictability and controllability and the differential involvement of neuronal networks (memory systems), is crucial for understanding the effects of CORT. The response patterns are primed by previous experience and genetic background, which may further contribute to the large interindividual differences. Acute stress has a clearly adaptive value. Likewise, chronic, stress-induced changes should be viewed initially as signs of an adaptive response, yet the potential for damage and pathology is increased.

In conclusion, there is ample support for the thesis that MR-mediated actions rapidly amplify attention, vigilance and appraisal processes and thus the onset of the behavioral stress response, whereas, via GR, CORT promotes management of the later adaptive phases that include recovery from the stressor, storage of the experience in memory and elimination of behaviors that are of no more relevance.

Mechanism: Responsive Ggene Patterns and Pathways

Gene expression profiling technology using SAGE and DNA microarrays has revealed highly differentiated gene networks that respond to either MR and/or GR activation in discrete regions of the hippocampus. Given the different functions of both receptors in HPA-axis regulation and neuroexcitability, it seems highly likely that parts of the MR- and GR-mediated effects are opposite in regulation of gene expression, either at the level of individual genes or of pathways. Despite the fact that MR and GR have an identical DNA binding domain, the majority of the hippocampal gene targets of MR and GR appear to be different at the individual gene level (Datson et al. 2001). Whether these MR- and GR-specific gene targets feed into the same pathways remains to be clarified, as does the functional consequence of this receptor-specific gene regulation. Interestingly, several genes with a U-shaped or inverted U-shaped regulation, depending on receptor activation, were identified in hippocampal neurons (Fig. 4), reminiscent of the well-known, U-shaped dose-response relationship to excitability of, for example, CA1 neurons in response to corticosteroid action (Joëls 2006).

Given the differential effects of MR and GR on gene expression, the local MR/GR balance within the hippocampus is relevant for the resulting gene expression pattern at a given level of corticosteroids. This pattern differs throughout the hippocampus: the CA3 region of the hippocampus is relatively devoid of GR expression, whereas MR expression is relatively constant throughout all subregions, and there are also a number of receptor variants that may convey differential signals (Lu and Cidlowski 2006). Not only does the MR/GR balance differ throughout the hippocampus (Fig. 4), but there are also large differences in overall gene expression patterns between hippocampal subregions (Lein et al. 2004; Datson et al. 2004), a fact that has consequences for the repertoire of available co-activators and co-repressors as well as the availability of transcription factors that can interact with GR, both important determinants in glucocorticoid signalling. Laser microdissection and expression profiling of specific hippocampal subregions under different glucocorticoid levels and in different contextual settings are necessary to increase our understanding of the complexity of glucocorticoid signalling.

Corticosteroid-responsive gene networks respond in a time- and context-dependent fashion. The dynamics of the transcriptional response to GR activation appears to be conserved between different neuronal substrates. Both in hippocampal explant slices and in neuronally differentiated PC12 cells, a rapid wave of exclusively downregulated genes was observed 1 hour after activating GR, followed by a second later wave of upregulated genes (Morsink et al. 2006a,b). This finding suggests that transrepression involving interactions with other transcription factors may be the predominant mode of corticosteroid action immediately after GR activation, followed by a later wave of transactivation. Since transrepression is an important route through which corticosteroid receptors can interact with other activated signalling pathways, this fast downregulation of genes may be of functional importance for the brain to rapidly fine-tune its response to environmental signals. It may be the preferred route, dampening initial stress reactions as part of the recovery phase from exposure to the stressor.

In conclusion, due to this context dependency, the transcriptional response and the repertoire of genes regulated by corticosteroids are highly diverse. This finding is reflected in the pleiotropy of functional gene classes known today to be under direct control of or interacting with GR signalling in brain, including energy metabolism,

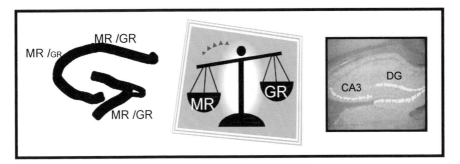

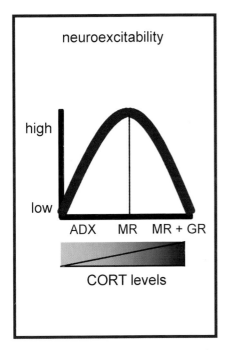
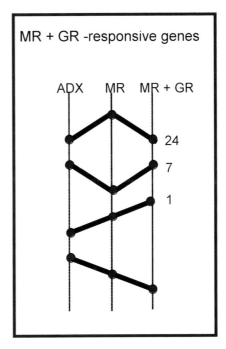

Fig. 4. CORT-dependent gene expression depends on the balance of MR- and GR-mediated actions and CORT levels. Circulating CORT levels (lower panel, *left*) and local MR/GR balance (top panel, *right*) are important determinants of CORT-dependent gene expression in the hippocampus. The MR/GR balance differs throughout the different subregions of the hippocampus (top panel, *left*), warranting specific isolation by laser microdissection and expression profiling of individual hippocampal subregions (top panel, *right*). Some functional properties of hippocampal CA neurons, including neuroexcitability, follow a U-shaped dose-response to CORT (lower panel, left; Joëls 2006). Several genes have been identified in the hippocampus with an (inverted) U-shaped pattern of expression, depending on CORT concentration and corresponding pattern of receptor activation (lower panel, *right*; the numbers of genes with a specific expression pattern are indicated; adapted from Datson et al. 2001)

signal transduction, neural cell adhesion, neuronal structure, vesicle dynamics, neurotransmitter turnover and oxidative stress (Datson et al. 2008). The specificity in the response is therefore directed by the context in which MR and GR signalling operates.

Diabetes as a Disease Model for Aberrant CORT

Peripheral and autonomous neuropathies are well-known and devastating complications of type 1 diabetes (T1D). However, T1D can also impact the integrity of the CNS, and the reason why T1D affects CNS integrity remains to be elucidated.

Diabetic animals show high circulating CORT levels and a poor shut-off of the stress response (Magarinos and McEwen 2000; Chan et al. 2001; McEwen et al. 2002), suggesting insensitivity to feedback mechanisms, which is consistent with the reported resistance to the dexamethasone suppression test (Scribner et al. 1993) and downregulation of GR levels in the hippocampus of streptozotocin (STZ) rats (De Nicola et al. 1976). Processes to adapt to the metabolic imbalance are created in T1D, involving poor glucose homeostasis, chronically elevated CORT levels, increased HPA axis reactivity, and metabolic adjustments. The conditions of aberrant CORT levels and extreme metabolic adjustments appear 1) to enhance the vulnerability to metabolic insults of brain areas showing a high degree of plasticity, such as the hippocampus, and 2) to underlie the impairment of cognitive performance.

In diabetic rodents, structural and functional abnormalities have been reported, in particular for the hippocampus, such as impaired LTP, synaptic alterations (dendritic spine densities and LTP), degeneration and neuronal loss (hamsters: Bestetti and Rossi 1980; rats: Gispen and Biessels 2000; Magarinos and McEwen 2000). Moreover, it has been demonstrated in the STZ-induced T1D mice that astrogliosis, increased apolipoprotein-E astrocyte number, neuronal activation (c-Jun and c-Fos immunoreactivity) and enhanced oxidative stress (NADPH-diaphorase increase), and decreased neurogenesis in the dentate gyrus (DG) occur. These results suggest a mild hippocampal neurodegeneration in the T1D mice (Fig. 5; Saravia et al. 2002, 2004; Revsin et al. 2005). The degenerative changes in brain morphology are paralleled by mild cognitive disturbances in spatial learning (Revsin et al. 2007). These changes in brain and behavior are also observed during chronic excess of glucocorticoids. Moreover, the degenerative cascade in this diabetes model can be exacerbated by glucocorticoids and chronic stress but attenuated by brief courses of anti-glucocorticoid treatment (Revsin et al. 2007; Beauquis et al. 2007)

In conclusion, the hippocampal disturbances manifested in this model of T1D may be among the primary basic mechanisms underlying the well-known brain alterations associated with diabetes. However, the factors that determine the variable onset and progression are not known, but exposure to chronic unpredictable stressors and hypercorticism per se can evoke a similar neurodegenerative cascade, suggesting a GR-mediated central role of CORT in diabetic neuropathology. Therefore, it is likely that T1D leads to a more fragile state of the brain in which the high levels of CORT may enhance the potential for damage and attenuate protective mechanisms, thus precipitating impairment in cognitive function.

Genetics and Early Experience

Genetic factors affect the MR/GR balance and the stress response. Individuals carrying the ER22/23EK SNP in exon 2 of the GR gene have a more favorable treatment outcome for depression (van Rossum and Lamberts 2004). Such individuals seem to have

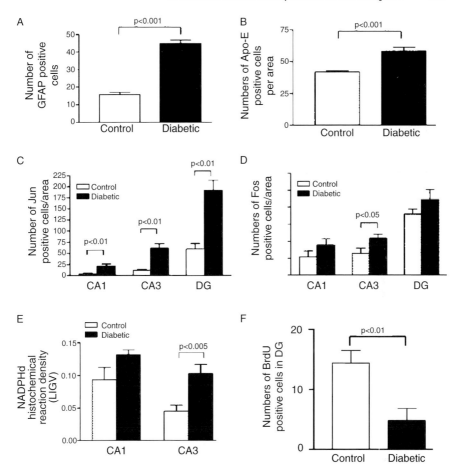

Fig. 5. Hippocampal alterations in STZ-induced type 1 diabetes mice (12-week-old c57Bl/6 mice, vehicle- or STZ-treated, control and diabetic, respectively). A) Number of immunoreactive GFAP-positive cells (per area of 65,310 mm^2) in hippocampal stratum radiatum region. B) Number of immunoreactive apolipoprotein-E (Apo-E)-positive cells per area in hippocampal stratum radiatum region. C) Number of c-Jun- and D) c-Fos-positive nuclei in CA1, CA3 and DG areas of the hippocampus. E) NADPH-diaphorase histochemistry in CA1 and CA3. F) Number of BrdU-positive cells in the subgranular cell layer of the dentate gyrus (DG). Quantitation was performed using computerized image analysis; values are expressed as mean ± SEM

a healthier metabolic profile and better cognitive function than the general population, and they appear to be relatively resistant to cortisol (van Rossum and Lamberts 2004). In contrast, individuals with other functional polymorphisms in the GR gene displayed a more enhanced ACTH and CORT response to a psychosocial stressor than did controls. Several SNPs have also been identified in the MR gene, and carriers of the common MR I180V variant showed enhanced CORT and heart-rate responses to a psychosocial challenge (deRijk et al. 2006). A weak association of this SNP with depression (geriatric depression scale; GDS) was found in the elderly population of 80 to

85 years of age (Kuningas et al. 2007). Moreover, patients carrying a specific mutation in the FKBP5 gene, which encodes a protein that interacts with the GR, responded much faster to antidepressants than did a comparison group who did not carry this mutation (Holsboer et al. 2000).

Animal studies showed that another factor determining the MR/GR balance and the stress response in later life is early experience. Rearing environment quality is a major concern for child welfare in modern societies. Adverse perinatal environments, particularly disruption in the mother-infant relationship, can greatly increase the susceptibility to psychiatric disorders later in life (Kendler et al., 2006). Subtler adverse childhood events, such as poor parenting (affectionless/distant), have also been reported to confer an enhanced risk for adult psychopathologies, in addition to behavioral and cognitive impairments (Coldwell et al. 2006). Although the mechanisms are unresolved, a large number of studies have emphasized the critical role of maternal care in the emergence of such phenomena.

The rodent maternal care model convincingly established that naturally occurring variations in maternal behavior can serve as a basis for non-genomic transmission of individual differences in adult traits (Meaney and Szyf 2005). The maternal care paradigm aims to mimic aspects of the early familial environment in humans and offers the unique advantage of examining the short- and long-term effects of a spectrum of parenting styles ranging from extremely high to extremely low maternal care. Among the variety of maternal behaviors scored, the amount of maternal licking and grooming (LG), a form of tactile stimulation, received early during the first week of life has been found not only to vary considerably across litters but to correlate with individual differences in neuroendocrine, emotional, and cognitive functioning in adult offspring. Specifically, rat offspring that received high amounts of LG during infancy display lower responsiveness to stress, both in term of endocrine (Fig. 6A) and behavioral patterns (Fig. 6B) as compared to offspring that received the lowest amount of LG.

Offspring that had experienced maternal care to a variable extent also showed profound differences in markers for brain plasticity. Thus infants that had received high amounts of LG exhibit greater hippocampal synaptogenesis, greater survival of newborn neurons, enhanced glutamatergic transmission, and greater synaptic functioning in the dentate gyrus of the hippocampus relative to offspring who received low amounts of LG (Meaney and Szy, 2005). These characteristics persist into adulthood and correlate with improved cognitive performance (Fig. 6C; Liu et al. 2000). The mechanisms underlying these effects are unclear, but one plausible explanation could be the level of hippocampal GR expression. Compared to low LG, high LG offspring display higher levels of hippocampal GR expression, a phenomenon accounted for by epigenetic modifications (Meaney and Szyf 2005; Fig. 6D). GR alterations have been proposed to be an important modulator of cell excitability in the hippocampus and thus could modulate cortisol negative feedback and cognitive functioning, especially in stressful situations (Champagne et al. 2008, in press).

Supporting this later contention is a recent study by Champagne et al. (2008, in press) showing that extreme differences in maternal care alter morphological and functional aspects of hippocampal synaptic plasticity depending on the degree of GR activation in later life. The authors report that while shorter dendritic branch length and lower spine density are observed in low-LG compared to high-LG offspring under resting conditions (low GR activation), dramatic effects on the ability to induce LTP

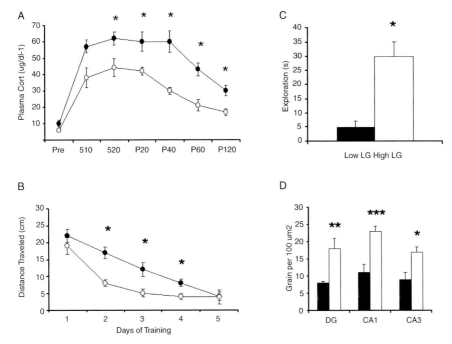

Fig. 6. An endocrine response to stress. Adult offspring of high licking and grooming (LG) mothers display lower corticosteroid (Cort) levels in response to acute restrain stress relative to low-LG offspring. S10 and S20 represent time points during stress; P20, P40, P60, and P120 represent time points post-stress (Figure adapted with permission from Liu et al., 1997). **B** Behavioral response to stress. Adult high-LG offspring spent a greater amount of time exploring the center of an open field compared to low-LG offspring. (Figure adapted with permission from Caldji et al. 1998) **C** Cognitive performance. Across days, adult high-LG offspring travelled shorter distances to a hidden platform during the Morris water maze task compared to low-LG offspring. (Figure adapted with permission from Liu et al. 1997) **D** Glucocorticosteroid receptor (GR) level in the hippocampus. GR mRNA levels were found to be higher in all subfields of the hippocampus in high- relative to low-LG offspring (Figure adapted with permission from Liu et al. 1997). Black bars and circles represent low-LG offspring; white bars and circles represent high-LG offspring. *= $p < 0.05$, **= $p < 0.01$, and ***= $p < 0.001$

were seen. In contrast to animals receiving high LG in infancy, LTP was significantly impaired in low-LG offspring under resting conditions but greatly enhanced in response to high CORT (stress-like condition and high GR activation). These changes were accompanied by lower levels of both hippocampal GR and MR in low-LG compared to high-LG offspring. These findings suggest that, while morphological alterations are likely to contribute to LTP differences under resting conditions, alterations in MR and GR protein levels may account for phenotypic differences in synaptic plasticity when CORT levels are high.

In conclusion, these results indicate that maternal effects may modulate optimal cognitive functioning in environments varying in degrees of stressfulness (i.e., GR activation) in later life whith offspring of high- and low-LG mothers "advantaged" under contexts of low and high stress, respectively.

Perspectives

This colloquium was devoted to hormones and social behavior in the healthy and diseased brain. This chapter has focussed on the action of stress hormones, particularly CORT, on mechanisms underlying resilience and vulnerability. Currently, three questions deserve attention:

First, gene variants and early experience can shape a vulnerable or resilient phenotype. Which phenotype is being expressed depends on the environmental context in later life, but how is this environmental context translated into a cellular and molecular mechanism?

Second, the environmental context in later life presents an interesting paradox. High CORT induced by exercise, food deprivation and, in general, rewarding stressors have an opposite influence on brain and behavior if compared with high CORT produced by chronic, uncontrollable and unpredictable psychosocial stressors. Thus, how can CORT action change from a protective to a damaging signal? What is the cause? What are the consequences?

Third, CORT acts on fast membrane and slower gene-mediated processes via MR and GR. Knowledge about these mechanisms and CORT-controlled pathways is rapidly increasing. However, CORT action is pleiotropic and has, therefore, an enormous diversity, making the context-dependent issue crucial for resolving questions about resilience and vulnerability. The finding that CORT is a hormone coordinating cell and organ function, and now also perhaps genomic and non-genomic regulations, is an important *Leitmotiv* for further experiments.

Acknowledgements. The support by the Royal Netherlands Academy of Arts and Sciences, the Top Institute of Pharmaceutical Sciences T5 #209, NWO Meervoud 836.06.010, NWO-DN95420 IRTG, Smartmix Senter Novem SSM06019 EU Lifespan (www.lifespannetwork.nl) is gratefully acknowledged. We thank Ms Ellen Heidema for editorial assistance.

References

Bestetti G, Rossi GL (1980) Hypothalamic lesions in rats with long-term streptozotocin-induced diabetes mellitus. A semiquantitative light- and electron-microscopic study. Acta Neuropathol (Berl) 52:119–127
Beauquis J, Roig P, Revsin Y, de Kloet ER, Homo-Delarche F, Saravia F, De Nicola AF (2007). El bloqueo del receptor para glucocorticoides (GR) restaura la neurogénesis en el hipocampo de ratones diabéticos. Sociedad Argentina de Investigación Clínica, Mar del Plata, Argentina. Abstract 0124
Bohus B, de Kloet ER (1981) Adrenal steroids and extinction behavior: antagonism by progesterone, deoxycorticosterone and dexamethasone of a specific effect of corticosterone. Life Sci 28:433–440
Brinks V, van der Mark MH, de Kloet ER, Oitzl MS (2007) Differential MR/GR activation in mice results in emotional states beneficial or impairing for cognition. Neural Plast 90163
Caldji C, Tannenbaum B, Sharma S, Francis D, Plotsky PM, Meaney MJ (1998) Maternal care during infancy regulates the development of neural systems mediating the expression of fearfulness in the rat. Proc Natl Acad Sci USA 95:5335–5340

Champagne D, van Hasselt F, Ramakers G, Meaney M, de Kloet ER, Joëls M, Krugers HJ (2006) Maternal care and hippocampal plasticity. J Neurosci (in press)

Chan O, Chan S, Inouye K, Vranic M, Matthews SG (2001) Molecular regulation of the hypothalamo-pituitary-adrenal axis in streptozotocin-induced diabetes: effects of insulin treatment. Endocrinology 142:4872–4879

Coldwell J, Pike A, Dunn J (2006) Household chaos–links with parenting and child behaviour. J Child Psychol Psychiat 47:1116–1122

Conway-Campbell BL, McKenna MA, Wiles CC, Atkinson HC, de Kloet ER, Lightman SL (2007) Proteasome-dependent down-regulation of activated nuclear hippocampal glucocorticoid receptors determines dynamic responses to corticosterone. Endocrinology. 148:5470–5477

Datson NA, van der Perk J, de Kloet ER, Vreugdenhil E (2001) Identification of corticosteroid-responsive genes in rat hippocampus using serial analysis of gene expression. Eur J Neurosci 14:675–689

Datson NA, Meijer L, Steenbergen PJ, Morsink MC, van der Laan S, Meijer OC, de Kloet ER (2004) Expression profiling in laser microdissected hippocampal subregions in rat brain reveals large subregion-specific differences in expression. Eur J Neurosci 20:2541–2554

Datson NA, Morsink MC, Meijer OC, de Kloet ER (2008) Central corticosteroid actions: search for gene targets. Eur J Pharmacol, 583:272–289

de Kloet ER, Sutanto W, van den Berg DTWM, Carey MP, van Haarst AD, Hornsby CD, Meijer OC, Rots NY, Oitzl MS (1993) Brain mineralocorticoid receptor diversity: functional implications. J Steroid Biochem Molecul Biol 47:1–6

de Kloet ER, Vreugdenhil E, Oitzl MS, Joëls M (1998) Brain corticosteroid receptor balance in health and disease. Endocr Rev 19:269–301

de Kloet ER, Oitzl MS, Joëls M (1999) Stress and cognition: are corticosteroids good or bad guys? Trends Neurosci 22:422–426

de Kloet ER, Joëls M, Holsboer F (2005) Stress and the brain: from adaptation to disease. Nat Rev Neurosci 6:463–475

de Kloet ER, Oitzl MS, Vermetten E (2007) Stress hormones and PTSD: basic studies and clinical perspectives. Progr Brain Res 167:1–320

De Nicola AF, Fridman O, Del Castillo EJ, Foglia VG (1976) The influence of streptozotocin diabetes on adrenal function in male rats. Horm Metab Res 8:388–392

de Quervain DJ, Roozendaal B, McGaugh JL (1998) Stress and glucocorticoids impair retrieval of long-term spatial memory. Nature 394:787–90

de Wied D (1997) The neuropeptide story. Geoffrey Harris Lecture, Budapest, Hungary, July 1994. Front Neuroendocrinol 18:101–113

DeRijk RH, Wüst S, Meijer OC, Zennaro MC, Federenko IS, Hellhammer DH, Giacchetti G, Vreugdenhil E, Zitman FG, de Kloet ER (2006) A common polymorphism in the mineralocorticoid receptor modulates stress responsiveness. J Clin Endocrinol Metab 91:5083–5089

Dupret D, Fabre A, Döbrössy MD, Panatier A, Rodríguez JJ, Lamarque S, Lemaire V, Oliet SH, Piazza PV, Abrous DN (2007) Spatial learning depends on both the addition and removal of new hippocampal neurons. PLoS Biol 5:e214

Ferguson D, Sapolsky R (2007) Mineralocorticoid receptor overexpression differentially modulates specific phases of spatial and nonspatial memory. J Neurosci 27:8046–8052

Gass P, Kretz O, Wolfer DP, Berger S, Tronche F, Reichardt HM, Kellendonk C, Lipp HP, Schmid W, Schütz G (2000) Genetic disruption of mineralocorticoid receptor leads to impaired neurogenesis and granule cell degeneration in the hippocampus of adult mice. EMBO Rep 1:447–451

Gispen WH, Biessels GJ (2000) Cognition and synaptic plasticity in diabetes mellitus. Trends Neurosci 23:542–549

Grootendorst J, de Kloet ER, Dalm S, Oitzl MS (2001a) Reversal of cognitive deficit of apolipoprotein E knockout mice after repeated exposure to a common environmental experience. Neuroscience 108:237–247

Grootendorst J, de Kloet ER, Vossen C, Dalm S, Oitzl MS (2001b) Repeated exposure to rats has persistent genotype-dependent effects on learning and locomotor activity of apolipoprotein E knockout and C57Bl/6 mice. Behav Brain Res 125:249–259

Holsboer F (2000) The corticosteroid receptor hypothesis of depression. Neuropsychopharmacology 23:477–501

Joëls M (1997) Steroid hormones and excitability in the mammalian brain. Front Neuroendocrinol 18:2–48

Joëls M (2006) Corticosteroid effects in the brain: U-shape it. Trends Pharmacol Sci 27:244–250

Joëls M, de Kloet ER (1989) Effects of glucocorticoids and norepinephrine on the excitability in the hippocampus. Science 245:1502–1505

Joëls M, de Kloet ER (1994) Mineralocorticoid and glucocorticoid receptors in the brain. Implications for ion permeability and transmitter systems. Prog Neurobiol 43:1–36

Joëls M, Pu Z, Wiegert O, Oitzl MS, Krugers HJ (2006) Learning under stress: How does it work? Trends Cogn Sci 10:152–158

Joëls M, Karst H, Krugers HJ, Lucassen PJ (2007) Chronic stress: implications for neuronal morphology, function and neurogenesis. Front Neuroendocrinol 28:72–96

Joëls M, Karst H, Derijk R, de Kloet ER (2008) The coming out of the brain mineralocrticoid receptor. Trends Neurosci 31:1–7

Karssen AM, Meijer OC, Berry A, Sanjuan Piñol R, de Kloet ER (2005) Low doses of dexamethasone can produce a hypocorticosteroid state in the brain. Endocrinology 146:5587–5595

Karst H, Joëls M (2007) Brief RU 38486 treatment normalizes the effects of chronic stress on calcium currents in rat hippocampal CA1 neurons. Neuropsychopharmacology 32:1830–1839

Karst H, Berger S, Turiault M, Tronche F, Schütz G, Joëls M (2005) Mineralocorticoid receptors are indispensable for non-genomic modulation of hippocampal glutamate transmission by corticosterone. Proc Natl Acad Sci USA 102:19204–19207

Kendler KS, Gardner CO, Prescott CA (2006) Toward a comprehensive developmental model for major depression in men. Am J Psychiat 163:115–124

Kiss JZ, Voorhuis TA, van Eekelen JA, de Kloet ER, de Wied D (1987) Organization of vasotocin-immunoreactive cells and fibers in the canary brain. J Comp Neurol 263:347–364

Krugers HJ, Goltstein PM, van der Linden S, Joëls M (2006) Blockade of glucocorticoid receptors rapidly restores hippocampal CA1 synaptic plasticity after exposure to chronic stress. Eur J Neurosci 23:3051–3055

Kruk MR, Halász J, Meelis W, Haller J (2004) Fast positive feedback between the adrenocortical stress response and a brain mechanism involved in aggressive behavior. Behav Neurosci 118:1062–1070

Kuningas M, de Rijk RH, Westendorp RG, Jolles J, Slagboom PE, van Heemst D (2007) Mental performance in old age dependent on cortisol and genetic variance in the mineralocorticoid and glucocorticoid receptors. Neuropsychopharmacology 32:1295–1301

Lein ES, Zhao X, Gage FH (2004) Defining a molecular atlas of the hippocampus using DNA microarrays and high-throughput in situ hybridization. J Neurosci 24:3879–3889

Levine S (2005) Developmental determinants of sensitivity and resistance to stress. Psychoneuroendocrinology 30:939–946

Liu D, Diorio J, Day JC, Francis DD, Meaney MJ (2000) Maternal care, hippocampal synaptogenesis and cognitive development in rats. Nature Neurosci 3:799–806

Liu D, Diorio J, Tannenbaum B, Caldji C, Francis D, Freedman A, Sharma S, Pearson D, Plotsky PM, Meaney MJ (1997) Maternal care, hippocampal glucocorticoid receptors, and hypothalamic-pituitary-adrenal responses to stress. Science 277:1659–1662

Lu NZ, Cidlowski JA (2006) Glucocorticoid receptor isoforms generate transcription specificity. Trends Cell Biol 16:301–307

Magarinos AM, McEwen BS (2000) Experimental diabetes in rats causes hippocampal dendritic and synaptic reorganization and increased glucocorticoid reactivity to stress. Proc Natl Acad Sci USA 97:11056–11061

McEwen BS (1999) Stress and hippocampal plasticity. Ann Rev Neurosci 22:105–122

McEwen BS (2007) Physiology and neurobiology of stress and adaptation: central role of the brain. Physiol Rev 87:873–904

McEwen BS, Magarinos AM, Reagan LP (2002) Studies of hormone action in the hippocampal formation: possible relevance to depression and diabetes. J Psychosom Res 53:883–890

McLaughlin KJ, Gomez JL, Baran SE, Conrad CD (2007) The effects of chronic stress on hippocampal morphology and function: an evaluation of chronic restraint paradigms. Brain Res 1161:56–64

Meaney MJ, Szyf M (2005) Maternal care as a model for experience-dependent chromatin plasticity? Trends Neurosci 28:456–463

Meijer OC, de Lange EC, Breimer DD, de Boer AG, Workel JO, de Kloet ER (1998) Penetration of dexamethasone into brain glucocorticoid targets is enhanced in mdr1A P-glycoprotein knockout mice. Endocrinology 139(4):1789–1793

Meijer OC, van der Laan S, Lachize S, Steenbergen PJ, de Kloet ER (2006) Steroid receptor coregulator diversity: what can it mean for the stressed brain? Neuroscience 138:891–899

Mikičs E, Barsy B, Barsvari B, Haller J (2005) Behavioral specificity of non-genomic glucocorticoid effects in rats: effects on risk assessment in the elevated plus-maze and the open-field. Horm Behav 48:152–162

Morsink MC, Joëls M, Sarabdjitsingh RA, Meijer OC, De Kloet ER, Datson NA (2006a) The dynamic pattern of glucocorticoid receptor-mediated transcriptional responses in neuronal PC12 cells. J Neurochem 99:1282–1298

Morsink MC, Steenbergen PJ, Vos JB, Karst H, Joëls M, De Kloet ER, Datson NA (2006b) Acute activation of hippocampal glucocorticoid receptors results in different waves of gene expression throughout time. J Neuroendocrinol 18:239–252

Nair SM, Karst H, Dumas T, Phillips R, Sapolsky RM, Rumpff-van Essen L, Maslam S, Lucassen PJ, Joëls M (2004) Gene expression profiles associated with survival of individual rat dentate cells after endogenous corticosteroid deprivation. Eur J Neurosci 20:3233–3243

Nottebohm F (2005) The neural basis of birdsong. PLoS Biol 3:e164

Oitzl MS, de Kloet, ER (1992) Selective corticoid-receptor antagonists modulate specific aspects of spatial orientation learning. Behav Neurosci 106:62–71

Oitzl MS, de Kloet ER, Joëls M, Schmid W, Cole TJ (1997) Spatial learning deficits in mice with a targeted glucocorticoid receptor gene disruption. Eur J Neurosci 9:2284–2296

Oitzl MS, Fluttert M, Sutanto W and de Kloet ER (1998) Continuous blockade of brain glucocorticoid receptors facilitates spatial learning and memory in rats. Eur J Neurosci 10:3759–3766

Oitzl MS, Reichardt HM, Joëls M, de Kloet ER (2001) Point mutation in the mouse glucocorticoid receptor preventing DNA binding impairs spatial memory. Proc Natl Acad Sci USA 98:12790–12795

Olijslagers JE, de Kloet ER, Elgersma Y, Joëls M, Karst H (2008) Rapid pre- and postsynaptic effect via membran mineralocorticoid receptors increase excitability in the hippocampal CA1 area. Eur J Neurosci (in press)

Peters A, Schweiger U, Pellerin L, Hubold C, Oltmanns KM, Conrad M, Schultes B, Born J, Fehm HL (2004) The selfish brain: competition for energy resources. Neurosci Biobehav Rev 28:143–80

Pu Z, Krugers HJ, Joëls M (2007) Corticosterone time-dependently modulates beta-adrenergic effects on long-term potentiation in the hippocampal dentate gyrus. Learn Mem 14:359–367

Reichardt HM, Kaestner KH, Tuckermann J, Kretz O, Wessely O, Bock R, Gass P, Schmid W, Herrlich P, Angel P, Schütz G (1998) DNA binding of the glucocorticoid receptor is not essential for survival. Cell 93:531–541

Revsin Y, Saravia F, Roig P, Lima A, de Kloet ER, Homo-Delarche F, De Nicola AF (2005) Neuronal and astroglial alterations in the hippocampus of a mouse model for type 1 diabetes. Brain Res 1038:22–31

Revsin Y, van Wijk D, Saravia FE, Oitzl M, De Nicola AF, de Kloet ER (2008) Adrenal hypersensitivity precedes chronic hypercorticism in Streptozotocin-induced diabetes mice. Endocrinology (in press)

Sandi C, Merino JJ, Cordero MI, Touyarot K, Venero C (2001) Effects of chronic stress on contextual fear conditioning and the hippocampal expression of the neural cell adhesion molecule, its polysialylation, and L1. Neuroscience 102:329–339

Sapolsky RM, Romero LM, Munck AU (2000) How do glucocorticoids influence stress responses? Integrating permissive, suppressive, stimulatory, and preparative actions. Endocr Rev 21:55–89

Saravia FE, Revsin Y, Gonzalez Deniselle MC, Gonzalez SL, Roig P, Lima A, Homo-Delarche F, De Nicola AF (2002) Increased astrocyte reactivity in the hippocampus of murine models of type 1 diabetes: the nonobese diabetic (NOD) and streptozotocin-treated mice. Brain Res 957:345–353

Saravia F, Revsin Y, Lux-Lantos V, Beauquis J, Homo-Delarche F, De Nicola AF (2004) Oestradiol restores cell proliferation in dentate gyrus and subventricular zone of streptozotocin-diabetic mice. J Neuroendocrinol 16:704–710

Scribner KA, Akana SF, Walker CD, Dallman MF (1993) Streptozotocin-diabetic rats exhibit facilitated adrenocorticotropin responses to acute stress, but normal sensitivity to feedback by corticosteroids. Endocrinology 133:2667–2674

Stienstra CM, Van Der Graaf F, Bosma A, Karten YJ, Hesen W, Joëls M (1998) Synaptic transmission in the rat dentate gyrus after adrenalectomy. Neuroscience 85:1061–1071

Tirard M, Almeida OFX, Hutzler P, Melchior F, Michaelidis (2007) Sumoylation and proteasomal activity determine the transactivation properties of the mineralocorticoid receptor. Mol Cell Endocr 268:20–29

Touyarot K, Venero C, Sandi C (2004) Spatial learning impairment induced by chronic stress is related to individual differences in novelty reactivity: search for neurobiological correlates. Psychoneuroendocrinology 29:290–305

van Rossum EFC and Lamberts SW (2004) Polymorphisms in the glucocorticoid receptor gene and their associations with metabolic parameters and body composition. Recent Prog Horm Res 59:333–357

Veldhuis JD, Keenan DM, Roelfsema F, Iranmanesh A (2005) Aging-related adaptations in the corticotropic axis: modulation by gender. Endocrinol Metab Clin North Am 34:993–1014, x–xi

Voorhuis TA, de Kloet ER, de Wied D (1988) The distribution and plasticity of [3H]vasopressin-labelled specific binding sites in the canary brain. Brain Res 457:148–153

Voorhuis TAM, Elands JPM, De Kloet ER (1990) Vasotocin target sites in the capsular region surrounding the nucleus robustus archistriatalis of the canary brain. J Neuroendocrinol 2:653–657

Voorhuis TA, de Kloet ER, de Wied D (1991) Effect of a vasotocin analog on singing behavior in the canary. Horm Behav 25:549–559

Wiegert O, Joëls M, Krugers H (2006) Timing is essential for rapid effects of corticosteroids on synaptic potentiation in the mouse hippocampus. Learn Mem 13:110–113

Yehuda R (2006) Advances in understanding neuroendocrine alterations in PTSD and their therapeutic implications. Ann NY Acad Sci 1071:137–166

Young EA, Abelson J, Lightman SL (2004) Cortisol pulsatility and its role in stress regulation and health. Front Neuroendocrinol 25:69–76

Zorawski M, Killcross S (2002) Posttraining glucocorticoid receptor agonist enhances memory in appetitive and aversive Pavlovian discrete-cue conditioning paradigms. Neurobiol Learn Mem 78:458–464

Aspects of Behavior in Pedophillic Sex Offenders Treated with Leuprolide Acetate

Justine Schober[1]

Summary

Testosterone-lowering agents, serotonin re-uptake inhibitors, surgical castration, and stereotaxic neurosurgery have been used to reduce libido, deviant sexual arousal and fantasy, and the frequency of deviant sexual behavior in pedophiles. Though classified as a psychosexual disorder, there are strong obsession and compulsion components that make incorporation of cognitive behavioral skills difficult. Medications that lower sex drive are thought to enhance voluntary control. Leuprolide acetate (LA) has been used for this type of therapy. It is one of several synthesized agonist analogs of luteinizing hormone-releasing hormone (LHRH, aka GnRH), the hypothalamic factor that stimulates gonadotropin release from the pituitary and produces a paradoxical effect on the pituitary, with initial stimulation of the release of luteinizing hormone (LH) and follicle-stimulating hormone (FSH) followed by inhibition after repeated administration. LA causes a reduction in testosterone release (a decrease in testicular steroidogenesis) that is probably secondary to a primary reduction in LH levels. With LA, testosterone levels are lower than those attained with other medications. Pedophiles were studied in a placebo-controlled, blinded, multidisciplinary study that detailed the objective effects of this drug on measurable aspects of the arousal response. One year of therapy on LA was followed by one year on a saline placebo. Testosterone levels were correlated with outcomes from polygraph testing, plethysmography (PPG) with audio and visual stimuli, viewing time for visual stimuli, and self report of urges and masturbatory frequency toward children. Testosterone levels on LA decreased to less than 50 ng/dl with sustained suppression of testosterone, FSH, and LH for the duration of treatment. On placebo, testosterone levels rose to approach baseline. The study subjects reported decreased sex drive, decreased pedophilic sexual urges, and decreased masturbation frequency when on LA. Modified visual reaction time and PPG indicated no consistent change in pedophilic interest preferences with LA. PPG verified self-reported claims of significant reductions in the magnitude of sexual arousal. LA reduced pedophilic fantasies, urges, and masturbation on self report with polygraph agreement.

[1] Hamot Medical Center, Erie, PA, Department of Neurobiology and Behavior, The Rockefeller University, New York, NY, e-mail: schobermd@aol.com

Pfaff et al.
Hormones and Social Behavior
© Springer-Verlag Berlin Heidelberg 2008

Introduction

Pedophilia is a persistent sexual interest in, and sexual arousal to, stimuli, in a variety of forms, involving prepubescent children. A contemporary definition of pedophilia as an enduring sexual preference for children may also lend a view of pedophilia as a sexual orientation (Langevin 2002). However, pedophillic behavior has been considered a manifestation of mental illness, a psychological condition, a criminal condition, and a condition due to an alteration in sexual orientation. There is much controversy surrounding the causality of this condition and its logical treatment. Among the disciplines of medicine, psychology, social sciences and law, agreement may be found that pedophilia is a disordered social behavior and that child sexual abuse is a widespread social problem.

Pedophilic behaviors are the actions that result from pedophilic thoughts, fantasies, urges, and arousal. Arousal may be either genital (peripheral) or central. In humans, much like other vertebrates, sexual behaviors include approach, creating situations that allow exposure to stimuli that are sexually relevant, i.e., a potential source of sexual gratification, as well as overt sexual activity (direct genital stimulation or contact). These behaviors, in the case of pedophilia, may include viewing child pornography, masturbating to images or thoughts of children, seeking out and interacting with children, and actual sexual activity with children. Obvious ethical principals limit the extent of behaviors a researcher may allow, and observe, with regards to pedophilia. Much of what is available in the literature to gauge response to therapy has relied on self report of these behaviors, but there are more objective means to help evaluate self report (polygraph), as well as means to help evaluate an individual's differential response to the stimuli (auditory and visual images) of variable sexual situations and targets (visual pause time, plethysmography).

The literature on treatment of pedophilia is broadly based, including behavioral, punitive, surgical and medical therapies. Each has been tried with variable degrees of response to a number of outcome measures (Hanson and Bussière 1998; McConaghy 1999; Hanson and Morton-Bourgon 2005). There is substantial scientific evidence to suggest a wide range of psychiatric comorbidity associated with paraphilias and sexual offense (Berger et al. 1999; Kraus et al. 1999; Berner and Karlick-Bolten 1986; McElroy et al. 1999; Blocher et al. 2001; Vaih-Koch et al. 2001; Smith and Taylor 1999). Empirically based treatments for these disorders involve treatment of impulsivity, anxiety and mood disorders and these treatments may also decrease sexual impulsivity. Another component of medical interventions for pedophilia includes substantial lowering of testosterone levels. Testosterone-lowering agents, surgical castration, and stereotaxic neurosurgery have also been used to reduce libido, deviant sexual arousal and fantasy, and the frequency of deviant sexual behavior. Pharmacotherapy has included testosterone-lowering agents such as medroxyprogesterone acetate (MPA), cyproterone acetate (CPA) and luteinizing hormone-releasing hormone (LHRH, aka GnRH) inhibitors, and gonadotropin-releasing hormone (GnRH) agonists, as well as selective serotonin reuptake inhibitors (SSRIs). Leuprolide acetate (LA) is one of several synthesized agonist analogs of LHRH (aka GnRH), the hypothalamic factor that stimulates gonadotropin release from the pituitary (Vance and Smith 1984). It produces a paradoxical effect on the pituitary, with initial stimulation of the release of luteinizing hormone (LH) and follicle-stimulating hormone (FSH) followed by inhibition after repeated administration (Belchetz et al. 1978; Bergquist et al. 1979; Evans et al. 1984; Vilchez-Martinez et al. 1974). LA causes a reduction in sex hormone release (a decrease in testicular steroidogenesis) that is probably secondary to a primary reduction in LH levels (Vance and Smith 1984). Agonist analogs have also been shown to decrease the number of LH receptors in Leydig's cells of hypophysectomized rats (Bambino et al. 1980; Vance and Smith 1984).

Materials and Methods

Pubmed was searched for all case reports, case control studies, clinical trials and other relevant studies detailing the treatment outcomes for pedophilia, sex offenders and paraphilias treated with LHRH agonists, under the following keywords: LHRH agonists, GnRH agonists, antiandrogens, pedophilia, paraphilia, and sex offender.

Five men age 50 years; range, 36 to 58) with a diagnosis of pedophilia (DSM-IV) and who admitted pedophilic behavior were recruited for this study and invited to participate on a voluntary basis. The study was conducted over a 26-month period in a medical research center in northwestern Pennsylvania. All subjects had normal testosterone levels and were in fair to good health. The study was reviewed and approved by the local Institutional Review Board. All subjects provided informed consent. Participation was not a condition of probation or parole. The subjects were informed that they would receive either a drug or placebo without an indication of duration of dose, the sequence, or if a sequence would occur. All had an IQ > 70. Four of the five participants reported having been sexually abused during their childhood. Four had served lengthy prison sentences (mean 7.8 years) following conviction of sexual crimes. All subjects had received previous treatment in penitentiary- or community-based sexual offender programs. Two had a history of major depression and two had a prior diagnosis of alcoholism. All fulfilled criteria for diagnosis of antisocial personality disorder and moderate to severe obsessive compulsive disorder. Two subjects reported bisexual pedophilic preferences, two had exclusively heterosexual preferences and one had exclusively homosexual preferences. Study design was a prospective, repeated-measures, nonrandomized, masked study. All subjects and investigators, except the principal investigator (PI), project director, and study coordinator, were masked.

The PI administered the drug or placebo, the PI and project director designed the study and were cognizant of the dosing schedule, and the coordinator was responsible for the supply of study drug. However, the PI, project director and coordinator were not involved in direct data collection or evaluation of the subjects. Subjects received weekly psychotherapy for 24 months and LA depot injection of 7.5 mg at baseline and 22.5 mg at months 1, 4, 7, and 10. Flutamide (250 mg TID for 14 days) was administered with the first injection. At baseline, one month after initiation of LA therapy, and then at 3-month intervals, subjects underwent Abel Assessment, Monarch Penile Plethysmography (PPG), polygraph, physical examinations, laboratory studies, and psychological testing.

Abel Assessment

Abel Assessment, a combination of self report and visual reaction time (VRT), was utilized according to manufacturer's instructions (Abel Screening, Inc., Atlanta, GA).

To assess VRT (the amount of time a subject viewed a picture), a slide projector was used to present still images of models onto a 12" computer screen. Models were clothed generally in swimsuits and none were in sexual positions. Twenty-one stimulus categories, with seven slides in each category, were viewed by the subject. Slides depicted Caucasian and African American males and females comprising preschool and school-age children, adolescents, and adults. Because of the large number of sexual preference choices generated by the Abel method, a modification was adopted. For this study, predominant sexual preference was defined as a relative visual reaction time z-score ≥ 1 SD. The number of times each stimulus was ≥ 1 SD was recorded. If only one or none of the SD were ≥ 1, the two highest scores were recorded. This modification resulted in an objective measure of only those selections that stimulated the longest VRT. Z-scores for each stimulus set were reported at baseline, on LA, and off LA.

Penile Plethysmography

Monarch PPG (Behavioral Technology, Inc., Salt Lake City, UT), along with the Monarch Adult Projective Audio Visual Set, Version 5 (Salt Lake City, UT), a commercially available set of standardized stimulus materials, was used to assess all subjects. The stimuli contained audio and visual depictions of males and females comprising preschool and grammar school children, teens, and adults. The audio scripts were based on a projective, rather than explicit, portrayal of sexual activity. Unlike most other PPG visual stimuli, the set contained clothed pictures of children (all child models were shown in bathing suits or underwear). No lewd or provocative poses were presented (Byrne 2000). During this procedure, the subject was seated in a reclining chair located in a private room equipped with an intercom. The audiovisual stimulus materials were presented via headphones and on a 14" television monitor. Stimulus presentation and collection of penile, galvanic skin response (GSR), and respiration data were recorded and coordinated by a microprocessor-based Monarch Data Recording Device (DRD; Behavioral Technology, Inc., Salt Lake City, UT). Penile circumference changes were measured using an indium gallium gauge supplied by Behavioral Technology, Inc. The signal from the indium gallium gauge was amplified by 1000; data retrieval was set at a rate of 10 samples per second. Each penile gauge was calibrated to a full range of 3.0 cm before each assessment to ensure that the correlation between circumference and deflection was linear. GSR electrodes and respiration belts also were used for deterrence and potential detection of faking or suppression attempts.

Data from the assessment were compiled and analyzed using Monarch Adult Male Software Version 3.22f. This software guided the collection, management, and initial analysis of the PPG data. The software analyzed the PPG data and provided maximum scores and area- under-the-curve scores for each of the 22 segments of the test. A maximum penile tumescence score was calculated for each subject for each category of stimuli. For the purposes of this study, maximum penile tumescence was defined as any response above 20 points (0.60 cm), which is 20% of the calibration of the gauge. Murphy and Barbaree (1994) argued that a minimum level for significance was 20%. To meet this requirement, a response was considered to be significant if it was at least 20/100-scaled units from the beginning of the stimulus detumesced level. Subject's PPG calibration and projected full-scale responding were set to 3.0 cm. Thus, the cutoff of 20 points for significant responding falls within the 20% minimum criterion for significant responding. A repeated measures ANOVA was performed on the PPG data to assess significant changes in arousal level throughout the study ($\alpha = 0.05$). To assess sexual preferences, raw data for each subject were transformed to z-scores. The z-scores for each stimulus were recorded at baseline, on LA, and off LA. All the responses ≥ 1 SD, or the two highest responses, were recorded. Finally, a subject's classification as pedophilic/nonpedophilic was determined by using a deviance differential (Harris et al. 1992), which was calculated using z-score data and taking the highest response to adults (male and female segments) minus the highest response to infants and children (male or female preschool or grammar school age). The adolescent segment was excluded from analysis. For the purposes of data analysis, deviance differential scores greater than 0 were classified as nonpedophilic and scores less than 0, pedophilic.

All subjects were assessed at baseline. One subject (#1) did not respond to a level of clinical significance (20 points). Further inspection revealed that this client did not obtain a significant response at any point during the two-year study. He was removed from the analysis of the PPG data (repeated measures ANOVA) because low-level data generated from a circumferential PPG transducer were not considered reliable (Kuban et al. 1999; Barbaree and Mewhort 1994).

Polygraph

An Axciton Computerized Polygraph System (Axciton Systems, Houston, TX) and the Lafayette Instrument LX-4000 (Lafayette Instrument Co., Lafayette, IN) were utilized. The examiner was certified by the Colorado Sex Offender Management Board. For purposes of score reliability and validity confirmation, the results were scored by hand and by using the Johns Hopkins Applied Physics Laboratory Polyscore computer scoring algorithm (Heil et al. 1999). Hand scoring is recognized by the American Polygraph Association as the most accurate and reliable method of scoring. It was the only method used to evaluate the data. The algorithm was used as a quality control check of the hand scoring method. Subjects provided a separate informed consent before the first polygraph examination. The polygraph was standardized by an American Polygraph Association approved test procedure and was administered by a single experienced examiner, who was masked to the dosing protocol. The polygraph examination process contained pretest and posttest components. The examiner worked closely with the psychotherapist in developing appropriate polygraph questions for confirmation of the disclosed number of victims and offenses, discovery of new offenses, and/or compliance with study conditions. This study examined past victim and offense admissions data, as well as responses evaluating 30 paraphilias. The pretest established which questions the examiner would ask based on the subject's self report of new admissions of past offending or the absence of accountability statements for known offending behaviors (identified in prison histories). The subject's cardiovascular, respiratory, and galvanic skin resistance were assessed in response to three specific key questions:

1. In the past three months, have you masturbated to sexual thoughts about anyone under the age of 18?
2. In the past three months, have you purposely withheld important sexual information from your therapist?

3. In the past three months, have you had strong urges to initiate sexual contact with anyone under 18 years old?

Psychotherapy

The psychotherapy program comprised cognitive and behavioral therapy. The weekly sessions were cofacilitated by a man and woman therapist. After establishing the rules for group therapy, psychotherapists guided participants through a basic group curriculum that included breaking down defense mechanisms, identifying the typology of sex offenders, and discussing the effects of sexual abuse on victims. The counseling component involved insight-oriented psychotherapy. Relapse prevention plans were constructed with and for each participant.

Results

A placebo-controlled, masked, multidisciplinary study of LA in pedophiles detailed the objective effects of this drug on measurable aspects of the arousal response. One year of therapy on LA followed by one year on a saline-placebo detailed testosterone levels during polygraph testing, plethysmography (PPG) with audio and visual stimuli, viewing time for visual stimuli, and self report of urges and masturbatory frequency toward children (Schober et al. 2005). Testosterone levels were reduced to castrate levels (less than 50 ng/dl) or one tenth the mean average level. By the second week of treatment, there was a sustained, profound suppression of testosterone, FSH, and LH that remained for the duration of treatment with LA. On saline placebo, testosterone levels rose slowly over a three-month period to approach baseline, which was the result of treatment with, and withdrawal of, LA.

When considering the impact on aspects of pedophilic behaviors, this study data distinguished genital and central arousal to pedophillic visual and auditory stimuli, masturbation to pedophilic stimuli, and urges to initiate contact with minors.

During the initial testosterone rise (first two weeks after LA administration), no patient reported an increase in pedophilic urges, sex drive, or masturbation. Subsequently, levels fell to a mean of 11.6 ng/dL one month after the initial injection and remained low until LA was withdrawn. After testosterone fell to castrate levels, the study subjects reported decreased sex drive, decreased pedophilic sexual urges, and decreased masturbation frequency. When LA was replaced with saline placebo, all subjects initially reported no increase in sex drive, pedophilic sexual urges, or masturbation frequency. After three months on placebo, testosterone averaged 195 ng/dL. Some subjects continued to report no increase in sex drive, pedophilic sexual urges, or masturbation frequency, but others expressed great distress that the medication was losing effectiveness and they were fearful of reoffense. At this time, the placebo was revealed to the distressed subjects only. All these chose to return to LA therapy.

Throughout the study, modified visual reaction time results detected the subject's self-reported choice of interest/preference and indicated no consistent change in pedophilic interest preference. Overall, interest preference, as measured by PPG, indicated no consistent change in pedophilic interest preferences with LA therapy. However, the degree to which subjects responded decreased significantly, demonstrating that LA significantly decreased arousal.

Penile plethysmography verified self-reported claims of lowered libido, in that LA therapy caused significant reductions in the magnitude of their sexual arousal pattern. Even with profound testosterone suppression, a complete suppression of arousal did not occur. Low levels of arousal and erectile ability persisted with sufficient tumescence to generate detectable levels on PPG. LA significantly reduced pedophilic fantasies, urges, and masturbation on the self-report portion of this study tool.

On all polygraphic assessments, at baseline, almost all responses were classified as deceptive. Deceptive responses about masturbation frequency, urges to initiate sexual contact, and sexual thoughts decreased dramatically with LA therapy and deceptive responses increased dramatically on placebo. A direct and readily apparent correlation existed between deceptive responses and LA injection. When urges and masturbation frequency decreased on LA, the polygraph indicated almost no deceptive responses.

While on LA, subjects indicated they were better able to focus on employment, relaxation activities, and life planning without continual interruptions by sexual thoughts. All subjects noted a decrease in anxiety, better ability to regulate or control their actions and increased motivation for work/school activities.

Discussion

Consideration of the use of antiandrogens as a clinical treatment for pedophilia is logical because androgens have been proposed to be the keystones of sexual arousal in men (Caldwell 2002; van Lunsen and Laan 1997; Dei et al. 1997; Money 1961; Anderson et al. 1992; Davidson et al. 1979). The physiologic systems that modulate and control genital arousability are similar to those that control arousability in the central nervous system. Both may be vulnerable to the effects of gonadal steroids. Cognitive perception of arousal, responses to arousal, control of impulses created by arousal, and socially appropriate behavior are variable human traits. Pedophilia might be described as altered sexual cognition, a response to inappropriate sexual stimuli and a lack of sexual impulse control leading to socially unacceptable sexual behaviors. Anomalous sexual targets and anomalous sexual activities are what define paraphilias.

In the case of pedophilia, it is personal distress or acting out on thoughts, fantasies and urges that produces a dysfunction requiring intervention or treatment. Historically, pedophilia has been treated with behavioral therapy, pharmacotherapy or both. Medication interventions that substantially lower serum testosterone show definite promise as a significant component of the treatment of paraphilias (Briken and Kafka 2007). Meta-analysis of behavioral therapy (psychotherapy) alone has not shown treatment effectiveness (Rice and Harris 2003). However, because of the profound effect of antiandrogen therapy on sexuality, the personal distress of subjects diagnosed and significant relationship of comorbidities, psychotherapy is always recommended as a component of treatment.

Testosterone levels attained with continued administration of LA were lower than those attained with other medications and may result in LA being a more potent inhibitor of erectile responses compared with other agents. Patients generally become sexually impotent when plasma testosterone levels are less than one quarter of their initial value, but erectile and ejaculatory function after LA administration has been found to be variable (Hill et al. 2003; Krueger and Kaplan 2001).

When considering differential pharmacological treatments, particularly those that lower testosterone as a mechanism to affect outcomes in behavior, analysis of the literature clearly favors LHRH agonists for efficacy when overt behavior is problematic (Hill et al. 2003; Krueger and Kaplan 2001). LA has shown good therapeutic effects in cases where other medications, including SSRIs, CPA and MPA. have failed. Most studies are limited to observational and self-report data, but even these detail sexual behaviors affected by antiandrogen medications as therapeutic effects that suppress sexual desire, fantasies, erections, ejaculation, and orgasm (a marked reduction of overall sexuality).

In our study, LA caused profound suppression of testosterone, with minimal side effects. LA was very effective for lowering pedophilic sexual urges and masturbation to pedophilic stimuli. Even with profound testosterone suppression, low levels of arousal and erectile ability persisted with sufficient tumescence to generate detectable levels of pedophilic interest with the Monarch PPG. The Abel Assessment likewise consistently identified pedophilic interest while subjects were on LA. Predominant sexual preference by z-score was consistent with the subjects' self-reported age and sex of victim(s).

Baseline testosterone levels were normal for all subjects. The occurrence of antici-pated mean testosterone rise two weeks after the initial injection caused no increase in pedophilic urges, sex drive, or masturbation as self-reported by the subjects. Although in this study flutamide was give to minimize the effects of a flare period, other studies have utilized CPA for the same purpose (Hill et al. 2003). Subsequently, testosterone levels fell to castrate level one month after the initial injection and remained low until LA was withdrawn. We noted the return of the testosterone level to approximate base-line, as have other studies. We also noted the return of pedophilic urges in a portion of our patients within the year of placebo treatment. In our study, those who did note these urges experienced a recurrence within three months of withdrawal of LA. This finding has been noted in other studies (Hill et al. 2003; Krueger and Kaplan 2001). The recurrence of symptomatology, and in some cases the time until recurrence, is variable from the time of withdrawal; this finding has been suggested to be dependent on the age of the patient and baseline testosterone level. The strength of sexual arousability in pedophiles and others has been found to be an inverse function of age (Blanchard and Barbaree 2005).

Most physical findings associated with testosterone suppression were anticipated, including weight gain, loss of testicular size, and decreased libido. Decreased volume of the testes with LA treatment has been documented by Rösler and Witztum (1998). Although previously undocumented in humans, a significant decrease in flaccid penile circumference was noted. This finding has been previously described in rats (Ichikawa et al. 1988). This decrease in penile circumference was important as it affected the Monarch PPG evaluation procedure and required changes in gauge size.

Osteopenia and/or osteoporosis are also concerns with long-term testosterone suppression therapy. Not all subjects had a bone scan, but the two that did had normal scans after 12 months of therapy. A 12-month treatment with LA may not be a long enough interval to manifest the expected bone changes from the drug. Others have noted osteopenia after several years of LA therapy (Hill et al. 2003; Krueger and Kaplan

2001; Saleh and Berlin 2003; Saleh and Guidry 2003). With prolonged treatment, a yearly assessment with bone scan is prudent.

Both Abel Assessment and Monarch PPG were efficacious in evaluating sexual preferences. The polygraph and Monarch PPG provided indicators of treatment response. Monarch PPG detected increases in arousabilty that paralleled increases in polygraph deceptive responses with even minimal rises in serum testosterone levels. Though these instruments are used as research tools, their limitations with regard to reliability and validity are well known (Freund 1989; Schouten 1992; Marshall 2000). In a review of the literature, a variety of stimulus sets have been used.

A readily apparent relationship existed between deceptive responses and LA treatment. When self report of urges and masturbation dramatically decreased on LA, the polygraph generally indicated almost no deceptive responses about behaviors, i.e., pedophilic urges, masturbation, and pedophilic contact. Almost all subjects had polygraph evidence of deception at baseline and on placebo, indicating discordance with self report. Because of these results, we concluded that self report alone was insufficient and thus a poor outcome measure to evaluate responses to treatment.

We believe the polygraph is, in general, a reliable monitor in these subjects both on and off testosterone suppression. Perhaps this was because the subjects were generally deceptive off testosterone suppression as they had information to hide; they were generally truthful on testosterone suppression as they had little to hide regarding masturbatory frequency and urges to engage in sexual activity. Certainly, data from a larger number of subjects could strengthen the findings.

Observed arousability, unchanged interest preferences and persistence of erectile capability in some subjects led us to believe that, even with profound testosterone suppression and cognitive-behavioral psychotherapy, persistent objective monitoring, such as testosterone measurement, polygraph examination, and Monarch PPG, were necessary to assess continued treatment efficacy. In terms of sexual arousal, the risk for reoffense was significantly lowered, but not eliminated. Supervision elements of treatment and law enforcement are still required.

Cognitive-behavioral psychotherapy alone is probably insufficient for long-term, ongoing control of pedophilic urges. The obsessive-compulsive nature of the paraphilia and the strong influence of sex drive make incorporation of cognitive behavioral skills difficult. Medications may enhance voluntary control by decreasing sex drive (Berlin 1983).

While on LA, subjects indicated they were better able to focus without continual interruptions by deviant sexual thoughts. The expressed feeling of relaxation from treated subjects has been mentioned in other studies (Briken et al. 2001). This effect was directly related to drug administration; withdrawal correlated with a return of obsessive thoughts and a sensation of distress in two of our five subjects.

The limitations of this study included a small sample size. The subjects did not represent the entire spectrum of men with pedophilia. As a group, they had normal intelligence though a tendency toward lower intelligence has been noted (Blanchard et al. 1999). Neuropsychiatric differences are a recent subject of interest, though this was not an obvious feature of the subjects studied in this group (Hall and Hall 2007).

We have observed initiators of sexual behaviors and limited aspects of sexual behavior with regards to pedophilic subjects. It must be recognized that cognitive perception of arousal is separate from measured genital arousal; genital arousal alone cannot fully explain an individual's level of sexual arousal (Caldwell 2002; Bancroft 1989; Everaerd 1993).

Future studies with greater numbers of subjects treated for longer periods are necessary to fully explore the potential of testosterone-suppressing therapy by LA for modification of pedophilic behaviors. Pharmacotherapy, cognitive-behavioral psychotherapy, and polygraph examination may have better efficacy than any single or dual modality in long-term control of pedophilic urges and behavior.

Acknowledgements. The author would like to acknowledge Peter M. Byrne, PhD, Phyllis J. Kuhn, Ph.D, Paul G. Kovacs, PhD, James H. Earle, PhD, and Ruth A. Fries, BS CIP, for their extensive contribution as a multidisciplinary team allowing production of this research.

References

Anderson RA, Bancroft J, Wu FC (1992) The effects of exogenous testosterone on sexuality and mood of normal men. J Clin Endocrinol Metab 75:1503–1507

Bambino TH, Schreiber JR, Hsueh AJ (1980) Gonadotropin-releasing hormone and its agonist inhibit testicular luteinizing hormone receptor and steroidogenesis in immature and adult hypophysectomized rats. Endocrinology 107:908–917

Bancroft J (1989) Human sexuality and its problems. Edinburgh, Churchill Livingstone

Barbaree HE, Mewhort DJ (1994) The effects of the z-score transformation on measures of relative erectile response strength: a re-appraisal. Behav Res Ther 32:547–558

Belchetz PE, Plant TM, Nakai Y, Keogh EJ, Knobil E (1978) Hypophysial responses to continuous and intermittent delivery of hypothalamic gonadotropin-releasing hormone. Science 202:631–633

Berger P, Berner W, Bolterauer J, Gutierrez K, Berger K (1999) Sadistic personality disorder in sex offenders: relationship to antisocial personality disorder and sexual sadism. J Personal Disord 13:175–186

Bergquist C, Nillius SJ, Wide L (1979) Intranasal gonadotropin-releasing hormone agonist as a contraceptive agent. Lancet 2:215–217

Berlin FS (1983). Sex offenders: A biomedical perspective and a status report on biomedical treatment. In: Greer JC, Stuart IR (eds) The sexual aggressor: current perspectives on treatment. New York, Van Nostrand Reinhold Company, pp 82–123

Berner W, Karlick-Bolten E (1986) Verlaufsformen der Sexualkriminalität [Development of sex offenders]. Stuttgart, Germany, Ferdinand Enke-Verlag

Blanchard R, Barbaree HE (2005) The strength of sexual arousal as a function of the age of the sex offender: comparisons among pedophiles, hebephiles, and teleiophiles. Sex Abuse 17:441–456

Blanchard R, Watson MS, Choy A, Dickey R, Klassen P, Kuban M, Ferren DJ (1999) Pedophiles: mental retardation, maternal age, and sexual orientation. Arch Sex Behav 28:111–127

Blocher D, Henkel K, Retz W, Retz-Junginger P, Thome J, Rösler M (2001) Symptoms from the spectrum of Attention-Deficit/Hyperactivity Disorder (ADHD) in sexual delinquents [German]. Fortschr Neurol Psychiatr 69:453–459

Briken P, Kafka MP (2007) Pharmacological treatments for paraphilic patients and sexual offenders. Curr Opin Psychiat 20:609–613

Briken P, Nika E, Berner W (2001) Treatment of paraphilia with luteinizing hormone-releasing hormone agonists. J Sex Marital Ther 27:45–55

Byrne PM (2000) The reliability and validity of a less explicit audio and "clothed" visual penile plethysmograph set with child molesters and nonoffenders. Unpublished doctoral dissertation, University of Utah, Salt Lake City, Utah.

Caldwell JD (2002) A sexual arousability model involving steroid effects at the plasma membrane. Neurosci Biobehav Rev 26:13–30

Davidson JM, Camargo CA, Smith ER (1979) Effects of androgen on sexual behavior in hypogonadal men. J Clin Endocrinol Metab 48:955–958

Dei M, Verni A, Bigozzi L, Bruni V (1997) Sex steroids and libido. Eur J Contracep Reprod Health Care 2:253–258

Evans RM, Doelle GC, Alexander AN, Uderman HD, Rabin D (1984) Gonadotropin and steroid secretory patterns during chronic treatment with a luteinizing hormone-releasing hormone agonist analog in men. J Clin Endocrinol Metab 58:862–867

Everaerd W (1993) Male erectile disorder. In: O'Donohue WT, Geer JH (eds) Handbook of sexual dysfunctions: assessment and treatment. Boston: Allyn and Bacon, pp 201–224

Freund K, Blanchard R (1989) Phallometric diagnosis of pedophilia. J Consult Clin Psychol 57:100–105

Hall RC, Hall RC (2007) A profile of pedophilia: definition, characteristics of offenders, recidivism, treatment outcomes, and forensic issues. Mayo Clin Proc 82:457–471

Hanson RK, Bussière MT (1998) Predicting relapse: a meta-analysis of sexual offender recidivism studies. J Consult Clin Psychol 66:348–362

Hanson RK, Morton-Bourgon KE (2005) The characteristics of persistent sexual offenders: a meta-analysis of recidivism studies. J Consult Clin Psychol 73:1154–1163

Harris GT, Rice ME, Quinsey VL, Chaplin TC, Earls C (1992) Maximizing the discriminant validity of phallometric assessment data. Psychol Assess 4:502–511

Heil P, Ahlmeyer S, Simons D, English K (1999) The impact of polygraphy on admissions of crossover offending behavior in adult sexual offenders. Paper presented at the meeting of The 18th Annual ATSA Research and Treatment Conference, Lake Buena Vista, Florida

Hill A, Briken P, Kraus C, Strohm K, Berner W (2003) Differential pharmacological treatment of paraphilias and sex offenders. Int J Offender Ther Comp Criminol 47:407–421

Ichikawa T, Akimoto S, Shimazaki J (1988) Effect of leuprolide on growth of rat prostatic tumor (R 3327) and weight of male accessory sex organs. Endocrinol Jpn 35:181–187

Kraus C, Berner W, Nigbur A (1999) Bezüge der Psychopathy Checklist-Revised (PCL-R) zu den DSM-II-R und ICD-10-Klassifikationen bei Sexualstraftätern [Relations between the Psychopathy Checklist-Revised (PCL-R) and the DSM-III-R and JCD-10 classifications in sexual offenders]. Mschr Krim 82:36–46

Krueger RB, Kaplan MS (2001) Depot-leuprolide acetate for treatment of paraphilias: a report of twelve cases. Arch Sex Behav 30:409–422

Kuban M, Barbaree HE, Blanchard R (1999). A comparison of volume and circumference phallometry: response magnitude and method agreement. Arch Sex Behav 28:345–359

Langevin R (2002) Yes, Virginia, there are real pedophiles: a need to revise and supervise, not eliminate, DSM. Peer Commentaries on Green (2002) and Schmidt (2002). DSM IV, p 488

Marshall WL, Fernandez YM (2000) Phallometric testing with sexual offenders: limits to its value. Clin Psychol Rev 20:807–822

McConaghy N (1999) Unresolved issues in scientific sexology. Arch Sex Behav 28:285–318

McElroy SL, Soutullo CA, Taylor P Jr, Nelson EB, Beckman DA, Brusman LA, Ombaba JM, Strakowski SM, Keck PE Jr (1999) Psychiatric features of 36 men convicted of sexual offenses. J Clin Psychiatry 60:414–420; quiz 421–422

Money J (1961) Components of eroticism in man. I. The hormones in relation to sexual morphology and sexual desire. J Nerv Ment Dis 132:239–248

Murphy WD, Barbaree HE (1994) Assessments of sex offenders by measures of erectile response: psychometric properties and decision making. Brandon, VT: Safer Society Press.

Rice ME, Harris GT (2003) The size and sign of treatment effects in sex offender therapy. Ann NY Acad Sci 989:428–440; discussion 441–445

Rösler A, Witztum E (1998) Treatment of men with paraphilia with a long-acting analogue of gonadotropin-releasing hormone. New Engl J Med 338:416–422

Saleh FM, Berlin FS (2003) Sex hormones, neurotransmitters, and psychopharmacological treatments in men with paraphilic disorders. J Child Sex Abus 12:233–253

Saleh FM, Guidry LL (2003) Psychosocial and biological treatment considerations for the paraphilic and nonparaphilic sex offender. J Am Acad Psychiatry Law 31:486–493

Schober JM, Kuhn PJ, Kovacs PG, Earle JH, Byrne PM, Fries RA (2005) Leuprolide acetate suppresses pedophilic urges and arousability. Arch Sex Behav 34:691–705

Schouten PG, Simon WT (1992) Validity of phallometric measures with sex offenders: comments on the Quinsey, Laws, and Hall debate. J Consult Clin Psychol 60:812–814

Smith AD, Taylor PJ (1999) Serious sex offending against women by men with schizophrenia. Relationship of illness and psychotic symptoms to offending. Br J Psychiat 174:233–237

Vaih-Koch SR, Ponseti J, Bosinski HAG (2001) ADHD und Störung des Sozialverhaltens im Kindesalter als Prädiktoren aggressiver Sexualdelinquenz? [ADHD and conduct disorder during childhood and predictors of sexual delinquency?]. Sexuologie 8:1–18

van Lunsen RH, Laan E (1997) Sex, hormones and the brain. Eur J Contracept Reprod Health Care 2:247–251

Vance MA, Smith JA Jr (1984) Endocrine and clinical effects of leuprolide in prostatic cancer. Clin Pharmacol Ther 36:350–354

Vilchez-Martinez JA, Coy DH, Arimura A, Coy EJ, Hirotsu Y, Schally AV (1974) Synthesis and biological properties of (Leu-6)-LH-RH and (D-Leu-6,desGly-NH210)-LH-RH ethylamide. Biochem Biophys Res Commun 59:1226–1232

The Brain, Androgens, and Pedophilia

Serge Stoléru[1]

Summary

Pedophilia is a major public health problem because of its frequency and its severe consequences on the mental health of victims. Estimates of the prevalence of child abuse vary from 7% to 53% in girls and from 3% to 37% in boys. The incidence of child sexual abuse in France and Germany has been estimated to be as high as 100 and 550 cases per day, respectively. Adults with a history of child sexual abuse have a substantially increased risk for developing a wide range of psychiatric disorders. In human beings, the brain is a major determinant of sexual orientation, sexual fantasy, sexual motivation and sexual behavior. Studies of healthy male volunteers and of hypogonadal patients have demonstrated that sexual fantasy, motivation and behavior are largely dependent on plasma testosterone. Although pedophilia is not characterized by increased levels of testosterone, reduction of plasma testosterone levels through antiandrogens or GnRH agonists has been shown to be effective in controlling sexual fantasy, sexual urges and sexual behavior in these patients. This pharmacological treatment is always used in combination with a psychotherapeutic approach and only in severe cases for which the latter approach is not sufficient to control the disorder. Antihormonal treatment of pedophilia is not, however, targeted to the etiology of the disorder. Future studies should focus on understanding the determinants of pedophilic orientation in an effort to develop improved preventive and therapeutic measures.

Introduction

According to DSM-IV-TR (American Psychiatric Association 2000), the diagnostic criteria of pedophilia are the following: 1) over a period of at least six months, recurrent, intense sexually arousing fantasies, sexual urges, or behaviors involving sexual activity with a prepubescent child or children (generally age $\leq$ 13); 2) the person has acted on these urges, or the sexual urges or fantasies cause marked distress or interpersonal difficulty; and 3) the person is at least 16 years old and is at least five years older than the child or children in criterion 1.

Sexual abuse committed on children is a major public health problem because of its frequency and its severe consequences on the mental health of victims. Estimates of the prevalence of child abuse vary from 7% to 53% in girls and from 3% to 37% in boys

[1] Inserm U742, 9 quai Saint-Bernard, 75005 Paris, France, e-mail: serge.stoleru@snv.jussieu.fr

Pfaff et al.
Hormones and Social Behavior
© Springer-Verlag Berlin Heidelberg 2008

(Salter et al. 2003). In the United States, there are an estimated 104,000 child victims of sexual abuse per year (US Department of Health and Human Services 2000). It has been estimated that in France 15% of girls and 2% of boys have been sexually abused by the time they reach the age of 18 (Lagrange and Lhomond 1997) and that 100 episodes of sexual molestation against minors occur each day (Observatoire de l'Action Sociale Décentralisée 1999; see http://www.innocenceendanger.org/index.php?id=677&L=3, website visited on February 26, 2008). According to estimates by German authorities, the incidence of child sexual abuse in Germany is as high as 550 cases per day (200,000 per year), though only every 20th case is recorded (Schiffer et al. 2007).

Sexual molestation of children is significantly associated with later severe psychopathological disorders in those children. A state of posttraumatic stress may appear immediately after the abuse. Frequently, symptoms appear, or reappear, months or years later. A population-based study of 1,411 female adult twins, where one sister had been sexually victimized, demonstrated that siblings with a history of child sexual abuse had a substantially increased risk for developing a wide range of psychopathology, including bulimia, alcohol and other drug dependence, depression, anxiety disorders, and the simultaneous occurrence of several of these disorders (Kendler et al. 2000). In these abused siblings, depending on the specific disorders, odds-ratios for various severe mental disorders were multiplied by 2.6 to 5.7.

It has been estimated that recidivism rates among pedophiles after one, two and five years of follow-up were 7%, 18% and 24%, respectively (Furby et al. 1989). In a study of 377 pedophiles, the mean number of acts of child molestation was 23.2 for pedophiles with non-incestuous female targets and 281.7 acts for pedophiles with non-incestuous male targets (Abel et al. 1987).

In spite of the difficulty of studying a topic such as pedophilia, the societal and public health problems generated by this condition are so important that it is mandatory to conduct rigorous scientific and ethical research on this disorder. It is only on the basis of such studies that public policy and therapeutic approaches can be improved.

The Brain Is a Major Determinant of Sexual Behavior

Animal studies have shown that the brain is involved in the whole behavioral chain of events, from the assessment of motivational relevance of sexual stimuli to the performance of sexual behavior; it is also involved in the inhibition of sexual arousal and the control of acting out (Meisel and Sachs 1994). In human beings, too, the brain is a major determinant of sexual motivation, sexual fantasy and sexual behavior. In recent years, neuroimaging studies – mainly functional Magnetic Resonance Imaging (fMRI) and Positron Emission Tomography (PET) – have greatly improved our knowledge of the brain regions involved in the control of sexual arousal. In light of regional activations and deactivations recorded through neuroimaging techniques in response to visual sexual stimuli, our group (Redouté et al. 2000) has proposed a four-component neurobehavioral model of the brain processes involved in sexual arousal, comprising cognitive, motivational, emotional and autonomic components. In addition, each component appears to be controlled by inhibitory processes. Briefly, the cognitive component comprises 1) a process of appraisal through which stimuli are categorized as sexual incentives and quantitatively evaluated as such, 2) increased attention to stimuli evaluated as sexual, and 3) motor imagery in relation to sexual behavior. We have interpreted the activation of the right lateral orbitofrontal cortex (Fig. 1), the right and the left inferior temporal cortices, the superior parietal lobules, and areas belonging to the neural network mediating motor imagery (inferior parietal lobules, left ventral premotor area, right and left supplementary motor areas, cerebellum; Fig. 2) as the neural correlates of this cognitive component of the model (Stoléru et al. 2003). The process of appraisal is postulated as being the earliest one, with other processes depending on it. Thus, cognitive appraisal of stimuli as sexual is not considered to precede sexual arousal but to be the first step in the whole process

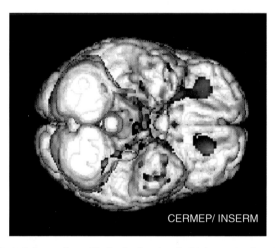

Fig. 1. A view of the inferior surface of the brain showing the higher activation of the orbitofrontal cortices of healthy males in response to sexually stimulating video clips than to humorous clips

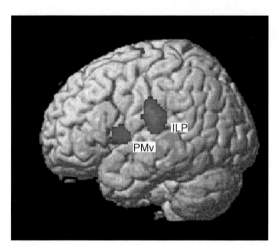

Fig. 2. Activation of the left inferior parietal lobule (IPL) and premotor ventral area (PMv) in response to visual sexual stimuli is higher in healthy subjects than in patients with hypoactive sexual desire disorder

166   S. Stoléru

of unfolding sexual arousal. The emotional component includes the specific hedonic quality of sexual arousal, i.e., the pleasure associated with rising arousal and with the perception of specific bodily changes, such as penile tumescence. We have interpreted the activation of the left secondary somatosensory cortex and of the right insula as neural correlates of this emotional component. The motivational component comprises the processes that direct behavior to a sexual goal, including the perceived urge to express overt sexual behavior. We have suggested that the activated caudal part of the left anterior cingulate gyrus (Fig. 3), right and left claustrum, and left nucleus accumbens were neural correlates of this motivational component. The autonomic and endocrinological components include various responses (e.g., cardiovascular, respiratory, genital) leading the subject to a state of physiological readiness for sexual behavior. We have proposed that the activation of the rostral portion of the anterior cingulate gyrus (Fig. 3) and of the posterior hypothalamus participate in the mediation of the autonomic responses of sexual arousal. These four components are conceived as closely interrelated and coordinated. For instance, the emotional component is partly based on the perception of bodily changes generated by the autonomic component. Finally, inhibitory processes comprise 1) processes that are active between periods of sexual arousal and that prevent its emergence; we have suggested that this type of inhibitory control is exerted by regions of the temporal lobes where activity decreases in response to visual sexual stimuli (Fig. 4); 2) cognitive processes that may – at least in patients with decreased sexual desire – devalue the sexual relevance of visual sexual stimuli; we have proposed that this type of control is mediated by the medial orbitofrontal cortex (Stoléru et al. 2003; Fig. 5); and 3) processes that control the overt behavioral expression of sexual aronsal, once it has begun to develop; we have proposed that the head of the right caudate nucleus participates in this function.

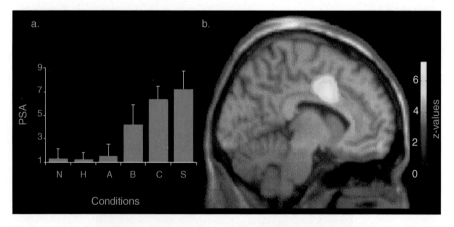

Fig. 3. Perceived sexual arousal (PSA) and regional cerebral blood flow in left anterior cingulate gyrus (Redouté et al. 2000). **a)** Means and standard deviations of PSA in each experimental condition: N = neutral clips, H = humorous clips, A = neutral photographs, B = moderately stimulating photographs, C = highly stimulating photographs, S = sexual clips. **b)** Parasagittal section (4 mm left of midline) showing the positive correlation between regional cerebral blood flow in the left anterior cingulate gyrus (Brodmann area 24) and PSA. Height threshold: z = 3.71, p < 0.0001, uncorrected. Anterior is to the right

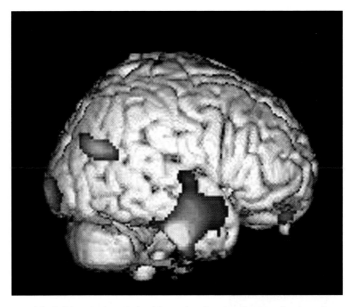

Fig. 4. A view of the left hemisphere in healthy males showing the deactivation of temporal areas and medial orbitofrontal cortex in response to visual sexual stimuli

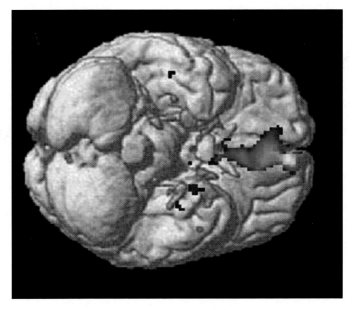

Fig. 5. Maintained activity in the left medial orbitofrontal cortex of patients with hypoactive sexual desire disorder in response to visual sexual stimuli, contrasting with a deactivation in controls

In a further study (Redouté et al. 2005), we purported to map the regions where the response to visual sexual stimuli was related to plasma testosterone. We used PET to investigate responses of regional cerebral blood flow to visual sexual stimuli in eight healthy males and in nine hypogonadal patients, untreated and during treatment. The regions that responded differentially both in untreated patients compared with controls and in untreated patients compared with themselves under treatment were the right orbitofrontal cortex (Fig. 6), insula and claustrum, where the activation was higher in controls than in untreated patients and where activation increased under treatment, and the left inferior frontal gyrus, which demonstrated a deactivation only in controls and in patients under treatment.

The brain plays a role in gender identity, and the conviction of being a male or a female has been investigated. Transsexuals have the strong feeling, often from childhood onwards, of having been born the wrong sex. Zhou et al. (1995) showed that the volume of the central subdivision of the bed nucleus of the stria terminalis (BSTc), a brain area that is essential for sexual behavior, is larger in men than in women. A female-sized BSTc was found in male-to-female transsexuals.

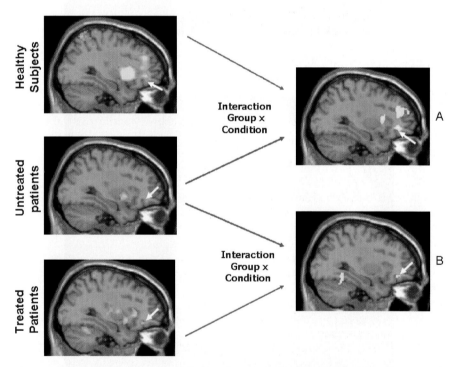

Fig. 6. Higher activation of right orbitofrontal cortex in healthy subjects (*A*) and in treated hypogonadal patients (*B*) than in untreated patients. Parasagittal sections, x = 32 mm right of midline. Front is to the right. The highlighted areas correspond to the clusters of voxels where a significant activation or a significant Group by Condition interaction was found both in response to sexually stimulating films and to sexually stimulating photographs. Height threshold: p < 0.001, uncorrected (Redouté et al. 2005)

Contradictory findings have been reported on brain regions that may mediate sexual orientation. The suprachiasmatic nucleus of the hypothalamus has been found to be 1.7 times larger in gay than in heterosexual men and to contain 2.1 times as many cells (Swaab and Hofman 1990). LeVay (1991) measured the third interstitial nucleus of the hypothalamus (INAH-3), a nucleus located in the preoptic area, in the autopsied brains of 19 gay men who had died of AIDS, 16 presumably heterosexual men (six had died of AIDS), and six presumably heterosexual women (one had died of AIDS). INAH-3 was more than twice as large in the heterosexual men as in the women. It was also, however, more than twice as large in the heterosexual men as in the homosexual men. The volume of the INAH-3 was similar in heterosexual women and gay men. Byne et al. (1991) reported a nonsignificant trend toward INAH-3 occupying a smaller volume in gay men (N = 14 HIV+) than in heterosexual men (N = 34; 25 HIV- and 9 HIV+), with no difference in the number of neurons within the nucleus. As pointed out by Mustanski et al. (2001), a limitation of these studies is the potential confound of AIDS serostatus, as reductions in testosterone levels have been documented in late stages of HIV infections. Another limitation is that these studies have not included homosexual women.

Brain lesions associated with changes of sexual behavior have led to some hypotheses about the neural basis of pedophilia. Mendez et al. (2000) reported two case studies of patients aged more than 60 years with late-life homosexual pedophilia. The first case met criteria for frontotemporal dementia; the second had bilateral hippocampal sclerosis. In both, 18-fluorodeoxyglucose PET revealed prominent right temporal lobe hypometabolism. Although the patients had different brain diseases, the right temporal lobe hypometabolism common to both patients seemed to implicate this area in their sexual behavior disturbance. Does the right temporal lobe dysfunction have a role in pedophilia, or does it facilitate the expression of the pedophilic orientation in persons with a predisposition?

Experimental work in nonhuman primates may help answer this question. In 1939, Klüver and Bucy described a behavioral syndrome following bilateral temporal lobectomy in rhesus monkeys (Klüver and Bucy 1939). This syndrome was characterized by complex behavioral symptoms, such as hypersexuality with repetitive attempts to copulate with non-receptive females, males, immature conspecifics, animals of other species and inanimate objects. This syndrome was also described in man (Terzian and Dalle Ore 1955). In a 19-year-old patient suffering from epilepsy, a bilateral removal of the temporal lobes brought about a lasting hypersexuality, with tendencies to exhibit himself and to masturbate in front of people and the onset of a homosexual orientation. Therefore, the temporal cortex seems to have an inhibitory influence on sexual behavior, an interpretation consistent with the deactivation of temporal areas reported above (Fig. 4). Concerning the two patients with late-life pedophilia, pre-existent latent pedophilic tendencies were probable (Mendez et al. 2000). The temporal lesions could have unmasked a pedophilic orientation hidden until that point.

However, heterosexual pedophilia with no previous history of the disorder appeared suddenly in a 40-year-old patient (Burns and Swerdlow 2003). Magnetic resonance imaging revealed an enhancing anterior fossa skull base mass that displaced the right orbitofrontal lobe and distorted the dorsolateral prefrontal cortex. Pedophilic symptoms resolved with the excision of the tumor. As with the temporal cortex, the medial orbitofrontal cortex seems to have an inhibitory influence on sexual behavior, an interpretation consistent with the deactivation of this area reported above (Figs. 4 and 5).

These studies suggest a particular role of frontal and temporal areas in pedophilic behavior. However, observed lesions were often complex and rarely limited to a single cortical area. In addition, the majority of the patients with frontal or temporal lesions do not present a pedophilic behavior, which decreases the significance of these results.

Two functional brain imaging studies performed in pedophilic patients aimed to identify brain areas involved in pedophilic sexual arousal, but with different techniques: one used PET, the other fMRI. Cohen et al. (2002) used PET to study seven pedophilic patients and seven healthy volunteers. Three conditions based on auditory stimuli were presented: a story describing a sexual encounter between an adult male and an 8- to 10-year-old girl; a story describing a sexual encounter between an adult male and a 30-year-old woman; and words read from the dictionary (neutral condition). Under the neutral condition, pedophilic subjects compared to controls had decreased glucose metabolism in the right inferior temporal cortex and superior ventral frontal gyrus. However, this result has to be considered carefully because the difference was no longer significant after Bonferroni correction. In addition, pedophilic subjects showed an erection under the neutral condition: they were not really in a baseline state. The fMRI study focused on a single case, a homosexual pedophile (Dressing et al. 2001). Three types of visual stimuli were shown in random order: photographs of adult women in swimsuit or underwear; photographs of 10- to 12-year-old boys in swimsuit or underwear; and non-figurative pictures matched in complexity and color intensity. By contrast with the two others conditions, the presentation of the photographs of young boys resulted in a significant increase in right orbitofrontal and prefrontal cortex activity. Neuroimaging studies have shown an activation of the orbitofrontal cortex in healthy volunteers during the presentation of visual sexually arousing stimuli (e.g., Redouté et al. 2000).

Based on a comparison between 13 pedophilic patients and 14 healthy controls, Walter et al. (2007) reported that, in response to the presentation of erotic photographs representing adult women, patients showed a lower activation of the hypothalamus, periacqueductal gray, and left dorsolateral prefrontal cortex. Walter et al. suggested that pedophilic patients remained unable to recruit key structures, which might contribute to an altered sexual interest of these patients toward adults.

Recently, using morphometric analysis techniques, Schiltz et al. (2007) compared the volume of various brain regions, including the amygdala, in patients with pedophilia and in age-matched controls. Pedophilic perpetrators showed a significant decrease in right amygdalar volume. This study also reported reduced gray matter in the hypothalamus (bilaterally), septal regions, substantia innominata, and bed nucleus of the striae terminalis. Smaller right amygdalar volumes were correlated with the propensity to commit uniform pedophilic sexual offenses exclusively, but did not correlate with age, which is inconsistent with a classic atrophic or degenerative process emerging over time. Smaller right amygdalar volumes might rather be explained by a developmental disorder or pre-existing hypoplasia.

In a study by Schiffer et al. (2007), whole brain structural T1-weighted MRI images from 18 pedophilic patients and 24 healthy age-matched control subjects were processed by using optimized automated voxel-based morphometry within multiple linear regression analyses. Compared to control subjects, pedophiles showed decreased gray matter volume in the ventral striatum, including nucleus accumbens, the orbitofrontal cortex and the cerebellum.

Human Sexual Behavior Is Largely Dependent on Plasma Testosterone

Studies of healthy male volunteers and hypogonadal patients have demonstrated that sexual fantasy, motivation and behavior are largely dependent on plasma testosterone. Studies on the localization of androgen receptors (Sarrieau et al. 1990; Puy et al. 1995; Tohgi et al. 1995; Beyenburg et al. 2000) and of aromatase (the enzyme converting androgens to estrogen; Stoffel-Wagner et al. 1999) in the human brain are sparse, so we depend on extrapolation from studies on nonhuman primates or rodents (Clark et al. 1988; Michael et al. 1989; Simerly et al. 1990; Finley and Kritzer 1999; Roselli et al. 2001). Androgen receptors have thus been demonstrated in the medial preoptic area, dorsomedial hypothalamus, ventromedial hypothalamus, arcuate nucleus, lateral mammillary area, bed nucleus of stria terminalis, amygdalas, septum, hippocampi, and the pararhinal cortex and orbitofrontal cortices.

In healthy volunteers, an acute and marked decrease of plasma testosterone induced by the experimental administration of a GnRH antagonist caused decreased sexual desire and fantasy as well as a decreased rate of sexual intercourse (Bagatell et al. 1994). Similarly, the great majority of men with primary hypogonadism reported markedly decreased sexual desire (e.g., Beumont et al. 1972; Salmimies et al. 1982; Gooren 1987). As shown by several controlled studies, sexual desire increased to normal levels with administration of exogenous androgens (Davidson et al. 1979; Skakkebaek et al. 1981). Testosterone increases not only erectile capacity but also sexual desire (Bancroft and Wu 1983; Burris et al. 1992).

In hypogonadal patients treated with exogenous androgens, there is a linear relationship between the level of plasma androgens and the level of sexual behavior. However, the level of sexual behavior reaches a plateau when the testosterone level approaches values observed in eugonadal subjects. Conversely, within three to four weeks after cessation of androgen administration, there is a decrease in the rate of sexual behavior (intercourse, masturbation) and of sexual thoughts and fantasies. Although pedophilia is not characterized by increased levels of testosterone, the dependence of sexual behavior of human males on the level of plasma testosterone has provided a rationale for antihormonal therapy in this disorder.

Antihormonal Therapy in Pedophilia

Antihormonal therapy should be reserved for severe or moderately severe cases of pedophilia, i.e., for patients who cannot control their sexual attraction to children and who do not show clinical improvement after psychotherapy and serotonin reuptake inhibitor antidepressant medication have been initiated (Bradford 2001; Briken et al. 2003). The use of antihormonal therapy should always be combined with psychotherapy adapted to pedophilia. Two categories of drugs, antiandrogens and GnRH agonists, have been used as antihormonal therapies in pedophilia. While the antiandrogens, medroxyprogesterone acetate and cyproterone acetate (CPA), were introduced as treatments for sexual offenders in the 1960s, the use of GnRH agonists in this indication started in the 1990s. In the US, among antiandrogens only medroxyprogesterone is being used in this indication, whereas in Europe and Canada both compounds are used. As the clinical efficacy of medroxyprogesterone acetate and CPA is similar (Cooper et al. 1992), we shall mainly focus here on CPA.

CPA and GnRH agonists induce a decrease in sexual desire and sexual potency, including frequent erectile dysfunction, but they have no effect on sexual orientation. At present, there is no pharmacological treatment able to selectively decrease pedophilic desire while leaving sexual orientation to adult partners unaffected. CPA (Cooper 1981, 1986; Bradford 1988; Neumann and Kalmus 1991), a progestational compound, acts via two mechanisms: on the one hand, as an antiandrogen it competes with endogenous androgens for binding to testosterone receptors; on the other hand, it decreases GnRH secretion, which lessens luteinizing hormone (LH) and testosterone secretions. CPA is usually taken orally and daily dosage varies between 50 mg and 200 mg. In about 80% of patients, sexual fantasies and behavior decrease and deviant behavior is suppressed within one month. When patients under CPA are presented with erotic videoclips corresponding to their sexual orientation, phallometry, i.e., penile plethysmography, a measure of sexual arousal, demonstrates a decreased erectile response, an effect that is more or less pronounced among individual patients (Cooper and Cernovsky 1992). Biological and behavioral effects are reversible within one month after treatment cessation. Side effects include liver toxicity, gynecomastia (about 20% of cases), tiredness, weight gain, depressive mood, and inhibition of spermatogenesis.

Prolonged exposure of pituitary gonadotropes to GnRH agonists results in profound suppression of gonadotropin release, known as down-regulation. Down-regulation of the gonadotropin-testicular axis induces a reversible inhibition of testicular secretion of testosterone, with plasma testosterone falling to castration levels. However, down-regulation is preceded by a two-week period of stimulation of gonadotropin secretion ("flare up"), resulting in a stimulation of testosterone secretion, which is countered by administering CPA. GnRH agonists are administered via subcutaneous or intramuscular injections. Five clinical trials of GnRH agonist treatment (Thibaut et al. 1993; Briken et al. 2001; Krueger and Kaplan 2001; Rösler and Witztum 1998; Schober et al. 2005) have yielded very encouraging results, with only one patient in these five studies reported as having relapsed while under treatment. Under leuprolide acetate (Schober et al. 2005), penile tumescence was significantly suppressed compared with baseline, but sufficient response remained to detect pedophilic interest. Besides relapse prevention, this treatment helps the social and professional rehabilitation of patients. These favorable results have been maintained over several years of treatment. Few side effects have been noted. They include nausea, vomiting, edema in extremities, headache, bone pain and decrease of bone density, tiredness, and hot flashes. Biological and hormonal changes are reversible within one to two months.

However, some obstacles impede antihormonal therapy. Many pedophiles refuse it because "chemical castration," as this therapy is commonly referred to, has a punitive rather than therapeutic connotation. On the clinical side, the more medically intensive antihormonal treatments, the need for injections, and their possible side effects require the involvement of a dedicated psychiatrist, medical/endocrinological backup, and a well-informed and highly motivated patient. Many psychiatrists are wary about the medical responsibility associated with the prescription of powerful drugs that they often do not know as well as psychotropic medications (Briken and Kafka 2007).

Finally, antihormonal treatment of pedophilia is not targeted to the etiology of the disorder. Future studies should focus on understanding the determinants of pedophilic orientation in an effort to develop improved preventive and therapeutic measures.

References

Abel GG, Becker JV, Mittelman M, Cunningham-Rathner J, Rouleau, JL, Murphy WD (1987) Self-reported sex crimes of nonincarcerated paraphiliacs. J Interpers Violence 2:3–25

American Psychiatric Association (2000) Diagnostic and statistical manual of mental disorders. 4th Edn. Text Revision. American Psychiatric Association, Washington, DC

Bagatell CJ, Heiman J, Rivier JE, Bremner WJ (1994) Effects of endogenous testosterone and estradiol on sexual behavior in normal young men. J Clin Endocrinol Metab 78: 711–716

Bancroft J, Wu FC (1983) Changes in erectile responsive during replacement therapy. Arch Sex Behav 12:59–66

Beumont PJV, Bancroft JH, Beardwood CJ, Russel GFM (1972) Behavioral changes after treatment with testosterone: Case report. Psychol Med 2:70–72

Beyenburg S, Watzka M, Clusmann H, Blümcke I, Bidlingmaier F, Elger CE, Stoffel-Wagner B (2000) Androgen receptor mRNA expression in the human hippocampus. Neurosci Lett 294:25–28

Bradford JM (2001) The neurobiology, neuropharmacology, and pharmacological treatment of the paraphilias and compulsive sexual behaviour. Can J Psychiat 46: 26–34

Bradford JMW (1988) Organic treatment for the male sexual offender. Ann NY Acad Sci 528:193–202

Briken P, Kafka MP (2007) Pharmacological treatments for paraphilic patients and sexual offenders. Curr Opin Psychiat 20:609–613

Briken P, Nika E, Berner W (2001) Treatment of paraphilia with luteinizing hormone-releasing hormone agonists. J Sex Marital Ther 27: 45–55

Briken P, Hill A, Berner W (2003) Pharmacotherapy of paraphilias with long-acting agonists of luteinizing hormone-releasing hormone: a systematic review. J Clin Psychiat 64:890–897

Burns JM, Swerdlow RH (2003) Right orbitofrontal tumor with pedophilia symptom and constructional apraxia sign. Arch Neurol 60:437–440

Burris AS, Banks SM, Carter CS, Davidson JM, Sherins RJ (1992) A long-term, prospective study of the physiologic and behavioural effects of hormone replacement in untreated hypogonadal men. J Andrology 13: 297–304

Byne W, Tobet S, Mattiace LA, Lasco MS, Kemether E, Edgar MA, Morgello S, Buchsbaum MS, Jones LB (2001) The interstitial nuclei of the human anterior hypothalamus: an investigation of variation with sex, sexual orientation, and HIV status. Horm Behav 40:86–92

Clark AS, MacLusky NJ, Goldman-Rakic PS (1988) Androgen binding and metabolism in the cerebral cortex of the developing rhesus monkey. Endocrinology 123:932–940

Cohen LJ, Nikiforov K, Gans S, Poznansky O, McGeoch P, Weaver C, King EG, Cullen K, Galynker II (2002) Heterosexual male perpetrators of childhood sexual abuse: a preliminary neuropsychiatric model. Psychiatr Quart 73: 313–336

Cooper AJ (1981) A placebo-controlled trial of the antiandrogen cyproterone acetate in deviant hypersexuality. Comprehensive Psychiat 22:458–465

Cooper AJ (1986) Progestogens in the treatment of male sex offenders: a review. Can J Psychiat 31:73–9

Cooper AJ, Cernovsky Z (1992) The effect of cyproterone acetate on sleeping and waking penile erections in pedophiles: possible implications for treatment. Can J Psychiat 37:33–39

Cooper AJ, Sandhu S, Losztyn S, Cernovovsky Z (1992) A double-blind placebo crossover trial of medroxyprogesterone acetate and cyproterone acetate with seven pedophiles. Can J Psychiat 37: 687–693

Davidson JM, Camargo C, Smith ER (1979) Effects of androgen on sexual behavior in hypogonadal men. J Clin Endocrinol Metab 48:955–958

Dressing H, Obergriesser T, Tost H, Kaumeier S, Ruf M, Braus DF (2001) Homosexuelle Pädophilie und funktionelle Netzwerke – fMRI-Fallstudie. Fortschritte Neurol Psychiatr 69:539–544

Finley SK, Kritzer MF (1999) Immunoreactivity for intracellular androgen receptors in identified subpopulations of neurons, astrocytes and oligodendrocytes in primate prefrontal cortex. J Neurobiol 40:446–457

Furby L, Weinrott MR, Blackshaw L (1989) Sex offender recidivism: a review. Psychol Bull 105: 3–30

Gooren LJ (1987) Androgen levels and sex functions in testosterone-treated hypogonadal men. Arch Sex Behav 16:463–473

Kendler KS, Bulik CM, Silberg JS, Hettema JM, Myers J, Prescott CA (2000) Childhood sexual abuse and adult psychiatric and substance use disorders in women. An epidemiological and cotwin control analysis. Arch Gen Psychiat 57:953–959

Klüver H, Bucy PD (1939) Preliminary analysis of functions of the temporal lobes in monkeys. Arch Neurol Psychiat 42:979–1000

Krueger RB, Kaplan MS (2001) Depot-leuprolide acetate for treatment of paraphilias: A report of twelve cases. Arch Sex Behav 30:409–422

Lagrange, H, Lhomond, B, eds (1997) L'entrée dans la sexualité. La Découverte, Paris

LeVay S (1991) A difference in hypothalamic structure between heterosexual and homosexual men. Science 253:1034–1037

Meisel RL, Sachs BD (1994) The physiology of male sexual behavior. In: Knobil E, Neill JD (eds) The physiology of reproduction. Raven Press, New York, Vol 2, pp 3–105

Mendez MF, Chow T, Ringman J, Twitchell G, Hinkin CH (2000) Pedophilia and temporal lobe disturbances. J Neuropsychiat Clin Neurosci 12:71–6

Michael RP, Rees HD, Bonsall RW (1989) Sites in the male primate brain at which testosterone acts as an androgen. Brain Res 502:11–20

Mustanski BS, Chivers ML, Bailey JM (2002) A critical review of recent biological research on human sexual orientation. Annu Rev Sex Res 13:89–140

Neumann F, Kalmus J (1991) Cyproterone acetate in the treatment of sexual disorders: pharma-cological base and clinical experience. Exp Clin Endocrinol 98:71–80

Observatoire National de l'Enfance en Danger (1999) Observatoire de l'enfance en danger en 1998. La Lettre de l'ODAS, n°10

Puy L, MacLusky NJ, Becker L, Karsan N, Trachtenberg J, Brown TJ (1995) Immunocytochemical detection of androgen receptor in human temporal cortex: characterization and application of polyclonal androgen receptor antibodies in frozen and paraffin-embedded tissues. J Steroid Biochem Mol Biol 55:197–209

Redouté J, Stoléru S, Grégoire MC, Costes N, Cinotti L, Lavenne F, Le Bars D, Forest M G, Pujol JF (2000) Brain processing of visual sexual stimuli in human males. Human Brain Mapping 11:162–177

Redouté J, Stoléru S, Pugeat M, Costes N, Lavenne F, Le Bars D, Dechaud H, Cinotti L, Pujol JF (2005) Brain processing of visual sexual stimuli in treated and untreated hypogonadal patients. Psychoneuroendocrinology 30:461–482

Roselli CE, Klosterman S, Resko JA (2001) Anatomic relationships between aromatase and andro-gen receptor mRNA expression in the hypothalamus and amygdala of adult male cynomolgus monkeys. J Comp Neurol 439:208–23

Rösler A, Witztum E (1998) Treatment of men with paraphilia with a long-acting analogue of gonadotropin-releasing hormone. New Engl J Med 338: 416–422

Salmimies P, Kockott G, Pirke KM, Vogt HJ, Schill WB (1982) Effects of testosterone replacement on sexual behavior in hypogonadal men. Arch Sex Behav 11:345–353

Salter D, McMillan D, Richards M, Talbot T, Hodges J, Bentovim A, Hastings R, Stevenson J, Skuse D (2003) Development of sexually abusive behaviour in sexually victimised males: a longitudinal study. Lancet 361:471–476

Sarrieau A, Mitchell JB, Lal S, Olivier A, Quirion R, Meaney MJ (1990) Androgen binding sites in human temporal cortex. Neuroendocrinology 51:713–716

Schiffer B, Peschel T, Paul T, Gizewski E, Forsting M, Leygraf N, Schedlowski M, Krueger TH (2007) Structural brain abnormalities in the frontostriatal system and cerebellum in pedophilia. J Psychiat Res 41:753–62

Schiltz K, Witzel J, Northoff G, Zierhut K, Gubka U, Fellmann H, Kaufmann J, Tempelmann C, Wiebking C, Bogerts B (2007) Brain pathology in pedophilic offenders: evidence of volume reduction in the right amygdala and related diencephalic structures. Arch Gen Psychiat 64:737–746

Schober JM, Kuhn PJ, Kovacs PG, Earle JH, Byrne PM, Fries RA (2005) Leuprolide acetate suppresses pedophilic urges and arousability. Arch Sex Behav 34:691–705

Simerly RB, Chang C, Muramatsu M, Swanson LW (1990) Distribution of androgen and estrogen receptor mRNA-containing cells in the rat brain: an in situ hybridization study. J Comp Neurol 294:76–95

Skakkebaek NE, Bancroft J, Davidson DW, Warner P (1981) Androgen replacement with oral testosterone undecanoate in hypogonadal men: a double blind controlled study. Clin Endocrinol 14:49–61

Stoffel-Wagner B, Watzka M, Schramm J, Bidlingmaier F, Klingmuller D (1999) Expression of CYP19 (aromatase) mRNA in different areas of the human brain. J Steroid Biochem Mol Biol 70:237–241

Stoléru S, Redouté J, Costes N, Lavenne F, Le Bars D, Dechaud H, Forest MG, Pugeat M, Cinotti L, Pujol JF (2003) Brain processing of visual sexual stimuli in men with hypoactive sexual desire disorder. Psychiat Res Neuroimaging 124:67–86

Swaab DF, Hofman MA (1990) An enlarged suprachiasmatic nucleus in homosexual men. Brain Res 537: 141–148

Terzian H, Dalle Ore G (1955) Syndrome of Klüver and Bucy reproduced in man by bilateral removal of temporal lobes. Neurology 5:373–380

Thibaut F, Cordier B, Kuhn JM (1993) Effects of long-lasting gonadotrophin hormone-releasing hormone agonist in six cases of severe male paraphilia. Act Psychiatr Scand 87:445–50

Tohgi H, Utsugisawa K, Yamagata M, Yoshimura M (1995) Effects of age on messenger RNA expression of glucocorticoid, thyroid hormone, androgen, and estrogen receptors in post-mortem human hippocampus. Brain Res 700:245–253

U.S. Department of Health and Human Services (2000) Child maltreatment 1998: Reports from the States to the National Child Abuse and Neglect Data System. US Government Printing Office, Washington, DC

Walter M, Witzel J, Wiebking C, Gubka U, Rotte M, Schiltz K, Bermpohl F, Tempelmann C, Bogerts B, Heinze HJ, Northoff G (2007) Pedophilia is linked to reduced activation in hypothalamus and lateral prefrontal cortex during visual erotic stimulation. Biol Psychiat 62:698–701

Zhou JN, Hofman MA, Gooren LJ, Swaab DF (1995) A sex difference in the human brain and its relation to transsexuality. Nature 378:68–70

Role of Alcohol and Sex Hormones on Human Aggressive Behavior

C.J. Peter Eriksson[1]

Summary

The promoting role of alcohol on human aggressive behavior is well established. This action may relate to the fact that alcohol is commonly consumed in situations where aggression in also initiated for other reasons: the reduction in the capacity to cognitively control the behavior or comprehend the situational context, facilitation due to expectancy factors, and effects on steroid hormone levels and other biological structures.

Positive associations have been reported between endogenous testosterone levels and both psychological and physical aggression in both men and women. Thus, possible effects of alcohol on testosterone levels are relevant for the expression of aggressive behavior. Recent investigations have demonstrated that alcohol may elevate testosterone levels in men, which may further affect aggressive behavior. In contrast, alcohol commonly elevates testosterone levels in women, especially during the use of oral contraceptives. This could have a major effect in promoting aggression in women under the influence of alcohol.

In comparison to androgens, little is known about the role of estrogens in human aggressive behavior. Recently, however, a positive association was demonstrated between plasma estradiol and emotional negotiation during interpersonal conflict situations. Furthermore, a negative association was observed between estradiol and testosterone-related physical, violent aggression in men with a history of alcohol-related aggression. On the other hand, estradiol, rather than testosterone, was positively associated with psychological aggression in both control men and in men with alcohol-related aggression.

The following conclusions may been drawn from the most recent studies: it seems that physical aggression itself is caused by factors other than testosterone but the underlying strength by which the aggression is expressed is related to testosterone.

Furthermore, endogenous female sex hormones may be related to empathic behavior and could, thus, represent a counter-balancing factor in alcohol-related male aggressive behavior. Overall, recent findings imply that estradiol-testosterone-related regulations may not only explain individual differences in men but may also explain part of the broader gender differences regarding empathic and aggressive behavior.

---

[1] Department of Mental Health and Alcohol Research, National Public Health Institute, POB 33, 00251 Helsinki, Finland, e-mail: peter.eriksson@ktl.fi

Pfaff et al.
Hormones and Social Behavior
© Springer-Verlag Berlin Heidelberg 2008

Introduction

Human aggression is a complex behavior that involves a number of components that, in turn, are regulated by both psychosocial and biological factors. The present survey will focus on psychological and physical aggression, which may lead to injury-inflicting violence. These forms of aggression are initiated by situation-mediated feelings or emotions of anger, the strength of which is regulated by the comprehension of the situational context and underlying biological structures. The expression of anger into subsequent forms of aggression is in turn highly controlled by cognitive factors.

Both alcohol and sex hormones, especially androgens, are well known to be associated with aggressive behaviors in both men and women and, thus, the general aspects of these interactions will only briefly be discussed in the present work. Instead, the main aim of the present work is to review new data regarding the specific roles of testosterone and estradiol in the actions of alcohol-related aggression with special emphasis on the influence of alcohol and gender differences.

Alcohol and Aggression

Alcohol is well known to be associated with aggression, and several comprehensive reviews on this topic have been written (Boyatzis 1977; Brown and Witherspoon 2002; Bushman 1997; Bushman and Cooper 1990; Chermack and Giancola 1997; Giancola 2002; Langhinrichen-Rohling 2005; Kantor and Straus 1987; Leonard 2002; Milgram 1993; Taylor and Chermack 1993; von der Pahlen 2005). Naturally, one main social contextual reason for the association between alcohol intake and interpersonal aggression relates to the fact that alcohol is commonly consumed in situations and events where aggression is also initiated for other reasons, e.g., in alcohol-licensed establishments (pubs, bars, restaurants, etc), at sporting events and at other different types of gatherings, especially among the younger generation. With and without the combination of the preceding social factors, the other main explanations for alcohol-related aggression include the loss of cognitive capacity to control the behavior and to comprehend the situational context leading to aggression, as well as aggression-related alcohol expectancy. Thus, individuals with underlying general dispositions for aggressive behavior would be especially susceptible to such actions of alcohol. (Fig. 1)

The anxiolytic and stimulatory effects of alcohol have also been proposed to explain alcohol-related aggression (Blanchard et al. 1993; Phil et al. 1993). These and other more direct effects of alcohol on the regulation of aggressive behavior have been associated with the GABA, neurosteroid and monoamine systems (Lavine 1997; Miczek et al. 1997, 2003).

Testosterone and Aggression

Androgens, especially testosterone, have been firmly established to promote aggression (at least in some form and in some conditions) in a number of animal species (Albert et al. 1992; Giammanco et al. 2005; Hau 2007; Sluyter et al. 1996; Soma 2006). However, regarding humans, the positive association between aggression and testosterone has mostly, albeit not absolutely consistently, been documented in correlation

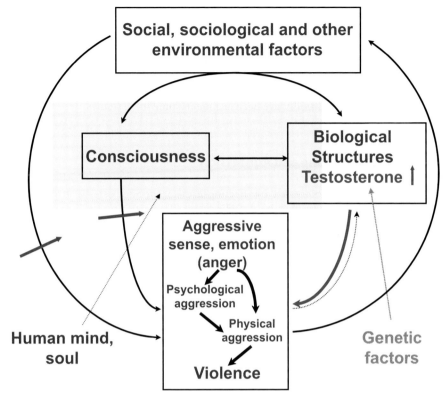

Fig. 1. The role of alcohol in the sociobiological regulation of aggression. The sites of alcohol actions are marked in red. Alcohol may promote aggression by the facilitation of social context-associated aggression, reduction of cognitive comprehension and control, and by the elevation of testosterone levels

studies involving both cross-sectional and selected populations and in group comparison studies usually comparing control and delinquent populations (Archer 1991, 2006; Christiansen 2001; Rubinow and Schmidt 1996, von der Pahlen 2005; Zitzmann and Nieschlag 2001). Also, objections to the meaning of the positive correlation between circulating testosterone levels and aggressive behavior have been raised based on observations of testosterone elevations as a consequence of aggression (Archer 1991; Christiansen 2001; Zitzmann and Nieschlag 2001). Although this effect may explain some of the positive associations, it seems unlikely that it would be the whole explanation for these relationships.

Intervention studies with exogenous testosterone administrations have displayed both significant (Finkelstein et al. 1997; Hermans et al. 2007; Kouri et al. 1995; Pope et al. 2000; van Honk et al. 2001) and non-significant (Anderson et al. 1992; O'Connor et al. 2002, 2004; Tricker et al. 1996; Yates et al. 1999) signs for, at least, prerequisites of aggressive behavior. One problem with the intervention experiments is that giving external testosterone immediately results in the cessation of the natural production of testosterone as a consequence of the feedback inhibition system. Thus, periodical testosterone elevations may have been followed by subsequent testosterone losses, which may have blurred the overall behavioral outcome. Without careful monitoring and determination of the circulating testosterone levels, which is the case in most of the above-mentioned studies, it is hard to evaluate the intervention results. The poor results from intervention studies may also be explained by the possibility that testosterone levels are only promoting aggression and the real situational reasons for initiating aggressive behavior have been lacking in some these studies.

Alcohol, Testosterone and Aggression

It is a challenging possibility that, by affecting testosterone homeostasis, alcohol could affect aggressive behavior. Two early studies showed no significant effects of alcohol on testosterone levels in male occasional drinkers (Ylikahri et al. 1978) and alcoholics (Huttunen et al. 1976). Other early studies displayed alcohol-mediated testosterone reductions with moderate to high alcohol doses in non-alcoholic men (Bertello et al. 1983; Dotson et al. 1975; Gordon et al. 1978; Mendelson et al. 1977, 1980; Rowe et al. 1974; Välimäki et al. 1984; Ylikahri et al. 1974). However, it has more recently been demonstrated that alcohol may also elevate testosterone levels in men during the intoxication (Sarkola and Eriksson 2003), which would fit with the notion of a promoting effect on aggressive behavior.

In contrast, alcohol commonly elevates testosterone levels in women, especially during the use of oral contraceptives (Eriksson et al. 1994; Frias et al. 2000, 2002; Sarkola et al. 2000, 2001). This could have a major effect in promoting aggression in women under the influence of alcohol.

An overall path-model of the proposed sociobiological regulation of alcohol and testosterone-mediated aggressive behavior is presented in Fig. 1. It is rather obvious that the high degree of alcohol intoxication constitutes a far too common condition during which the ratio between senses and sensibilities is too high for an individual to prevent the derivation and expression of regrettable aggression.

Role of Estradiol in Alcohol- and Testosterone-related Aggression

Early Findings on Estradiol and Aggression

An early review of aggressive behavior in hamsters (Floody and Pfaff 1974) concluded that endogenous estradiol facilitates aggressive behavior in females and that exogenous estradiol facilitates aggressive behavior in castrated males and in ovariectomized females. On the other hand, it was also concluded that exogenous estradiol may counteract male behaviors by interference with production, activity or both of testicular androgens. A later review concluded that the essential hormones for full manifestation of aggression in female rats appear to be both testosterone and estradiol (Albert et al. 1992). More recently, in line with previous conclusions, it was reported that estradiol itself, in addition to testosterone, may produce aggressive behavior also in male birds

(Wingfield et al. 2001). Finally, an elaborate study using CYP19 knockout male mice with an inborn lack of the aromatase P450, which is responsible for the conversion of androgens to estrogens, demonstrated that there was an absolute requirement for exogenous estradiol during the neonatal stages of life for the development of the potential for aggression observed in adulthood (Toda et al. 2001).

In comparison to androgens and the results on experimental animals, almost nothing has been reported about the role of estrogens in human aggressive behavior. Originally, estrogens were used with some success to suppress violent sexual aggression, but their use has been limited because of side effects such as nausea, vomiting, and feminization (Bradford 1983). The discussion about these and other ethical problems regarding this form of current "voluntary" treatment of sexual offenders continues (Berlin 2003).

Estrogen treatments of aggressive behavior in both male and female geriatric patients have resulted in some improvements, especially regarding sexual and physical aggression (Kyomen et al. 1991; Kay et al. 1995; Lothstein et al. 1997; Shelton and Brooks 1999; Wiseman et al. 1997). It is notable that no improvements were achieved regarding the suppression of verbal aggression (Kyomen et al. 1991; Shelton and Brooks 1999). Another problem may be the rebound aggression effect after the treatment (Hall et al. 2005). The overall benefits of this form of treatment are yet to be evaluated.

Estrogens have also been linked to empathic behavior in a study in which fatherhood elevated estradiol levels, post-birth compared with pre-birth, or compared with controls (Berg and Wynne-Edwards 2001). The results were interpreted as possible signs of paternal responsiveness.

Recent Findings Regarding the Relative Roles of Testosterone and Estradiol in Alcohol-related Aggression

Recently in Finland, a case-control study was performed in which a randomized male population (AGG−) was compared with men having a history of alcohol-related aggression (AGG+; Eriksson et al. 2003). The aim of the study was to explore the relationship between aggression and endogenous testosterone and estradiol levels. The CTS2 (revised Conflict Tactics Scale; Straus et al. 1996), which in addition to scales for psychological and injury-inflicting physical aggression contained scales for emotional negotiation, was chosen as the primary validated questionnaire.

The results were the following: 1) endogenous testosterone levels (adjusted for estradiol variation) correlated significantly positively with physical aggression and injury-inflicting violent aggression in the AGG+ group, but no significant correlations were found with psychological aggression and with the emotional negotiation scores in both groups of men; 2) although no significant group differences in testosterone levels were observed between the two groups of men, the injury-inflicting behavior occurred only at elevated testosterone levels in the AGG+ men; 3) endogenous estradiol levels (adjusted for testosterone variation) correlated significantly positively with psychological aggression and with emotional negotiation in the control group; and 4) in spite of no group differences in testosterone levels, significantly lower (about 25%) estradiol levels were detected in the violent AGG+ compared with the AGG− men.

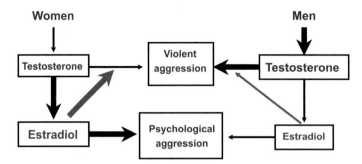

Fig. 2. The role of testosterone and estradiol in human aggression in a broader gender perspective. Red arrows depict inhibitory actions that may involve altruistic mechanisms

Conclusions

Testosterone is more likely to provide the underlying force for physical aggressive behavior than being the instigator of this behavior. Likewise, estradiol may provide the force for psychological aggression.

Earlier results on testosterone associations with less violent forms of aggression need to be re-evaluated for the possible role of estradiol. The dissection of aggression into components, and the use of estradiol as a covariate, will be helpful in producing reliable future studies on the relationship between testosterone and aggression.

Estradiol counteracts testosterone-related violent aggression in men and probably also in women. This effect may be related to estrogen-related altruistic behavior.

The present estradiol-testosterone results may not only explain individual differences in men but may also account for part of the broader gender differences regarding empathic and aggressive behavior (see path-model in Fig. 2).

References

Albert DJ, Jonik RH, Walsh ML (1992) Hormone-dependent aggression in male and female rats: experimental, hormonal, and neuronal foundations. Neurosci Biobehav Rev 16:177–192

Anderson RA, Bancroft J, Wu FC (1992) The effect of exogenous testosterone on sexuality and mood of normal men. J Clin Endocrinol Metab 75:1503–1507

Archer J (1991) The influence of testosterone on human aggression. Br J Psychol 82:1–28

Archer J (2006) testosterone and human aggression: an evaluation of the challenge hypothesis. Neurosci Biobehav Rev 30:319–345

Berg SJ, Wynne-Edwards KE (2001) Changes in testosterone, cortisol, and estradiol levels in men becoming fathers. Mayo Clin Proc 76:582–592

Berlin FS (2003) Sex offender treatment and legislation. J Am Acad Psychiat Law 31:510–513

Bertello P, Gurioli L, Faggiuolo R, Veglio F, Tamagnone C, Angeli A (1983) Effect of ethanol infusion on the pituitary-testicular responsiveness to gonadotropin releasing hormone and thyrotropin releasing hormone in normal males and in chronic alcoholics presenting with hypogonadism. J Endocrinol Invest 6:413–420

Blanchard RJ, Magee L, Veniegas R, Blanchard DC (1993) Alcohol and anxiety: ethopharmacological approaches. Prog Neuropsychopharmacol Biol Psychiat 17:171–182

Boyatzis RE (1977) Alcohol and interpersonal aggression. Adv Exp Med Biol 85B:345–375

Bradford JM (1983) Research on sex offenders. Recent trends. Psychiatr Clin North Am 6:715–731

Brown JD,Witherspoon EM (2002) The mass media and American adolescents' health. J Adolesc Health Suppl 31:153–170

Bushman BJ (1997) Effects of alcohol on human aggression. Validity of proposed explanations. Recent Dev Alcohol 13:227–243

Bushman BJ, Cooper HM (1990) Effects of alcohol on human aggression: an integrative research review. Psychol Bull 107:341–354

Chermack ST, Giancola PR (1997) The relation between alcohol and aggression: an integrated biopsychosocial conceptualization. Clin Psychol Rev 17:621–649

Christiansen K (2001) Behavioural effects of androgen in men and women. J Endocrinol 170:39–48

Dotson LE, Robertson LS, Tuchfeld, B (1975) Plasma alcohol, smoking, hormone concentrations and self-reported aggression. A study in a social-drinking situation. J Stud Alcohol 36:578–586

Eriksson CJP, Fukunaga T, Lindman R (1994) Sex hormone response to alcohol. Nature 369:711

Eriksson CJP, von der Pahlen B, Sarkola T, Seppä K (2003) Oestradiol and human male alcohol-related aggression. Alcohol Alcohol 38:589–596

Finkelstein JW, Susman EJ, Chinchilli VM, Kunselman SJ, D'Arcangelo MR, Schwab J, Demers LM, Liben LS, Lookingbill G, Kulin HE (1997) Estrogen or testosterone increases self-reported aggressive behaviors in hypogonadal adolescents. J Clin Endocrinol Metab 82:2423–2438

Floody OR, Pfaff DW (1974) Steroid hormones and aggressive behavior: approaches to the study of hormone-sensitive brain mechanisms for behavior. Res Publ Assoc Res Nerv Ment Dis 52:149–185

Frias J, Rodriguez R, Torres JM, Ruiz E, Ortega E (2000) Effects of acute alcohol intoxication on pituitary gonadal axis hormones, pituitary adrenal axis hormones, beta-endorphin and prolactin in human adolescents of both sexes. Life Sci 67:1081–1086

Frias J, Torres JM, Miranda MT, Ruiz E, Ortega E (2002) Effects of acute alcohol intoxication on pituitary-gonadal axis hormones, pituitary-adrenal axis hormones, beta-endorphin and prolactin in human adults of both sexes. 37:169–173

Giammanco M, Tabacchi G, Giammanco S, Di Majo D, La Guardia M (2005) Testosterone and aggressiveness. Med Sci Monit 11:RA136–145

Giancola PR (2002) Alcohol-related aggression during the college years; theories, risk factors and policy implications. J Stud Alcohol Suppl Mar:129–139

Gordon GG, Southern AL, Lieber CS (1978) The effects of alcoholic liver disease and alcohol ingestion on sex hormone levels. Alcohol Clin Exp Res 2:259–263

Hall KA, Keks NA, O'Connor DW (2005) Transdermal estrogen patches for aggressive behavior in male patients with dementia: a randomized, controlled trial. Int Psychogeriatr 17:165–178

Hau M (2007) Regulation of male traits by testosterone: implications for the evolution of vertebrate life histories. Bioessays 29:133–144

Hermans EJ, Ramsey NF, Honk JV (2008) Exogenous testosterone enhances responsiveness to social threat in the neuronal circuitry of social aggression in humans. Biol Psychiat 63:263–270

Huttunen MO, Härkönen M, Niskanen P, Leino T, Ylikahri R (1976) Plasma testosterone concentrations in alcoholics. J Stud Alcohol 37:1165–1177

Kantor GK, Straus MA (1987) The 'drunken bum' theory of wife beating. Soc Probl 34:213–231

Kay PAJ, Yurkow J, Forman LJ, Chopra A, cavalieri T (1995) Transdermal estradiol in the management of aggressive behaviors in male patients with dementia. Clin Gerontol 15:54–58

Kouri EM, Lukas SE, Pope HG Jr, Oliva PS (1995) Increased aggressive responding in male volunteers following the administration of gradually increasing doses of testosterone cypionate. Drug Alcohol Depend 40:73–79

Kyomen HH, Nobel KW, Wei JY (1991) The use of estrogen to decrease aggressive physical behavior in elderly men with dementia. J Am Geriatr Soc 39:1110–1112

Langhinrichsen-Rohling J (2005) Top 10 greatest "hits": important findings and future directions for intimate partner violence research. J Interpers Violence 20:108–118

Lavine R (1997) Psychopharmacological treatment of aggression and violence in the substance using population. Psychoactive Drugs 29:321–329

Leonard KE (2002) Alcohol's role in domestic violence: a contributing cause or an excuse? Acta Psychiatr Scand 106 Suppl 412:9–14

Lothstein LM, Fogg-Waberski J, Reynolds P (1997) Risk management and treatment of sexual disinhibition in geriatric patients. Conn Med 61:609–618

Mendelson JH, Mello NK, Ellingboe J (1977) Effects of acute alcohol intake on pituitary-gonadal hormones in normal human males. J Pharmacol Exp Ther 202:676–682

Mendelson JH, Ellingboe J, Mello NK (1980) Ethanol induced alterations in pituitary gonadal hormones in human males. Adv Exp Med Biol 126:485–497

Miczek KA, DeBold JF, van Erp AM, Tornatzky W (1997) Alcohol. GABAA- benzodiazepine receptor complex, and aggression. Recent Dev Alcohol 13:139–171

Miczek KA, Fish EW, DeBold JF (2003) Neurosteroids, GABAA receptors, and escalated aggressive behavior. Horm Behav 44:242–257

Milgram GG (1993) Adolescents, alcohol and aggression. J Stud Alcohol 11 Suppl:53–61

O'Connor DB, Archer J, Hair WM, Wu FC (2002) Exogenous testosterone, aggression, and mood in eugonadal and hypogonadal men. Physiol Behav 75:557–566

O'Connor DB, Archer J, Wu FC (2004) Effects of testosterone on mood, aggression, and sexual behavior in young men: a double-blind, placebo-controlled, cross-over study. J Clin Endocrinol Metab 89:2837–2845

Pihl RO, Peterson JB, Lau MA (1993) A biosocial model of the alcohol-aggression relationship. J Stud Alcohol 11 Suppl:128–139

Pope HG Jr, Kouri EM, Hudson JI (2000) Effects of supraphysiologic doses of testosterone on mood and aggression in normal men: a randomized controlled trial. Arch Gen Psychiat 57:133–140

Rowe PH, Racey PA, Shenton JC, Ellwood M, Lehane J (1974) Effects of acute administration of alcohol and barbiturates on plasma luteinizing hormone and testosterone in man. J Endocrinol 63:50–51

Rubinow DR, Schmidt PJ (1996) Androgens, brain, and behavior. Am J Psychiat 153:974–984

Sarkola T, Eriksson CJP (2003) Testosterone increases in men after a low dose of alcohol. Alcohol Clin Exp Res 27:682–685

Sarkola T, Fukunaga T, Mäkisalo H, Eriksson CJP (2000) Acute effect of alcohol on androgens in premenopausal women. Alcohol Alcohol 35:84–90

Sarkola T, Adlercreutz H, Heinonen S, von der Pahlen B, Eriksson CJP (2001) The role of the liver in the acute effect of alcohol on androgens in women. J Clin Endocrinol Metab 86:1981–1985

Shelton PS, Brooks VG (1999) Estrogen for dementia-related aggression in elderly men. Ann Pharmacother 33:808–812

Sluyter F, van Oortmerssen GA, de Ruiter AJ, Koolhaas JM (1996) Aggression in wild mice: current state of affairs. Behav Genet 26:489–496

Soma KK (2006) Testosterone and aggression: Berthold, birds and beyond. Neuroendocrinology 18:543–551

Straus MA, Hamby SL, Boney-McCoy S, Sugarman DB (1976) The revised conflict tactic scales. Development and preliminary psychometric data. J Fam Issues 17:283–316

Taylor SP, Chermack ST (1993) Alcohol, drugs and human physical aggression. J Stud Alcohol 11 Suppl:78–88

Toda K, Saibara T, Okada T, Onishi S, Shizuta Y (2001) A loss of aggressive behaviour and its reinstatement by oestrogen in mice lacking the aromatase gene (Cyp19). J Endocrinol 168:217–220

Tricker R, Casaburi R, Storer TW, Clevenger B, Berman N, Shirazi A, Bhasin S (1996) The effects of supraphysiological doses of testosterone on angry behavior in healthy eugonadal men – a clinical research center study. J Clin Endocrinol Metab 81:3754–3758 van Honk J, Tuiten A, Hermans E, Putman P, Koppeschaar H, Thijssen J, Verbaten R, van Doornen L (2001) A single administration of testosterone induces cardiac accelerative responses to angry faces in healthy young women. Behav Neurosci 115:238–242

von der Pahlen B (2005) The role of alcohol and steroid hormones in human aggression. Vitam Horm 70:415–437

Wingfield JC, Lynn S, Soma KK (2001) Avoiding the 'costs' of testosterone: ecological bases of hormone-behavior interactions. Brain Behav Evol 57:239–251

Wiseman EJ, Souder E, Liem PH (1997) Estrogen use and psychiatric symptoms in women with dementia. Clin Gerontol 18:81–83

Välimäki M, Härkönen M, Eriksson CJP, Ylikahri R (1984) Sex hormones and adrenocortical steroid in men acutely intoxicated with ethanol. Alcohol 1:89–93

Yates WR, Perry PJ, MacIndoe, Holman T, Ellingrod V (1999) Psychosexual effects of three doses of testosterone cycling in normal men. Biol Psychiat 45:254–260

Ylikahri R, Huttunen M, Härkönen M, Seuderling U, Onikki S, Karonen S-L, Adlercreutz H (1974) Low plasma testosterone values during hangover. J Steroid Biochem 5:655–658

Ylikahri RH, Huttunen MO, Härkönen M, Leino T, Helenius T, Liewendahl K, Karonen S-L (1978) Acute effects of alcohol on anterior pituitary secretion of the tropic hormones. J Clin Endocrinol Metabol 46:715–720

Zitzmann M, Nieschlag E (2001) Testosterone levels in healthy men and the relation to behavioural and physical characteristics: facts and constructs. Eur J Endocrinology 144:183–197

Social Neuroscience: Complexities to Be Unravelled

Donald Pfaff[1] and Ralph Adolphs[2]

Summary

The use of hormone actions to help unravel brain mechanisms for behavior has led to several striking successes in analyzing neural circuits and cellular mechanisms for social behaviors. This success has prompted us to look forward and speculate about the essential nature of the most complex social behaviors. We propose that there are several aspects that distinguish social neuroscience from neuroscience more generally. One notion is that the nature of human social behavior is qualitatively different from that of any other species and was perhaps a key driving force behind the evolution of the human mind and brain. Other speculations involve the normative aspects of social behaviors, both prosocial and antisocial. Bringing complex social behaviors into the laboratory for systematic analysis will pose one of the major challenges for experimenters in our field.

Introduction

Science usually proceeds from the simple to the complex. In neuroscience, for example, some of the most brilliant forays of the last century involved discovering the stimulus properties of neuronal response requirements in the visual system, by David Hubel and Torsten Wiesel, and in the somatosensory system, by Vernon Mountcastle. On the subject of motor response regulation, the spinal cord reflexology of Charles Sherrington followed by the synaptologic analyses of John Eccles would provide two of the most famous illustrations. An extremely simple social behavior, lordosis behavior, was explainable both in terms of neural mechanisms and in terms of functional genomics, in part because of its hormonal dependency (Pfaff 1999). Then, without discarding any of these ambitions regarding stimulus processing and motor control, scientists have made considerable progress analyzing *states* of the CNS. Thus, mechanisms underlying stress (McEwen 2007), sleep/wake cycles (McCarley 2007), circadian biology (Young and Kay 2001) and fundamental brain arousal (Pfaff 2006) have been investigated. We note that these state changes are of considerable importance to medicine and public health, having implications for a variety of mood disorders and for cognitive functions

[1] The Rockefeller University Box 275, Department of Neurobiology and Behavior, 1230 York Avenue, NY 10021-6399 New York, USA, e-mail: pfaff@rockefeller.edu
[2] California Institute of Technology, 331B Baxter Hall, CA 91125 Pasadena, USA

Pfaff et al.
Hormones and Social Behavior
© Springer-Verlag Berlin Heidelberg 2008

involving attention. In all these cases, wherever there is a hormone dependency, the use of our knowledge of the molecular mechanisms of hormone action makes progress easier.

Now, using the hormonal dependencies revealed by chemical endocrinology and molecular endocrinology whenever possible, neuroscientists are attacking problems having to do with complex social behaviors, that is, they are invading territory that formerly concerned social psychologists. In fact, a journal, Social, Cognitive and Affective Neuroscience (SCAN), is entirely devoted to such research. These scientific developments seem somewhat amazing because of the astounding complexity of such behaviors. Chains of responses by two animals might be represented by quantitative

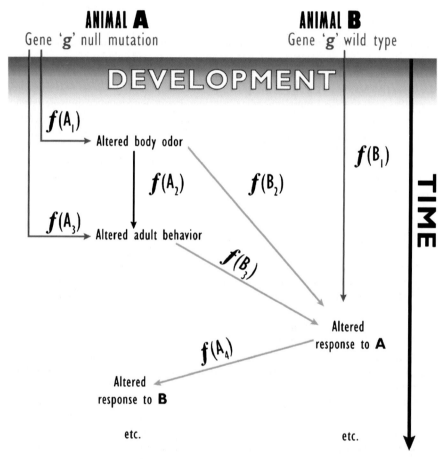

Fig. 1. Genomic effects on social behaviors are potentially complex in the extreme. If we think of just the fragment of an example sketched above quantitatively, as an equation, then it would be composed of at least seven functions, four for animal A and three for animal B. Are these functions multiplicative? Exponential? Note that Kavaliers et al. (2004) have shown that some of the behavioral dynamics of the estrogen receptor-alpha knockout mouse are due to its altered body odors – its properties as an olfactory stimulus to the other animal in the dyad

functions in which the two sets of behaviors are multiplicative or even exponential functions of each other. Indirect routes of causation abound. For example, when we talk about gene/behavior relations, we usually are considering that gene's impact on nerve cells in the relevant neural circuits of the very animal in which the gene has been altered. However, one recent paper (Kavaliers et al. 2004) indicates that removal of an estrogen receptor gene alters the stimulus properties (odors) of the knockout animal, thereby affecting the behavior of other mice (Fig. 1). Further aspects of the complexities of gene/behavior relations – applying to simple behaviors as well as to social behaviors – include pleitropy of gene action, redundancies of functions among different genes, and the incomplete penetrance of some dominant genes. These are illustrated in Fig. 2.

With respect to positively valenced social behaviors, we would stand, as did Claude Kordon (this volume), with the renowned evolutionary biologist Ernst Mayr, who considered sexual behavior to be at "the leading edge of evolutionary change." Mating behavior sets the *bauplan*, the initial organizing structure, for a variety of social behaviors and has been the subject of extensive neural, endocrine and genomic research (Pfaff 1999). With respect to negatively valenced behaviors, mechanisms for learned fear have been analyzed (LeDoux 2000) and have emphasized the crucial participation of nerve cells in the lateral amygdala.

In this brief chapter, we would like to take the opportunity to consider whether there are any unique, abstract issues that we will face, as special problems or opportunities, as we continue to study mechanisms for social behaviors in animals and humans. Is current work in social neuroscience just one more example of lab science pushing into domains that used to be part of the humanities or social sciences? We think not.

The Social Brain

We propose that there are several very interesting aspects that distinguish social neuroscience from neuroscience more generally. One notion is that the nature of human social behavior is qualitatively different from that of any other species and was perhaps a key driving force behind the evolution of the human mind and brain; so, the social aspects might be a lot of what make humans different from other species.

The "social brain hypothesis" has argued that the expansion of the human brain and the cognitive capacities that have resulted were driven by the need to adapt to an environment that was becoming more socially complex (Byrne and Whiten 1988; Dunbar 1998; Dunbar and Shultz 2007a). Precisely what it is about social behavior that makes it more complex and in need of more substantial cognitive capacity, and what it is about the brain whose evolution can adapt to this challenge, are still matters of some debate (Healy and Rowe 2007). There is good evidence for a correlation between neocortex volume, in particular, and the size of social groups; but social group size has been argued, on the basis of detailed path analyses, to be a proxy for "social group complexity," which is defined as the number and kind of social relationships that an individual must keep track of to successfully negotiate social transactions in its group (Dunbar and Shultz 2007b). While it seems clear that many or most brain regions must evolve in tandem to support any increase in one region in particular, sectors of the prefrontal cortex have received the most attention, as that region of the brain has

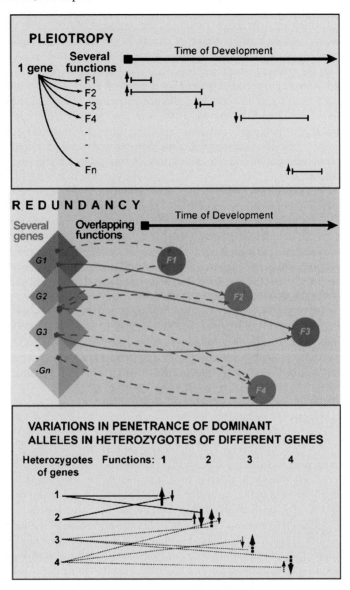

Fig. 2. Some of the reasons for complexity in gene/behavior relationships have to do with pleiotropy, redundancy and incomplete expression of dominant genes in heterozygotes (adapted from Pfaff 2001)

expanded the most specifically in human evolution. Prefrontal cortex as a whole is not larger in humans than it is in the great apes (relative to whole brain size; Semendeferi et al. 2002), but very anterior regions within it (Semendeferi et al. 2001), as well as white matter interconnecting its diverse sectors (Schoenemann et al. 2005) do seem to have expanded disproportionately in human evolution. Moreover, much of the expansion of the human brain has occurred quite recently in evolution. We assign importance to this expansion being coupled to the highly altricial (developing over a long period of time, and late developing) brain that human neonates have compared to those of other primate species (Coqueugnlot et al. 2004).

A related point of great public importance is that understanding the neural underpinnings of human social behavior has the potential to address what are arguably the most pressing issues for the future survival of our species. A pressing case concerns intergroup conflict. The most devastating examples would be instances of attempted genocide. Even during the relatively short time since the Holocaust, there have been five cases: Kosovo, Rwanda, Somalia, Cambodia and Darfur. Scientists may, in the future, be able to understand what is going on in such cases and may help in learning how to prevent such man-made disasters.

On the other hand, we all are aware of examples in which people have acted entirely unselfishly and helped others, at times with great danger or loss of life to themselves. In fact, one of us has argued that our brains are "wired for altruism" (Pfaff 2007). Such exemplary pro-social behavior appears to be exactly at the opposite end of the spectrum from the conflicts mentioned above that often make the headline news, but how can it be explained? Concerning perhaps one of the most exciting areas in social science and social neuroscience, several theoretical reasons have been given as to why non-reciprocally altruistic behaviors might evolve (Nowak and Sigmund 2005) and how the altruistic behaviors of even a small number of individuals could spread in a society and render it better adapted (Gintis et al. 2003). Aspects of prosocial behavior are now being investigated with techniques ranging from functioning neuroimaging (deQuervain et al. 2005) to pharmacology (Kosfeld et al. 2005). The mechanisms that would enable such behaviors are precisely the ones that would contribute to the "social complexity" factor we noted above and that would have contributed to the evolution of cognitive abilities and brain regions that could subserve them.

Social neuroscience looks at issues that are very important to us from a normative point of view, assigning positive or negative evaluations on any given set of acts. Since we are such an intensely social species, often living in crowded environments, the morality of our behaviors towards each other takes on overwhelming importance. One person living alone in a forest does not have such problems, but we presently are living in times when a very small number of people can do harm to a very large number of people. The psychological and neural underpinnings of moral judgment and moral reasoning are intense topics of recent research (Hauser 2006; Moll et al. 2005), as reviewed in Hauser's chapter in this volume. How to study actual moral behavior in an ecologically valid setting remains a challenge.

Social Experience Driving High Levels of Self Awareness?

A final point would be very speculative: that ultimately an understanding of how social information is processed in the brain will also yield insight into the nature of conscious experience. At least it seems plausible that much of the nature of human conscious experience depends on being embedded in a complex social environment. Consider that the tremendous expansion of the human cerebral cortex permits a human to use large numbers of facial muscles to express emotions and to emit grammatical speech, and correspondingly our powerful cortex leads to the human receiver's ability to recognize emotional expressions and to understand speech. In these ways, our social communication is associated with our highest nervous and mental capacities. It is notable that neurologists use the ability of a patient to initiate social communication and to respond to social signals as a sign that the patient has emerged from a vegetative state into a conscious state (Posner et al. 2007; Schiff et al. 2007).

While conscious experience remains one of the most difficult phenomena to approach scientifically, amounting to one of the "hardest" problems in science, it is also true that we can observe intriguing correlations between the richness (or even the presence) of conscious experience and social behavior. To make any such correlations causal, we will need to know much more about the processes and the neural structures that underlie both conscious experience and social cognition. There are some leads. Consider, for instance, the finding that similar network of brain structure is engaged when we construct episodic thoughts (either about our autobiographical past or the imagined future) and when we engage in self-referential thinking of any kind (Buckner and Carroll 2007). This network is also likely engaged when we think about the minds of other people. One direction in which the causality could run is from social to conscious experience. This idea would propose that complex social behavior promoted the evolution of higher cognitive functions required for large and episodic memory stores, for counterfactual and recursive thinking, in short, for outsmarting others, and that this collection of cognitive abilities provided much of the content, if not the state/level, of human conscious experience. But one could also see the causal chain running in the other direction. One strategy by which it is thought that humans figure out what other people believe and intend to do is by simulating aspects of what is going on in their minds at a conscious level. "Simulation" theories of how we predict and interpret other people's behavior seem to put emphasis on the simulation engaging conscious experience (although this is usually not made explicit in the theories), for instance in the form of conscious experiences of emotion when we empathize with another person we observe to be in pain (Singer et al. 2004). In summary, social cognition may have enabled (aspects of) the nature of human conscious experience or conscious experience may have enabled (e.g., simulation aspects of) social cognition.

All of these issues are extremely "high-level" in the sense that they are difficult to investigate experimentally in the laboratory. Self awareness and consciousness are hard subjects. We can make a start by defining and assaying generalized CNS arousal and working on its cellular and molecular mechanisms (Pfaff 2006). Beyond this humble start, certainly, the more abstract among these questions are the ones that neuroscience is barely beginning to study. We feel, however, that eventually they will be seen to be grounded in, and require a detailed understanding of, neuroscientific mechanisms. We expect that these mechanisms serve the more basic aspects of emotional and social information processing in humans, as well as aspects of emotional and social information processing in other animals. Indeed, there are now a number of findings showing the effects of specific neurotransmitters on social cognition (Chiavegatto et al. 2001; Clarke et al. 2004; Harmer et al. 2003; Kosfeld et al. 2005), the engagement of structures involved in emotion and reward processing (deQuervain et al. 2005; Eisenberger et al. 2003; Singer et al. 2006), and even the influence of specific genes (Good et al. 2003; Pezawas et al. 2005). The key question will be how these more basic mechanisms, taken together, can add up to and explain the full richness of social cognition.

Outlook

While some of the most solid work on mechanisms of social behaviors in animals and humans has made clever use of hormone actions on nerve cells, the very success of such neuroendocrine experiments on simple behaviors encourages speculations about the essential nature of still more complex social behaviors. As a result of such speculations, we do not consider that social neuroscience is just like neuroscience more generally, only more complex. Instead, it is distinguished qualitatively by giving special insight into how we (and other species) evolved, how we may survive as a species in the future, and how we experience the world. It remains an important challenge for future investigations to carve out precisely which domain, at the process level, is at the core of "social cognition," or which domains social cognition is most related to. There are certainly some abstract, and complex, operations that social cognition shares with other cognitive domains: for instance, recursion is a feature both of complex social interactions and language; causal reasoning may be related to complex tool use (Johnson-Frey 2003) and to counterfactual reasoning; and domains like language and social behavior may be related in other ways as well, such as that shared language influences social group membership (Kinzler et al. 2007). As we noted above, an intriguing recent observation is that there appears to be a common neutral substrate for self-reflective thought, for reasoning about other people's minds, and for retrospective and prospective episodic thinking (episodic memory and episodic future planning and anticipation; Buckner and Carroll 2007). All these abilities are certainly "complex" in some sense, requiring high-level inferential and counterfactual thinking (Gilbert and Wilson 2007), and it is intriguing to speculate that they might be related and perhaps driven by the need to be able to track and predict complex social interactions.

This book began at a high integrative level by considering prosocial, moral behavior as a natural product of the human mind and by presenting experimental data on trust and altruism shown by human subjects Then, brain mechanisms were analyzed in reductionistic experiments with animals, including hormones, neurotransmitters and neuropeptides. As far as antisocial behavior is concerned, we recognize that pathologies of social behavior abound. Some of the best-understood pathologies have to do with the human amygdala and the prefrontal cortex. We rush to acknowledge that not all causes of abnormal social behavior, such as violence are, ab initio, derived from the offender's central nervous system; humiliation of young men by huge disparities of wealth, mistreatment of children during critical periods such as the neonatal and pubertal periods, rendering children anonymous by virtue of overwhelmingly large schools and failing to provide children with positive visions of their roles in society all can play a part (Devine et al. 2004). This volume, however, is limited strictly to biological considerations, even while realizing that they are not the entire story. These chapters give multiple examples of the intimate relations between alterations in hormone levels and alterations in social behaviors.

In terms of public health, the most important aspects of hormones and social behaviors will deal with attempts to reduce the most damaging aspects of human behavior. Two structures linked to pathologies of social behavior, the amygdala and prefrontal cortex, are known to be involved in aspects of emotion processing: the amygdala in Pavlovian fear conditioning (LeDoux 2000) and in mediating emotional autonomic responses (Chapman et al. 1954) and the prefrontal cortex in aspects of autonomic response as well as in emotion regulation and self-control (Beauregard et al. 2001; Ochsner et al. 2002). There is even evidence at the circuit level implicating the prefrontal cortex in regulating the amygdala's participation in emotion processing (Jackson and Moghaddam 2001) as well as conversely (Garcia et al. 1999). Both structures are also well known to participate in social behavior. In the case of the prefrontal cortex, the classical case of Phineas Gage (Damasio et al. 1994) and modern lesion studies showing the critical role of this region in social decision-making (Damasio 1994) and moral judgment (Koenigs et al. 2007) are clear examples. In the case of the amygdala, the story is somewhat more subtle; it is clearest for recognizing social cues such as certain emotions (Adolphs et al. 1994) or trustworthiness (Adolphs et al. 1998) from viewing faces. It is interesting to note that, at least in the case of the amygdala, the basic mechanisms that seem to explain impaired social perception may not be specifically social at all but rather reflect more abstract attentional mechanisms. For instance, the amygdala's role in recognizing emotional facial expressions appears to result from its role in assigning saliency to particular features within faces, notably the eyes (Adolphs et al. 2005), and this attentional role appears to extend to processing unpredictable and potentially salient stimuli that are not in any way social or emotional, such as unpredictable sequences of tones (Herry et al. 2007). These findings provide substantial detail about the mechanisms whereby certain brain structures participate in social cognition, but they bring us back to some of the questions we raised earlier: what is left of the domain specificity of social cognition? Is it comprised entirely of a collection of non-social processing modules? These are important open questions for the future.

References

Adolphs R, Tranel D, Damasio H, Damasio A (1994). Impaired recognition of emotion in facial expressions following bilateral damage to the human amygdala. Nature 372:669–672

Adolphs R, Tranel D, Damasio AR (1998) The human amygdala in social judgment. Nature 393:470–474

Adolphs R, Gosselin F, Buchanan TW, Tranel D, Schyns P, Damasio AR (2005). A mechanism for impaired fear recognition after amygdala damage. Nature 433:68–72

Beauregard M, Levesque J, Bourgouin P (2001) Neural correlates of conscious self-regulation of emotion. J Neurosci 21(RC165):RC1–6

Buckner RL, Carroll DC (2007) Self-projection and the brain. Trends Cogn Sci 11:49–57

Byrne R, Whiten A (eds) (1988) Machiavellian intelligence: social expertise and the evolution of intellect in monkeys, apes, and humans. Oxford, Clarendon

Chapman WP, Schroeder HR, Geyer G, Brazier MAB, Fager C, Poppen JL, Solomon HC, Yakovlev PI (1954) Physiological evidence concerning importance of the amygdaloid nuclear region in the integration of circulatory function and emotion in man. Science, 120:949–950

Chiavegatto S, Dawson VL. Mamounas LA, Koliatsos VE, Dawson TM, Nelson RJ (2001) Brain serotonin dysfunction accounts for aggression in male mice lacking neuronal nitric oxide synthase. Proc Natl Acad Sci USA 98:1277–1281

Clarke HF, Dalley JW, Crofts HS, Robbins TW, Roberts AC (2004) Cognitive inflexibility after prefrontal serotonin depletion. Science 304:878–880

Coqueugnlot H, Hublin J-J, Vellon F, Houet F, Jacob T (2004) Early brain growth in Homo erectus and implications for cognitive ability. Nature 431:299–232

Damasio AR (1994) Descartes' error: emotion, reason, and the human brain. New York, Grosset/Putnam

Damasio H, Grabowski T, Frank R, Galaburda AM, Damasio AR (1994) The return of Phineas Gage: clues about the brain from the skull of a famous patient. Science 264:1102–1104

de Quervain D-J, Fischbacher U, Treyer V, Schellhammer M, Schnyder U, Buck A, Fehr E (2005) The neural basis of altruistic punishment. Nature 305:1254–1258

Devine J, Gilligan J, Miczek K, Shaikh R, Pfaff D (eds) (2004) Scientific approaches to the prevention of youth violence. Ann NY Acad Sci 1036

Dunbar R (1998) The social brain hypothesis. Evol Anthropol 6:178–190

Dunbar RI, Shultz S (2007a) Evolution in the social brain. Science 317(5843):1344–1347

Dunbar RI, Shultz S (2007b) Understanding primate brain evolution. Philos Trans R Soc Lond B Biol Sci 362:649–658

Eisenberger NI, Lieberman MD, Williams KD (2003) Does rejection hurt? An fMRI study of social exclusion. Science 302:290–292

Garcia R, Vouimba R-M, Baudry M, Thompson RF (1999) The amgdala modulates prefrontal cortex activity relative to conditioned fear. Nature 402:294 296

Gilbert DT, Wilson TD (2007) Prospection: experiencing the future. Science 317:1351–1354

Gintis H, Bowles S, Boyd R, Fehr E (2003) Explaining altruistic behavior in humans. Evol Human Behav 24:153–172

Good CD, Lawrence K, Thomas NS, Price CJ, Ashburner J, Friston KJ, Frackowiak RS, Oreland L, Skuse DH (2003) Dosage-sensitive X-linked locus influences the development of amygdala and orbitofrontal cortex, and fear recognition in humans. Brain 126:2431–2446

Harmer CJ, Bhagwagar Z, Perrett DI, Vollm BA, Cowen PJ, Goodwin GM (2003) Acute SSRI administration affects the processing of social cues in healthy volunteers. Neuropsychopharmacology 28:148–152

Hauser MD (2006) Moral minds: how nature designed our universal sense of right and wrong. New York, Harper Collins

Healy SD, Rowe C (2007) A critique of comparative studies of brain size. Proc Roy Soc B 274:453–464

Herry C, Bach DR, Esposito F, DiSalle F, Perrig WJ, Scheffler K, Lüthi A, Seifritz E (2007) Processing of temporal unpredictability in human and animal amygdala. J Neurosci 27:5958–5966

Jackson ME, Moghaddam B (2001) Amygdala regulation of nucleus accumbens dopamine output is governed by the prefrontal cortex. J Neurosci 21:676–681

Johnson-Frey SH (2003) What's so special about human tool use? Neuron 39:201–204

Kavaliers M, Ågmo A, Choleris E, Gustafsson JA, Korach KS, Muglia LJ, Pfaff DW, Ogawa S (2004) Oxytocin and estrogen receptor alpha and beta knockout mice provide discriminably different odour cues in behavioural assays. Genes Brain Behav 3:189–195

Kinzler KD, Dupoux E, Spelke ES (2007) The native language of social cognition. Proc Natl Acd Sci USA 104:12577–12580

Koenigs M, Young L, Adolphs R, Tranel D, Cushman F, Hauser M, Damasio A (2007) Damage to the prefrontal cortex increases utilitarian moral judgments. Nature 446:908–911

Kosfeld M, Heinrichs M, Zak PJ, Fischbacher U, Fehr E (2005) Oxytocin increases trust in humans. Nature 435:673–676

LeDoux J (2000) Emotion circuits in the brain. Ann Rev Neurosci 23:155–184

McCarley R (2007) Neurobiology of REM and NREM sleep. Sleep Med 8:302–330

McEwen BS (2007) Stress; definitions and concepts. Encyclopedia of stress. Oxford, Elsevier

Moll J, Zahn R, de Oliveira-Souza R, Krueger F, Grafman J (2005) The neural basis of human moral cognition. Nature Rev Neurosci 6:799–809

Nowak MA, Sigmund K (2005) Evolution of indirect reciprocity. Nature 437:1291–1298

Ochsner K, Bunge SA, Gross JJ, Gabrieli JDE (2002) Rethinking feelings: an fMRI study of the cognitive regulation of emotion. J Cogn Neurosci 14:1215–1229

Pezawas L, Meyer-Lindenberg A, Drabant EM, Verchinski BA, Munoz KE, Kolachana BS, Egan MF, Mattay VS, Hariri AR, Weinberger DR (2005) 5-HTTLPR polymorphism impacts human cingulate-amygdala interactions: a genetic susceptibility mechanism for depression. Nature Neurosci 8:828–834

Pfaff D (1999) Drive. Cambridge, The M.I.T. Press

Pfaff D (2006) Brain arousal and information theory. Cambridge, Harvard University Press

Pfaff D (2007) The neuroscience of fair play. Washington, Dana Press

Posner J, Saper C, Schiff N, Plum F (2007) Plum and Posner's diagnosis of stupor and coma. 4th ed. Oxford, Oxford University Press

Schiff ND, Giacino JT, Kalmar K, Victor JD Baker K, Gerber M, Fritz B, Eisenberg B, O'Connor J, Kobylarz EJ, Farris S, Machado A, McCagg C, Plum F, Fins JJ, Rezai AR (2007) Behavioral improvements with thalamic stimulation after severe traumatic brain injury. Nature 448:600–603

Schoenemann PT, Sheehan MJ, Glotzer LD (2005). Prefrontal white matter volume is disproportionately larger in humans than in other primates. Nature Neurosci 8:242–252

Semendeferi K, Armstrong E, Schleicher A, Zilles K, Van Hoesen GW (2001). Prefrontal cortex in humans and apes: a comparative study of area 10. Am J Phys Anthropol 114:224–241

Semendeferi K, Lu A, Schenker N, Damasio H (2002) Humans and great apes share a large frontal cortex. Nature Neurosci 5:272–277

Singer T, Seymour B, O'Doherty J, Kaube H, Dolan RJ, Frith CD (2004) Empathy for pain involves the affective but not sensory components of pain. Science 303:1157–1162

Singer T, Seymour B, O'Doherty J, Stephan KE, Dolan RJ, Frith CD (2006) Empathic neural responses are modulated by the perceived fairness of others. Nature 439:466–469

Young MW, Kay SA (2001) Time zones: a comparative genetics of circadian clocks. Nature Rev Genet 2:702–15

Subject Index

Previous titles in the book series
Research and Perspectives in Endocrine Interactions

C. Kordon, I. Robinson, J. Hanoune, R. Dantzer, Y. Christen (eds) (2003)
Brain Somatic Cross-Talk and the Central Control of Metabolism
ISBN 978-3-540-00090-7

P. Chanson, J. Epelbaum, S. Lamberts, Y. Christen (eds) (2004)
Endocrine Aspects of Successful Aging: Genes, Hormones and Lifestyles
ISBN 978-3-540-40573-3

C. Kordon, R.C. Gaillard, Y. Christen (eds) (2005)
Hormones and the Brain
ISBN 978-3-540-21355-0

J.-C. Carel, P.A. Kelly, Y. Christen (eds) (2005)
Deciphering Growth
ISBN 978-3-540-26192-6

M. Conn, C. Kordon, Y. Christen (eds) (2006)
Insights into Receptor Function and New Drug Development Targets
ISBN 978-3-540-34446-9

S. Melmed, H. Rochefort, P. Chanson, Y. Christen (eds.) (2008)
Hormonal Control of Cell Cycle
ISBN 978-3-540-73854-1

Printing: Krips bv, Meppel, The Netherlands
Binding: Stürtz, Würzburg, Germany